TAKING
SELF-CARE FOR YOU AND YOUR FAMILY
CARE

Michael B. Jacobs, M.D.,
and Select Faculty of Stanford University School of Medicine

Random House
New York

Taking Care: Self-Care for You and Your Family is a valuable resource that can help readers work more effectively with their doctors and make wise health care choices. However, you should not rely on it to replace necessary medical consultations to meet your individual health care needs. Not all treatments mentioned in this book are covered by all health plans. Check with your health plan regarding coverage of service.

Copyright © 2002 by Optum®

This is a revised, expanded and updated edition of *Taking Care: Self-Care for 100 Common Symptoms and 20 Long-Term Ailments,* copyright © 1997 by Random House Inc.

Library of Congress Cataloging-in-Publication Data is available.
ISBN 0-375-75990-5

Illustrated by Rolin Graphics Inc.
Icons illustrated by Chris Murphy

Random House Web site address: http://www.atrandom.com

Printed in the United States of America on acid-free paper

98765432

2002 Updated Edition

Taking Care: Self-Care for You and Your Family

Michael B. Jacobs, M.D.

Professor of Medicine, Stanford University; Clerkship Director, Ambulatory Internal Medicine,
Division of General Internal Medicine, Stanford University

Stanford University Medical Consultants

Jane A. Morton, M.D., Clinical Professor of Pediatrics, Stanford University;
Partner and Staff Physician, Palo Alto Medical Foundation, Palo Alto, California

Peter Pompei, M.D., Associate Professor of Medicine, Stanford University; Director, Fellowship
in Geriatric Medicine, Stanford University and the V.A. Palo Alto Health Care System

Maurice Druzin, M.D., Chief, Division of Maternal-Fetal Medicine, Dept. of Gynecology and
Obstetrics, Stanford University; Associate Dean for Academic Affairs, Stanford University

Optum® Medical Consultants

Robert G. Harmon, M.D., M.P.H., F.A.C.P.M.
Phyllis DeCarlo Cross, M.D., M.P.H.
Mindy S. Ring, L.P.C., M.A.C., C.E.A.P.
Bonnie J. Morcomb, R.N., M.S.
Marcie Parker, Ph.D., C.F.L.E.
Nancy M. Berryman, R.N.
Nancy E. Camp R.N., M.S.
Jane F. Omodt, R.N.
Martha L. Desrosiers, B.S.R.N., A.N.P.-B.C.
Melanie R. Polk, M.M.Sc., R.D., F.A.D.A.

Editor

Sara Fitzgerald Sonntag

Writers

Anne Brinser
Heather M. Pierce
Larissa Popchuk
Contributing Writer: Susan Perry

Senior Art Director

Angelique Larsen Carmello

Designers

Kristine A. Mitchell
Keun Yoo

Senior Communications Manager

Nancy Larson-Knott

Senior Product Manager

Renee L. Pietrzak

Table of Contents

Chapter 7: Long-Term Conditions 251

A Note to Our Readers

When it comes to good health and peace of mind, it really is true that knowledge is power. The more you know, the more confident you'll feel about taking care of your health.

It's natural to feel worried and uncertain about what to do when illnesses or injuries arise. It even may be difficult to know what questions to ask your doctor. At times like these, it can be comforting to have a simple, yet valuable resource to help you sort it all out.

Taking Care: Self-Care for You and Your Family was developed for that very purpose. The practical information throughout these pages can help you choose an appropriate level of care for your situation. Learn how and when to use self-care measures. Prepare questions to ask your nurse information service or doctor. Become more knowledgeable about symptoms—and make the most of every health care appointment.

Use this book as a handy reference when specific health questions come up. Or, just browse through it to learn more about healthy lifestyle choices or long-term concerns that may be important to you.

Above all, our wish is that you and your family enjoy this book in the best of health!

Michael B. Jacobs, M.D.

First Aid and Emergencies

Illness and injury often require quick action. Knowing what to do in an emergency sometimes can mean the difference between life and death.

But, don't forget your own safety. Stay alert when providing first aid—don't put yourself or anyone else in danger.

Know What's an Emergency

Learn to recognize emergencies so that you'll know when to call for immediate medical assistance. These are warning signs of medical emergencies:

- Difficulty breathing, shortness of breath
- Pain or pressure in the chest or upper abdominal area
- Fainting
- Sudden dizziness, weakness or change in vision
- Sudden change in mental status— such as unusual behavior, confusion or difficulty waking up
- Severe pain anywhere in the body
- Bleeding that won't stop after several minutes of direct pressure
- Severe or persistent vomiting
- Coughing up or vomiting blood
- Suicidal or homicidal feelings

Most importantly, trust your instincts. If you're alarmed by unusually severe symptoms that you think may indicate an emergency, call for help immediately.

Call for Help

In order to act quickly, know your local emergency number and post it near every phone. In most areas, this number is 911.

Provide the following information:

- The exact address of the emergency. You also may need to give nearby intersections, local landmarks, the floor of the building, or the apartment or room number.
- Your name and the phone number from which you're calling
- What happened
- The condition of the victim(s)
- What help currently is being given

Stay on the line. The emergency operator may tell you what to do until help arrives. Don't hang up until you're told to do so.

Listen carefully. The emergency operator may ask questions to help determine the exact medical problem.

While you're waiting for help to arrive:

- Stay calm. Reassure the patient that help is on the way.
- Follow the emergency operator's instructions.
- Don't move someone who is injured unless he or she is in imminent danger.
- Make the patient as comfortable as possible.

- If you can, send someone to meet the responding emergency personnel and direct them to you.
- If you determine that the person isn't breathing or doesn't have signs of circulation, perform CPR (see Page 3)—**but only if you've been trained in this technique.**

Before an Emergency Occurs

Being prepared before an emergency occurs can make a difference.

- Keep all emergency numbers—including your Poison Control Center number—near each phone.
- Teach your children how and when to call 911. Make sure they know their address and phone number.
- Discuss action plans for various emergency situations with your family. Develop a fire escape plan.

See Page 28 for more safety tips.

Your First-Aid Kit

A well-stocked, first-aid kit can be very helpful in emergencies. Consider taking a first-aid class to be well prepared.

Your first-aid kit should include:

- Adhesive bandages—an assortment including butterfly bandages
- Sterile gauze squares or dressings in various sizes
- Rolls of gauze
- Antiseptic wipes

- Disposable surgical gloves
- Calamine lotion
- Adhesive tape
- Sharp scissors with rounded tips
- Triangular cloth bandages for slings
- Safety pins
- Saline solution
- Antibiotic ointment
- Cotton balls and swabs
- Elastic bandage
- Tweezers
- Hydrocortisone cream
- Cold packs
- Pain relievers such as acetaminophen, ibuprofen or naproxen sodium
- Aspirin for sudden, severe chest pain
- Syrup of ipecac
- Thermometer
- Flashlight
- Saline eye drops and an eye wash kit
- Matches
- First-aid guide
- Important information—including a list of allergies and medications for each household member, as well as emergency phone numbers

Keep these items easily accessible. Store your first-aid kit in a clean, dry place—out of the reach of children. Consider keeping a kit in your home and another in your car.

Check your first-aid kit regularly to ensure that all contents are present, in good condition and not expired.

CPR— Cardiopulmonary Resuscitation

IMPORTANT: This brief description of CPR is not a replacement for training from the American Red Cross or the American Heart Association (AHA). To find a CPR course near you, contact your local American Red Cross chapter, or contact the AHA at (800) 242-8721 or www.americanheart.org.

CPR is administered when someone's breathing or circulation (or both) stops. When both stop, sudden death has occurred. This may have many possible causes—poisoning, drowning, choking, suffocation, electrocution or smoke inhalation—but the most common is cardiac arrest. The following steps can help you resuscitate someone who needs help.

Check responsiveness. Tap or gently shake the shoulder of the person who has collapsed. Shout, "Are you OK?" Anyone who is unresponsive needs emergency care.

Call 911 or your local emergency number immediately. If possible, have someone else call for help so you can begin CPR.

For infants and children ages 8 years or younger, have someone else call for help. If no one else is available, perform one minute of CPR before leaving the person to call for help. If the child is small and not injured, you may carry him or her to the phone when you make the call.

Perform CPR. Before you begin CPR, make sure you aren't in any physical danger—such as in traffic after an accident—when you help.

Remember the **ABCs: Airway, Breathing and Circulation.**

Step 1: Airway

Open the airway. Carefully place the person on his or her back. Then open the airway by gently tilting the head back (see figure 1). If you suspect a head, neck or back injury, pull the jaw forward without moving the head or neck.

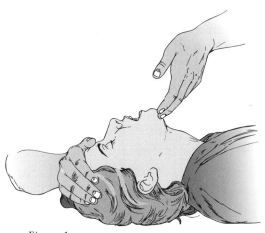

Figure 1

Be careful when handling an infant. Tilting the head too far back can close off the airway.

Step 2: Breathing

Check for breathing. Place your ear close to the person's nose and mouth. For five seconds, listen and feel for breathing, and look for chest movement.

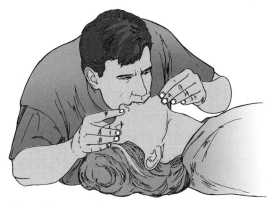

Figure 2

If there's no breathing, give two puffs of breath. Pinch the person's nostrils closed and give two breaths into his or her mouth (see figure 2). The chest should rise with each breath you give. If it doesn't, re-position the head and repeat this step.

Don't pinch an infant's nose. Place your mouth over the infant's nose and mouth at the same time.

4

Step 3: Circulation

Check circulation. Look for signs of circulation such as normal breathing, coughing or movement in response to stimulation.

If there's no sign of circulation, give compressions. Place the heel of your hand two finger-widths above the lowest notch of the person's breastbone (see figure 3). Place the heel of your other hand directly over the heel of the hand already in place. Don't let your fingers touch the person's chest. Lock your elbows straight, lean over your hands and firmly press straight down about 2 inches. Give 15 compressions. You should be providing a total of 80 to 100 compressions per minute. Counting aloud may help you establish a rhythm, "One and, two and, three and..."

> For children ages 8 years or younger, use the heel of one hand—not two—on the lower half of the breastbone. Give five compressions. You should be providing a total of 100 compressions per minute.
>
> For infants, use two or three fingers on the breastbone about one finger-width below the infant's nipple line. Provide at least 100 compressions per minute—120 compressions per minute for newborns.

Provide 15 compressions for every two breaths. Repeat this sequence four times, then check for breathing and signs of circulation.

> For infants and children ages 8 years or younger, provide five compressions for every one breath.

If there's no sign of circulation, continue providing 15 compressions for every two breaths. Check the person after every four cycles. Repeat until breathing resumes or help arrives.

> For infants and children, continue providing five compressions for every one breath until breathing resumes or help arrives.

If breathing resumes, place the person in a recovery position. Roll the person onto his or her side, taking care to move the body as a whole unit. Don't place a person into the recovery position if you suspect a neck, spine or back injury.

Remember, these steps aren't meant to substitute for a certified CPR class. Learn CPR and encourage your family and friends to join you.

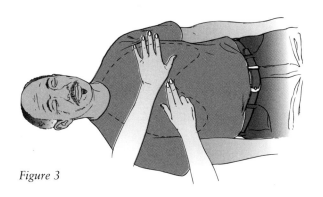

Figure 3

Choking

Choking occurs when a foreign object—often food—becomes lodged in the throat or airway. It's a life-threatening situation that requires quick action.

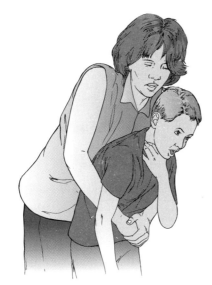

Figure 4

What to Look For

A person who is choking may:

- Grab at his or her throat
- Panic
- Gasp for breath
- Turn blue
- Become unconscious

What to Do

- Ask, "Are you choking?"
- If the person can cough or speak, he or she is getting enough air. Don't interfere.

If an infant is choking:

- Place the infant face down across your forearm, with your arm resting on your leg or lap. Support the infant's head with your hand.
- Give five forceful blows to the back, between the shoulder blades, with the heel of your hand.
- If the object isn't dislodged, turn the baby over. Give five forceful thrusts with two fingers to the infant's chest—in the center just below the nipple line.
- Alternate between back blows and chest thrusts until the object is coughed out.
- If the infant becomes unresponsive, check for breathing and signs of circulation. Perform CPR (see Page 3), if needed.

- If the person can't cough or speak, have someone call 911 or your local emergency number immediately.
- Begin the Heimlich maneuver to dislodge the object (see figure 4). If the person choking is pregnant, ask the emergency operator for special instructions. For conscious adults and children—but not infants age 1 year or younger:
  - Stand behind the person and place one foot between his or her feet.
  - Wrap your arms around the person's waist.

- Make a fist with one hand, thumb pointing toward the ground. Place it just above the person's belly button but below the rib cage. Cover your fist with your other hand.

- Pull up and back toward you with quick, forceful thrusts.

- Continue thrusts until the person coughs up the object, becomes unconscious, or emergency help arrives.

■ If the person becomes unresponsive, check to see if he or she is breathing and has signs of circulation. Check the airway—if you see an object, carefully remove it.

■ For unconscious adults and children, carefully follow the instructions of the emergency operator.

If you're choking and alone:

■ Stay calm.

■ Try to cough vigorously.

■ Give yourself abdominal thrusts (see figure 5). You can use your fist or lean over the back of a chair or railing and thrust yourself on it with quick, forceful movements.

■ Repeat until you've dislodged the object.

Cold Emergencies

Frostbite occurs when body tissue freezes. It can cause permanent damage. Fingers, toes and ears most often are affected. Hypothermia is a potentially

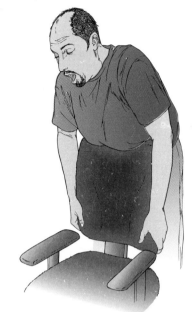

Figure 5

fatal condition in which the body's core temperature falls to a dangerous level. Seek emergency help.

Frostbite

What to Look For

■ Hard, pale and cold skin

■ Numbness in the affected areas

■ As frostbite progresses, the skin may turn from red, to white, to yellow or blue-white.

What to Do

■ Get out of the cold.

■ Warm your hands by tucking them under your armpits. Warm your nose, ears and face by covering them with dry, gloved hands.

- Don't rub frostbitten body parts.
- Don't use a hot water bottle, heating pad, hair dryer or heat lamp to warm body parts. Excessive heat and rapid rewarming can cause more damage.
- Call 911 or your local emergency number if numbness doesn't go away during warming.
- If help isn't immediately available, warm severely frostbitten hands or feet in warm—not hot—water.
- Don't smoke or drink beverages with alcohol or caffeine. These can alter blood flow.

Hypothermia

What to Look For

- Body temperature below 94° F
- Shivering—if hypothermia is severe, shivering may no longer occur
- Cold, pale skin
- Slurred speech
- Abnormally slow rate of breathing
- Loss of coordination
- Disorientation or confusion
- Drowsiness, exhaustion or apathy

What to Do

- Move the person out of the cold. If going indoors isn't possible, provide shelter from wetness and wind.
- Handle the person gently.

- Remove wet clothing. Provide a warm, dry covering—such as a blanket.
- Call 911 or your local emergency number.
- Monitor the person's breathing. Perform CPR (see Page 3), if needed.
- If help isn't immediately available, warm the person in a bath of warm—not hot—water. If this isn't possible, try to insulate the person by sharing body heat.
- Don't give the person alcohol. Offer warm, nonalcoholic drinks only if the person isn't vomiting.

Drowning

When trying to help a possible drowning victim, it's important that you avoid danger. Don't attempt a rescue beyond your abilities.

What to Look For

- Pale, cool skin
- Difficult or absent breathing
- Decreased level of consciousness
- Skin that looks pale or blue
- Weak or absent pulse

What to Do

- Stay calm.
- Get the person out of the water.
- Call 911 or your local emergency number immediately.

- Check to see if the person is breathing and has signs of circulation.
- Perform CPR (see Page 3), if needed.
- Treat hypothermia (see Page 8), if present.
- Treat neck and spine injuries (see Page 12), if present.

Near drowning can harm the respiratory system. On recovery, someone who nearly drowned may develop a buildup of fluid in the lungs. Anyone who has experienced near drowning must seek emergency help.

Electrical Shock

Be extremely careful around victims of electrical shock. Take care to avoid getting shocked yourself.

What to Look For
- Difficult or absent breathing
- Absent, weak or irregular pulse
- Evidence of burns
- Evidence of fractures
- Entrance and exit wound burns
- Unconsciousness

What to Do
- Stay calm.
- Call 911 or your local emergency number immediately.
- Don't touch an electrical shock victim!
- Disconnect the appliance or turn off the power if a person is being shocked.

- If you can't turn off the power, use a piece of wood, such as a wooden broom handle, to separate the person from the power source.
- If the person is touching a high voltage wire, don't try to move him or her. Wait for emergency help to arrive.
- Check to see if the person is breathing and has signs of circulation.
- Perform CPR (see Page 3), if needed.
- Treat for shock (see Page 15), if needed.
- Cover electrical burns with a sterile dressing. Don't apply grease or oil to the burns.

Head Injuries

Many head injuries are minor and don't require medical attention. But some, including concussions, can be serious. Seek emergency medical help for any severe head injury.

What to Look For
- Severe head or facial bleeding
- Change in level of consciousness— even if temporary
- Black and blue marks below the eyes or behind the ears
- Blood or clear fluid draining from the ears or nose
- Difficult or absent breathing
- Unequal-sized pupils, eyes crossed or not moving together

- Nausea or vomiting
- Restlessness, irritability or confusion
- Blurred or double vision
- Difficulty walking
- Dizziness
- Slurred speech

What to Do

- Stay calm.
- Call 911 or your local emergency number immediately.
- Check to see if the person is breathing and has signs of circulation.
- Perform CPR (see Page 3), if needed. Remember, there are special techniques to open the airway when spinal injuries are suspected.
- Keep the person still—lying down. Avoid moving the head or neck.
- Stop any bleeding with gauze or a clean cloth.

Some symptoms of a severe head injury may not appear immediately. If someone has suffered a head injury that doesn't seem serious at first, watch the person for one to two hours to be sure his or her level of consciousness doesn't change. Then monitor the person closely every two hours during the next 24 hours to make sure his or her pupils are of equal size, he or she awakens easily and has no problem walking. Continue to check on the person at increasing intervals for the next 48 hours.

Head, neck and spinal injuries are all related. Any person with a head injury who has an altered level of consciousness may have sustained a neck injury, as well. Keep the person still until emergency help arrives.

Heart Attack

Knowing the signs of a heart attack can help you take quick, appropriate action. Getting help promptly is crucial. Don't dismiss possible heart attack symptoms as indigestion or another minor problem. Seek emergency help immediately.

What to Look For

- Severe pain or uncomfortable pressure, fullness, squeezing or heaviness in the center of the chest that lasts several minutes
- Pain that spreads to the shoulders, neck, lower jaw or arms
- Lightheadedness
- Shortness of breath
- Nausea or vomiting
- Fainting
- Sweating

Some people, especially women, may not experience typical heart attack symptoms. Also look for:

- Unusual chest, stomach or abdominal pain
- Dizziness

- Unexplained anxiety, weakness or fatigue
- Palpitations, cold sweat or pale skin

Not all of these symptoms occur in every heart attack. If you notice one or more of these signs, seek emergency help immediately.

What to Do

- Stay calm.
- If you think you're having a heart attack, don't drive yourself to the hospital!
- Call 911 or your local emergency number immediately.
- If the person doesn't have an aspirin allergy or intolerance, have him or her chew one aspirin of any dose.
- Check to see if the person is breathing and has signs of circulation.
- Perform CPR (see Page 3), if needed.
- If the person is conscious, keep him or her in a comfortable position— preferably sitting. Loosen any tight-fitting clothing, especially around the neck.
- Offer reassurance.

If you've been diagnosed with angina (see Page 76), a condition that can cause symptoms similar to a heart attack, carefully follow your doctor's instructions about taking your medication.

Heat Emergencies

Heat exhaustion is due to dehydration— usually caused by fluid loss due to exertion in heat and high humidity. If not treated, heat exhaustion can lead to heatstroke. When this occurs, the body's normal mechanisms for dealing with heat—such as sweating and temperature control—fail. Heatstroke is potentially fatal. It requires immediate action to avoid coma or death.

Heat Exhaustion

What to Look For

- Pale, cool, moist skin
- Rapid breathing
- Profuse and prolonged sweating
- Muscle cramps
- Thirst
- Nausea or vomiting
- Headache
- Weakness and lightheadedness

What to Do

- Have the person lie down in the shade or an air-conditioned room. Elevate his or her feet slightly.
- Remove unnecessary clothing.
- Cool the person by placing cool, wet cloths on the skin. Place cold compresses on the neck, groin and armpits.

- Offer cool water to sip slowly—about one-half cup every 15 minutes.
- If symptoms don't improve, seek emergency help.

Heatstroke

What to Look For

- Fever
- Dry, hot, red skin
- Person is no longer sweating
- Irritability or confusion
- Fainting
- Rapid, shallow breathing
- Rapid, weak pulse
- Seizures

What to Do

- Call 911 or your local emergency number immediately.
- Place the person in the shade or an air-conditioned room. Elevate his or her feet slightly.
- Remove unnecessary clothing.
- Place cool, wet cloths on the person's skin. Place cold compresses on the neck, groin and armpits. Use fans to increase cooling.
- Offer cool water to sip slowly—about one-half cup every 15 minutes. Don't give water if the person isn't fully conscious and alert.
- Treat for shock (see Page 15), if needed.
- Perform CPR (see Page 3), if needed.

Neck and Spine Injuries

If you suspect a neck or spine injury, don't move the person. Permanent paralysis or other serious complications can result.

What to Look For

- Evidence of a head injury
- An injury that involved a strong force or blow to the back or head
- Severe pain in the neck or back
- Weakness, numbness or paralysis
- Loss of bladder or bowel control
- Neck or back that is oddly positioned
- Symptoms of shock (see Page 15)

What to Do

- Stay calm.
- Don't move the person.
- Call 911 or your local emergency number immediately.
- Check to see if the person is breathing and has signs of circulation.
- Perform CPR (see Page 3), if needed. Remember, there are special techniques to open the airway when spinal injuries are suspected.
- Keep the person still.
- Stabilize the neck with a heavy towel or other soft, bulky material.
- Treat any wounds you can—without moving the person's head or neck.
- Treat for shock (see Page 15), if needed.

12

- Reassure the person that help is on the way.

Poisoning

If you think someone has been poisoned, call your local Poison Control Center immediately. If you don't know your local number, call (800) 222-1222 to be connected with a Poison Control Center in your area. Keep this number near your phone.

Suspect poisoning if someone suddenly becomes sick for no apparent reason. Poisonings may occur through ingestion, inhalation or skin contact. Because there are so many types of poison, reactions—as well as proper treatment—can vary widely.

What to Look For
- Abdominal pain
- Bluish lips
- Burns around the mouth—may result from drinking certain poisons
- Chest pain
- Chills
- Confusion
- Cough
- Depressed mood
- Diarrhea
- Dizziness
- Double vision
- Drowsiness

- Fever
- Headache
- Heart palpitations
- Irritability
- Loss of appetite
- Loss of bladder control
- Muscle twitching
- Nausea or vomiting
- Numbness and dryness of the nose or mouth
- Pale, cool, moist skin
- Pupils that are dilated or constricted
- Rapid, weak or irregular pulse
- Seizures
- Shortness of breath
- Skin rash or burns
- Unconsciousness
- Unusual breath odor
- Weakness

What to Do
- Stay calm.
- If chemicals or household products have been swallowed, follow the first-aid instructions on the label.
- Call your Poison Control Center, 911 or your local emergency number.
- Have the product label ready when you call for help.
- Be prepared to tell the emergency operator the following information, if known:

- The person's age and weight
- Existing health conditions or problems
- The substance involved and how the person came in contact with it—such as inhaled, swallowed or skin contact
- Amount of substance involved and approximate time the poisoning occurred
- Any first aid that may have been given
- If the person vomited
- Your location

- Follow the instructions you're given.
- Don't induce vomiting unless advised to do so.
- Don't give anything by mouth unless advised to do so.
- Check to see if the person is breathing and has signs of circulation.
- Perform CPR (see Page 3), if needed.

Seizures

A seizure is a sudden, violent contraction and relaxation of the muscles. Seizures have many causes, including epilepsy, alcohol or drug use, high fever—especially in children, head injury, poisoning, heart disease or stroke.

What to Look For

- Vigorous muscle spasms with twitching and jerking limbs

- Brief blackout or period of confused behavior
- Drooling or frothing at the mouth
- Grunting and snorting
- Local tingling or twitching on one side of the body
- Loss of bladder or bowel control
- Sudden falling or loss of consciousness
- Temporary absence of breathing

What to Do

- Stay calm and be reassuring.
- Protect the person from injury. If possible, lay the person on his or her side on the ground in a safe area.
- Don't restrain the person.
- Don't place anything in the person's mouth.
- Try to loosen any tight clothing, especially around the neck.
- If vomiting occurs, try to turn the head so that the vomited material drains out the side of the mouth.
- Once the seizure has ended, check to see if the person is breathing and has signs of circulation.
- Perform CPR (see Page 3), if needed.

Many people will sleep after a seizure. This is OK. The person may be disoriented after waking up.

Many people, especially those with epilepsy—who have brief, self-limited seizures—may need only to call their doctors, and not go to the hospital.

14

However, call 911 or your local emergency number if:

- The seizure lasts longer than two minutes.
- There is more than one seizure in a 24-hour period.
- The person doesn't wake up between seizures.
- The person is sick, injured or intoxicated.
- The person has never had a seizure before.
- The person has diabetes or high blood pressure.
- The person is pregnant.
- The person had a seizure in water.
- The person seems weak and feverish after the seizure has stopped.
- You're concerned about the person's welfare for any reason.

Shock

Shock occurs when the body's cells aren't getting enough oxygen and nutrients. It's a life-threatening condition. Shock can have many causes, including trauma, heat, allergic reaction (called anaphylaxis), severe infection, bleeding, heart attack or poisoning.

What to Look For

- Pale, cool, clammy skin
- Thirst
- Rapid, shallow breathing
- Rapid, weak pulse
- Nausea or vomiting
- Fever
- Collapse and unconsciousness

What to Do

- Call 911 or your local emergency number immediately.
- Check to see if the person is breathing and has signs of circulation.
- Perform CPR (see Page 3), if needed.
- Control any bleeding.
- If conscious, the person should be placed on his or her back with legs elevated.

Anaphylaxis

People with strong allergies to certain substances may experience anaphylactic shock—a severe allergic reaction to an allergen. Anaphylactic shock is life-threatening and requires immediate action and emergency medical care. If you observe an allergic reaction with signs of shock:

- Call 911 or your local emergency number immediately.
- Check to see if the person is carrying medication—usually injectable epinephrine—to counter the effects of an allergic attack. Help the person administer his or her medication.
- Check to see if the person is breathing and has signs of circulation.
- Perform CPR (see Page 3), if needed.

- If unconscious, the person should be placed in a stable side position with support under the legs to elevate them.
- Keep the person warm and comfortable. Loosen tight clothing and cover the person with a blanket.
- Don't give the person anything to eat or drink.
- Treat any visible injuries.
- Offer reassurance.

Stroke

A stroke occurs when the blood supply to the brain is interrupted. It should be treated with the same degree of seriousness as a heart attack. If you notice symptoms of a stroke in yourself or someone else, seek emergency help.

What to Look For

- Sudden weakness or numbness in the face, arm or leg on one side of the body
- Slurred speech or difficulty talking
- Partial or total loss of vision, or double vision
- Confusion
- Dizziness
- Fainting
- Loss of balance or coordination
- Sudden, severe headache

What to Do

- Stay calm.
- Call 911 or your local emergency number immediately.
- Check to see if the person is breathing and has signs of circulation.
- Perform CPR (see Page 3), if needed.
- Place the person in a comfortable position, making sure the airway doesn't become blocked by drool or mucus.
- Offer reassurance. Talk to the person, even if he or she is unconscious.

Staying Healthy

2

Making healthy lifestyle choices is one of the most important things you can do to protect your health. For starters, you can reduce the risk of disease and live longer. You're also more likely to have the energy you need to achieve your goals, care for your family and enjoy life. And, when you feel better, your whole outlook can improve, too.

But, maybe you've been putting off starting your new lease on good health. You're not alone. Day-to-day life often is so busy—just the thought of making lifestyle changes can seem like one more thing you don't have time for. But, it may be easier than you think.

Start small—but start today. Taking small steps can result in big health benefits.

Start by being honest with yourself about what you eat, how much exercise you get and other habits that may be holding you back. Don't beat yourself up. Instead, resolve to begin making changes today.

Even if you haven't been the model of healthy living, it's never too late to start. With simple changes, you can strengthen your heart, lower your blood pressure and maintain a healthy weight.

Eat Well

Variety really is the spice of life. By choosing a wide range of foods, you're more likely to get the nutrients your body needs. Use the Food Guide

Pyramid (see Page 20) to plan balanced meals and healthy snacks.

Get your fruits and veggies. Consume at least five a day. It's not too hard to do. Sip fruit juice instead of soda, slice a banana on your cereal, grab dried fruit instead of chips, and toss all sorts of veggies into your dinner salad.

Add whole grains. Choose 100 percent whole-grain bread for more fiber and B vitamins. Cook brown rice instead of white. Eat whole-grain cereal instead of a doughnut for breakfast.

Select lean meats. Skinless chicken and turkey are good low-fat choices. They're versatile in recipes, too. If you prefer beef, choose the leanest cuts.

Enjoy seafood. The omega-3 fatty acids found in some seafood are believed to lower the risk of heart attack and stroke. Oily, deep-water fish, such as sardines, salmon, mackerel, tuna, herring or fresh-water rainbow trout, are good sources.

Keep the calcium. But, lose the fat found in many dairy products. There are lots of low-fat and fat-free versions of cheese, yogurt and sour cream. Look for calcium-fortified foods, too. Calcium is essential for keeping your bones and teeth strong throughout your life. If you have lactose intolerance (see Page 122), or trouble digesting dairy-based foods, look for lactose-free products. Also, talk with your doctor about over-the-counter calcium supplements.

Control your cholesterol. High-density lipoproteins (HDLs) can lower your risk of heart disease. Low-density lipoproteins (LDLs), or "bad cholesterol," can increase your risk. Fiber such as oats and beans can lower your total cholesterol. Soy products such as soymilk, tofu and tempeh can, too. Exercise and weight control are key to raising HDLs.

Limit all fats. Strive for a diet low in overall fat. In particular, limit saturated fat—found in meats, dairy products, and coconut and palm oil. Monounsaturated fat—found in canola, olive and peanut oils—can lower total cholesterol. Avoid trans-fatty acids. They can increase LDLs. Some margarines and hydrogenated vegetable oils are high in trans-fatty acids.

Drink plenty of water. Staying hydrated is important. Remember to drink more in hot weather or when you're physically active.

Portion Control Is Key

How much you eat can be just as important as what you eat. Plates piled high can cause extra pounds to add up quickly. Restaurant portions often are oversized. Try eating only half and taking the rest home for another meal.

At home, avoid the temptation of a second helping. Change the proportion of what's on your plate—spoon out less mashed potatoes and more broccoli. Make that slice of cake a sliver. If you can't resist those cookies, take two instead of a handful. Don't go into automatic. Try to think about all of your food choices—including the amount.

Go to the Source

Most people can get many of the nutrients they need from the foods they eat. However, some people may have special nutritional requirements. For instance, those with certain health conditions, pregnant women, smokers and older adults may benefit from supplements. Talk with your doctor about your individual health needs.

Nutrient	Good Food Sources
Vitamin A	Winter squash; sweet potatoes; dark green, leafy vegetables such as collard greens, mustard greens and kale; liver
Vitamin B-6	Whole grains, brown rice, nuts, beans, chicken, fish, lean pork
Vitamin B-12	Fish, meats, eggs, dairy products
Vitamin C	Citrus fruits, melons, strawberries, mangoes, bell peppers, broccoli, cauliflower, cabbage, dark green, leafy vegetables
Vitamin D	Fatty fish such as herring, salmon and tuna; fortified dairy products; fortified cereals
Vitamin E	Fortified cereals, whole grains, wheat germ, sunflower seeds, nuts, grain oils
Vitamin K	Spinach, turnip greens and other dark green, leafy vegetables, cabbage, broccoli, liver, green tea, cheese, oats, eggs
Calcium	Dairy products, dark green, leafy vegetables, canned salmon with edible bones, sardines, almonds
Folate (folic acid)	Liver, beans, beets, avocados, eggs, dark green, leafy vegetables, nuts, oranges, wheat germ, enriched grains
Iodine	Iodized salt, seafood, kelp
Iron	Red meat, chicken, seafood, dark green, leafy vegetables, whole grains, nuts, dried fruit, fortified cereals
Magnesium	Dark green, leafy vegetables, nuts, whole grains, beans
Niacin	Fish, peanut butter, poultry, liver, beef, beans
Phosphorus	Meat, poultry, fish, dairy products, eggs, nuts
Protein	Meat, fish, dairy products, poultry, dried beans, nuts, eggs, soy products
Riboflavin	Enriched bread, cheese, yogurt, eggs, soy products
Selenium	Whole grains, garlic, eggs, seafood
Thiamin	Whole grains, fortified cereals, lean pork
Zinc	Lean meat, seafood, eggs, soy products, cheese, peanuts

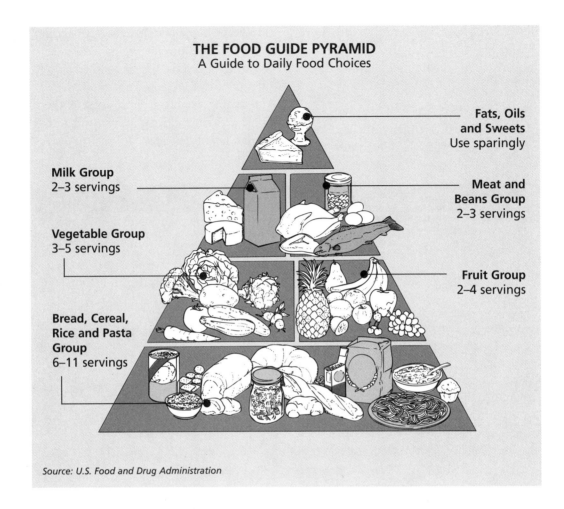

THE FOOD GUIDE PYRAMID
A Guide to Daily Food Choices

Fats, Oils and Sweets
Use sparingly

Milk Group
2–3 servings

Meat and Beans Group
2–3 servings

Vegetable Group
3–5 servings

Fruit Group
2–4 servings

Bread, Cereal, Rice and Pasta Group
6–11 servings

Source: U.S. Food and Drug Administration

Exercise and Energize

Is there a magic formula for better health? No—but exercise comes close. By adding exercise to your lifestyle, you'll feel some benefits right away. Your energy and stamina will get a boost, you'll sleep better, and your weight control efforts may be more successful. Exercise also can help you manage stress. Your whole attitude may change as you begin to feel stronger.

If that's not enough incentive to dust off your walking shoes, just think of the long-term benefits. Getting 30 minutes of exercise, five days a week can lower your risk of heart disease, stroke, diabetes and some cancers. Weight-bearing activity, in part, can help prevent osteoporosis. Overall, exercise also can raise your HDLs—or good cholesterol—and lower your blood pressure.

It All Adds Up

Think you just can't squeeze in 30 minutes of exercise? Think again. Walking for 10 minutes, three times a day is one of the easiest ways to fit exercise into your routine. Walk whenever you can. Park farther than usual from your workplace. Walk around the block a few times during lunch. Take the stairs instead of the elevator. Or, start taking a walk after dinner each evening.

There's no doubt that it may be tough to get yourself moving at first. But, once you do, it'll become easier each day. In fact, you'll actually start looking forward to it because exercise really does make you feel good.

Start Off on the Right Foot

If you haven't exercised for a while, have a chronic health condition, or if you're age 40 or older, talk with your doctor about which activities are right for you.

Start slowly. Warm up and cool down with some gentle stretching. In time, gradually pick up the pace and the frequency of your workouts. Develop a balanced exercise program with these activities:

- **Aerobic activity** strengthens your heart and lungs. There are lots of options—walking, running, biking, dancing and swimming are just a few.
- **Strength training** builds muscles, and helps keep your bones and joints healthy. Building muscle can speed up your metabolism, which helps control your weight. You can lift weights or use strength-training equipment.
- **Stretching** improves flexibility, balance and coordination. Use smooth, steady movements. Yoga and tai chi offer gentle but effective workouts (see Page 336).

Will a membership at the gym motivate you? Are you more comfortable at home with a fitness video? Or, do you prefer to run around the park with Fido? Be true to your own style—and you'll be more likely to keep moving toward better health.

Maintain a Healthy Weight

Healthy weight control is a struggle for many of us. But, it's a battle worth fighting because it's critical to your health. Those extra pounds can put you at risk for diabetes, high blood pressure, heart disease and other serious health conditions.

However, the struggle isn't just about reaching an ideal body weight. It's also about figuring out what's realistic and healthy. We're bombarded by messages in the media—telling us that we can't be too skinny, and weight loss is just a phone call and credit charge away. And, the pressure we sometimes put on each other about dieting can make things worse.

Back to Basics

It's time to listen to the most important voice of all—your own. Turn the focus of your weight control toward better health, higher energy and a sense of accomplishment.

Talk with your doctor. Ask what is a healthy weight for you, based on your age and health history. Discuss the best way to lose weight, including how quickly or slowly.

Rely on the dynamic duo. Good nutrition and exercise are an unbeatable team. Watching what you eat is important but isn't enough. Add movement to help you build muscle and shed pounds.

Take one day at a time. Set daily goals in addition to your long-term objectives. Reward yourself for the small victories. Take a long walk with a friend, buy a new CD, watch your favorite movie or pick up that new best seller from the library.

Plan for success. Is chocolate your downfall? Is pasta irresistible? Make a plan to counter your cravings. If you need to—get rid of those foods you just can't say, "No" to. Make healthy snacking easy. Cut up veggies for easy munching. Bring low-fat, whole grain crackers to work instead of snacking from the vending machine.

Choose restaurants wisely. You still can enjoy eating out, but be sure to do your homework first. Find out which restaurants offer heart-healthy options. Avoid cream dressings and fried foods. Watch those portions.

Forgive yourself if you slip. Do the best you can. Don't turn a slip into a reason for giving up.

Get support. Having someone to talk with can really help. Enlist support from family and friends. Ask your doctor about support groups. Some weight loss programs can help motivate you. Shop around for one that focuses on good health and respects your self-esteem.

Measure Your Waist

Those extra pounds around your waist can be an indicator of your risk of developing serious health problems. How does your waist measure up? Wrap a tape measure around the smallest part of your waist. Relax. Don't pull in your stomach.

You may be at increased risk of heart disease, diabetes and other concerns if:

- You're male and your waist measures more than 40 inches.

- You're female and your waist measures more than 35 inches.

Your risk is even greater if you also have a BMI of 25 or more (see Page 24). Call your nurse information service or doctor to learn about making healthy changes.

Beware the Fad-Diet Trap

The old adage, "If it seems too good to be true, then it probably is," really applies to fad diets. Most require some extreme action such as eliminating one or more food groups, or consuming very low amounts of calories. You may lose some weight at first, but in the long run you may jeopardize your health.

Fad diets can leave you feeling run down. Any weight you lose likely will return. Basic good nutrition and exercise might not seem glamorous, but they're healthier, more dependable and longer lasting.

Body Mass Index

The Body Mass Index (BMI) chart (see Page 24) lets you see if your weight falls within a healthy range. Use this as a guide only. Work closely with your doctor to develop a weight control plan that's right for you.

If your weight or height doesn't fall within the limits of the chart in this book, use this formula to calculate your BMI—multiply your weight by 703, then divide that number by your height in inches, squared:

$$BMI = \frac{\text{Weight (pounds) X 703}}{\text{Height (inches)}^2}$$

Special Weight Concerns

Some weight concerns may result in serious health risks and, at times, emotional distress. It's critical to seek appropriate health care and compassionate support.

Obesity. Generally, a Body Mass Index (BMI) of 30 or higher indicates obesity. Excessive weight puts your health in jeopardy and even may put your life in danger. Talk with your doctor about lifestyle changes, medication or surgical procedures that may help.

Eating disorders. A disproportionate concern with body weight combined with unusual eating behaviors is called an eating disorder (see Page 333).

Anorexia nervosa is dieting to the point of starvation. This is a common eating disorder. Another is bulimia, which is binge eating followed by purging— forced vomiting or intentional overuse of laxatives. Women and teen-age girls are most vulnerable to eating disorders, but men and boys can develop them, too. Self-care isn't appropriate for these serious health concerns. Without professional treatment, they can lead to death. If you think you—or someone you love— has an eating disorder, seek professional help right away.

Underlying health concerns. If you have any unexplained weight gain (see Page 242) or weight loss (see Page 244), call your doctor. It may be a symptom of a serious health condition.

Body Mass Index Chart

	Normal						Overweight					Obese									
BMI	19	20	21	22	23	24	25	26	27	28	29	30	31	32	33	34	35	36	37	38	39
Height (inches)								**Body Weight (pounds)**													
58	91	96	100	105	110	115	119	124	129	134	138	143	148	153	158	162	167	172	177	181	186
59	94	99	104	109	114	119	124	128	133	138	143	148	153	158	163	168	173	178	183	188	193
60	97	102	107	112	118	123	128	133	138	143	148	153	158	163	168	174	179	184	189	194	199
61	100	106	111	116	122	127	132	137	143	148	153	158	164	169	174	180	185	190	195	201	206
62	104	109	115	120	126	131	136	142	147	153	158	164	169	175	180	186	191	196	202	207	213
63	107	113	118	124	130	135	141	146	152	158	163	169	175	180	186	191	197	203	208	214	220
64	110	116	122	128	134	140	145	151	157	163	169	174	180	186	192	197	204	209	215	221	227
65	114	120	126	132	138	144	150	156	162	168	174	180	186	192	198	204	210	216	222	228	234
66	118	124	130	136	142	148	155	161	167	173	179	186	192	198	204	210	216	223	229	235	241
67	121	127	134	140	146	153	159	166	172	178	185	191	198	204	211	217	223	230	236	242	249
68	125	131	138	144	151	158	164	171	177	184	190	197	203	210	216	223	230	236	243	249	256
69	128	135	142	149	155	162	169	176	182	189	196	203	209	216	223	230	236	243	250	257	263
70	132	139	146	153	160	167	174	181	188	195	202	209	216	222	229	236	243	250	257	264	271
71	136	143	150	157	165	172	179	186	193	200	208	215	222	229	236	243	250	257	265	272	279
72	140	147	154	162	169	177	184	191	199	206	213	221	228	235	242	250	258	265	272	279	287
73	144	151	159	166	174	182	189	197	204	212	219	227	235	242	250	257	265	272	280	288	295
74	148	155	163	171	179	186	194	202	210	218	225	233	241	249	256	264	272	280	287	295	303
75	152	160	168	176	184	192	200	208	216	224	232	240	248	256	264	272	279	287	295	303	311
76	156	164	172	180	189	197	205	213	221	230	238	246	254	263	271	279	287	295	304	312	320

Source: Adapted from Clinical Guidelines on the Identification, Evaluation and Treatment of Overweight and Obesity in Adults: The Evidence Report

Taking Care: Self-Care for You and Your Family

Quit Your Tobacco Habit

Chances are, you probably already know that using tobacco can damage your health. But quitting isn't easy. Maybe you've tried and weren't successful. Whether you use cigarettes, cigars, pipes, snuff or chewing tobacco, it's time to try quitting again.

Quitting can dramatically lower your risk of emphysema, heart disease, and lung, mouth and throat cancers. Not enough to motivate you? When you quit, you'll smell better and develop fewer wrinkles. That yellow will fade from your teeth and nails. And, food will taste better.

If you can't seem to do it for yourself, do it for your family and friends. Spare them the respiratory problems that secondhand smoke can cause. Quitting also will help you live longer for the people who love you.

But How?

The first step is to stop thinking that there's no point quitting. From the moment you quit—no matter how long you've used tobacco—your body starts healing itself.

Some people quit on their own. Others do it with the help of tobacco cessation programs. Many of these are offered through hospitals, health organizations and, sometimes, even employers. Ask your doctor about programs in your area.

Take one day at a time. Don't be too discouraged if you slip. Most successful quitters had to try more than once to become tobacco free. Try these tips:

- Set a date to give up tobacco and stick with it.
- Make a list of your reasons for wanting to quit. Carry it with you and refer to it when you feel a craving.
- Plan ahead for handling tobacco urges. Take a walk, practice deep breathing exercises, nibble on pretzels or carrot sticks, or call a "stop smoking" buddy.
- Avoid places and habits that make you want to use tobacco.
- Tell family and friends you're quitting—and enlist their support.
- Watch your tobacco money build up. Spend it on something special as a well-deserved reward.

Some people may benefit from smoking cessation medications or aids such as nicotine gum or patches. They can help minimize withdrawal symptoms. Ask your doctor if they're right for you. Be sure to check your health plan for coverage.

If You Drink, Do So in Moderation

Drinking alcohol is part of many traditions in our lives. We may make toasts at weddings and holidays. Our cultural heritage may call for wine with dinner.

Do You Have a Drug or Alcohol Problem?

- Do you believe you must use drugs or alcohol in order to have fun?

- Have you tried to stop using drugs or alcohol but couldn't?

- Have you had trouble at school, work or home because of your use of drugs or alcohol?

- Has a friend, relative, co-worker or medical professional expressed concern about your use of drugs or alcohol?

- Do you use drugs or alcohol to help you get through the day or when you're feeling angry, tense or sad?

- Do you drink or use drugs when you're alone?

- Do you need more drugs to get the same effect you used to get with smaller amounts?

If you answered, "Yes" to any of these questions, you may have a problem with drugs or alcohol. Seek help from your doctor or a mental health professional.

Source: Adapted from the National Institute on Alcohol Abuse and Alcoholism

Because alcohol is socially acceptable, it's all the more important to drink responsibly and in moderation.

- Don't mix alcohol and drugs. This can be a deadly combination, even with over-the-counter medications or supplements. Ask your doctor or pharmacist how alcohol interacts with the medications you take.

- Don't drink and drive. And, never ride with a driver who's been drinking. Even one drink can impair judgment and slow reaction time.

- Don't drink at all if you're pregnant— alcohol can harm your baby. Neither men nor women who are trying to conceive should drink alcohol.

- Don't engage in binge drinking.

There has been much discussion about whether alcohol offers positive health benefits. Most experts agree that the possible negative effects from long-term alcohol use outweigh possible benefits.

Alcohol is a powerful drug that can be abused easily. If you drink nearly every day at the same time, or rely on alcohol to help you deal with stress, you may have an alcohol abuse problem (see Page 328). Seek professional help. Your health, relationships and life may depend on it.

Don't Abuse Drugs

When you think of drug abuse, you probably think of illegal drugs, such as marijuana, cocaine and heroin. But any drug—even prescription medications and over-the-counter products—can be misused.

Drug abuse can destroy your life, from your physical health to your relationships with family and friends. It can impair your judgment and alter your personality. You may be more likely to harm yourself or others, find yourself in legal trouble and jeopardize your job. If you think that you or someone you love may have a drug abuse problem, get help right away (see Page 328). The longer the abuse continues, the harder it will be to break free.

Let Yourself Sleep

Does a good night's sleep seem like a luxury? When life is hectic, it may seem that way. However, sleep is essential to your health. Each person's sleep requirements are different, but most people need between eight and nine hours a night. However, some—especially teens—may need even more. But the reality is, most of us aren't even close to getting what we need.

Adequate rest improves your health and your mood; allows you to accomplish more; sharpens your memory; and decreases the likelihood of accidents. So, start thinking of sleep as an investment in your well-being and peace of mind. Make time for those ZZZs you need to feel your best.

Try these tips for a better night's sleep:

- Don't use tobacco. Nicotine is a stimulant and can keep you awake.
- Avoid caffeine at least six hours before bedtime—including coffee, tea, caffeinated soft drinks and chocolate.

- Say, "No" to that nightcap. Alcohol will give you a fitful sleep.
- Don't exercise too close to bedtime.
- Sleep and wake at the same time each day—even on weekends.
- Try not to nap.
- Keep your room dark, cool and as quiet as possible.
- Set up a relaxing, pre-sleep ritual. Take a warm bath, meditate or listen to soothing music. Read a book, but save the thriller for another time.

About Sleep Apnea

Some people suffer from sleep problems due to a disorder called sleep apnea. This is a condition in which the person's breathing is interrupted many times during sleep. The effects can range from annoying to life-threatening (see Page 94).

People with sleep apnea may not be aware they have it. Excessive daytime sleepiness can be a sign. This condition is complex, so if you think you have it—or if your partner notices abnormal snoring or breathing patterns when you sleep—see your doctor.

Everyone has trouble sleeping now and then. However, if you regularly toss and turn or have trouble staying awake during the day, talk with your doctor. He or she may recommend a medication to help you sleep. If so, follow all instructions carefully—including how long you can take it safely.

Reduce Stress

We experience stress when we react to the pressure that life sometimes puts on us. A little stress can be good. It can keep us motivated to do new things. But, too much stress can cause health problems ranging from headaches to heart conditions. It also can throw your emotions off balance, affect your relationships and just plain wear you down.

Are You Under Too Much Stress?

- Do minor problems and disappointments upset you excessively?

- Do the small pleasures of life fail to satisfy you?

- Are you unable to stop thinking about your worries?

- Do you feel inadequate or suffer from self-doubt?

- Are you constantly tired?

- Do you experience flashes of anger over situations that never bothered you before?

- Have you noticed a change in sleeping or eating patterns?

- Do you suffer from chronic pain, headaches or backaches not due to injury or physical illness?

If most of your answers are, "Yes," you may be under too much stress. Talk with your doctor or a mental health professional about how to manage your stress.

Source: National Mental Health Association

The stress in your life may run the gamut from minor aggravations to serious problems that you're facing. It's impossible to eliminate stress completely. But, these tips can help you learn how to manage the effect it has on you:

- **Take care of yourself.** You can handle stress better if you eat nutritious food, exercise and get enough sleep. Avoid caffeine, alcohol and tobacco.

- **Set limits.** Trying to do too much will add to your stress. Focus on what's most important and learn to say, "No" to the rest.

- **Use relaxation techniques each day.** Do some breathing exercises, gentle stretching or meditation. Listening to music, taking some quiet time for yourself or even picking up an old hobby can help, too.

- **Let it go.** Often we feel stressful about things we just can't change. Tell yourself that sometimes it's OK to just "let it go." Acceptance is wisdom, not defeat.

- **Get support.** Whether you turn to family, friends, a counselor, your doctor or a support group, sharing your feelings really can relieve your stress.

Adopt Safe Habits

Investing time and effort in preventing accidents and injuries can help keep you and your family safe.

Personal Safety

- Reduce your risk of infectious diseases. Wash your hands often with soap and warm running water—especially before cooking or eating, and after using the bathroom or handling animals.

- Reduce your risk of skin cancer. Use a sunblock with a sun protection factor (SPF) of 15 or higher, with both UVA and UVB protection. Reapply often.

- Wear sunglasses that block UVA and UVB rays.

- Prevent injuries. Wear protective gear during sports—consider helmets, elbow and knee pads, and eye protection, as appropriate.

Vehicle Safety

- Wear your seatbelt. Insist that everyone in the car do the same.

- Place infants and children in appropriate car seats—in the back seat. Follow manufacturer installation instructions carefully.

- Have your brakes, lights and windshield wipers checked regularly.

- Keep safety items in your trunk—include a first-aid kit (see Page 2), blanket, flares and reflectors.

- Don't drive aggressively. If an angry driver follows you, drive to a nearby police station or other safe place. Don't drive directly home.

- Don't use your cell phone while driving. Pull over to make or answer calls.

If You Own a Gun...

- Store it safely—unloaded and locked up.

- Lock and store ammunition separately.

- Hide the keys from your children and their friends.

- Take a gun-safety course.

- Teach your children about gun safety.

Be sure to ask if there are guns in the homes your children visit.

Prevent Accidents

- Keep hallways and staircases well lit and clear of clutter.

- Remove small throw rugs or secure them with double-sided tape.

- Use nightlights in bathrooms and hallways.

- Use nonslip mats in the bathtub and in shower stalls.

- Make sure window screens are secure.

- Don't let window-blind cords dangle low enough for a child to reach or get caught on.

Fires

- Install smoke detectors outside every bedroom—or inside, if you sleep with your bedroom door closed—and on every level of your house. Check the batteries monthly and replace them twice a year.

- Keep a fire extinguisher in the kitchen.
- Have a fire escape plan, and a designated spot to meet. Practice, and make sure everyone knows two ways out of every room.

Carbon Monoxide

- Install carbon monoxide detectors in your home and garage to detect this odorless gas.
- Have a qualified technician inspect and clean your heating system and chimney annually.

Poison Dangers

- Keep the number of your local Poison Control Center near the phone. If you don't know your local number, call (800) 222-1222 to be connected with a Poison Control Center in your area.
- Keep poisonous items such as household cleaning products, antifreeze, paints, solvents and insecticides locked up. Keep these items away from children and pets.
- Keep your purse out of children's reach if you keep medication in it.
- Store all medications in their original containers. Keep them locked up.
- Be aware of indoor and outdoor plants that may be poisonous to children and pets.

Environmental Concerns

- Use nontoxic cleaning products and insecticides around your home.
- Keep your children and pets off lawns that recently have been treated with pesticides.
- Have your house tested for radon. This odorless gas comes from uranium deposits in the soil. It's been linked to lung cancer. Your local environmental agency or health department can recommend how to test for radon. They also can tell you how to eliminate it from your home.
- Test your home for lead paint and asbestos before remodeling. Check with your local environmental agency or health department about proper removal procedures.

30

Prevention and Early Detection

There are some simple—but powerful—tools that can help you prevent illness and detect diseases in their earliest stages. Take a proactive approach to your health with regular health exams, immunizations, preventive screenings, self-exams and home health tests.

Regular health exams. It's natural to think about seeing your doctor when you're sick. But, it's important to see him or her when you're well, too. Some health problems don't have symptoms that you can feel or see. This is true for high blood pressure, diabetes, glaucoma and some cancers, for instance. When you get regular health exams, your doctor can help you stay healthy.

Based on your age and health history, your doctor will determine how often you should have checkups. Ask which immunizations, screenings and healthy lifestyle changes are right for you. See Page 344 for handy health forms.

Immunizations. They prevent diseases and save lives. Immunizations are crucial to infants, children and adults. The charts in this chapter—based on Centers for Disease Control and Prevention recommendations—can serve as a guide. Ask your doctor which immunizations are right for your family. Follow his or her recommendations.

Preventive screenings. A broad range of screenings can help children and adults

Immunizations—Birth to 24 Years

Immunization	What It's For	When and How Often	
		Ages 10 Years and Younger	*Ages 11 to 24 Years*
DTaP or DT (ages 7 years or younger) Tetanus-diphtheria (Td) (older than age 7)	Diphtheria, tetanus and pertussis (whooping cough)	Five immunizations (DTaP is preferred for all doses in the series) at the following ages: 2, 4 and 6 months, between 15 and 18 months, and between 4 and 6 years	Booster of Td between ages 11 and 16 years, and then every 10 years*
Polio (inactivated)	Polio	Four immunizations at the following ages: 2 and 4 months, between 6 and 18 months, and between 4 and 6 years	Not needed unless not previously immunized
Pneumococcal conjugate (Prevnar) †	Bacterial meningitis, blood and ear infections	Four immunizations at the following ages: 2, 4 and 6 months, and between 12 and 15 months; fifth dose at age 24 months for children who socialize with others	Not necessary
MMR	Measles, mumps and rubella (German measles)	Two immunizations at the following ages: between 12 and 15 months, and between 4 and 6 years	Second dose required if not yet received
H. influenzae type B (Hib)	Bacterial meningitis	Three to four immunizations (depending on the vaccine) at the following ages: 2, 4 and 6 months, and between 12 and 15 months	Not required after age 5 years
Hepatitis B	Hepatitis B	Three immunizations: birth, ages 1 and 6 months; or between birth and 2 months, one to two months later, and between ages 6 and 18 months; or for older children, by doctor's recommendation	If not previously immunized, three immunizations at the following schedule: next doctor visit, one month later and six months later, or by doctor's recommendation
Hepatitis A	Hepatitis A	In selected areas, two immunizations separated by six to 18 months, from ages 2 years and older	If not previously immunized, in selected areas, two immunizations separated by six to 18 months
Varicella	Chickenpox	One immunization between ages 12 and 18 months, or older if child has no history of chickenpox	If not previously immunized and no history of chickenpox, one dose between ages 11 and 12 years; or, two doses separated by four to eight weeks for ages 13 years and older
Influenza	Influenza	Annually for children age 6 months and older at high risk	Annually for those at high risk
Meningococcal	Meningococcal meningitis	Not necessary	One dose for college students living on campus

* *Discuss frequency with your doctor.*
† *Ask your doctor if you're at risk for pneumococcal disease—you may need additional preventive care.*
Immunization guidelines are continuously updated. Ask your doctor about the latest recommendations.

Immunizations—Ages 25 Years and Older†

Immunization	What It's For	When and How Often	
		Adults 25 to 64	**Adults 65 and older**
Rubella serology or vaccination history	Rubella (German measles)	Recommended once for all susceptible females of child-bearing age	Not necessary
Tetanus-diphtheria (Td)	Tetanus and diphtheria	Boosters every 10 years, or as recommended*	Boosters every 10 years or as recommended*
Pneumococcal	Pneumonia	Once for people with chronic illness**; some may require a second dose after five years	Once for most people; some may require a second dose after five years
Influenza	Flu	Annually for people ages 50 and older, or at high risk**	Annually

*   *Discuss frequency with your doctor.*
** *Check with your doctor.*
†   *Adults who haven't had basic childhood immunizations should discuss their status with their doctors.*

stay healthy. These charts are based on the recommendations of the U.S. Preventive Services Task Force. They offer general guidelines for people not at high risk. Talk with your doctor about which screenings your family needs— and how often you should have them.

Not all health plans cover all screenings. Check with your health plan regarding coverage.

Self-exams. While the effectiveness of self-exams isn't yet proven, they can help you take an active role in your health. Staying aware of any changes in your body can help you gather information to discuss with your doctor.

■ **Skin cancer.** When found early, skin cancer is very treatable. Examine your skin on all parts of your body carefully in a brightly lit room. Ask a

Screenings—Birth to 10 Years

Screening	What It Checks For	When and How Often
Height and weight	General development	Throughout infancy and childhood*
Blood pressure	General health	Periodically*
T4 and TSH	Hypothyroidism—a thyroid condition; if untreated, it can affect growth and brain development	Between day 2 and 6; or before leaving the hospital
Phenylalanine level	Phenylketonuria (PKU)—a rare condition; if untreated, it can cause brain damage	At birth

* *Discuss frequency with your doctor.*

Screenings—Ages 11 to 24 Years

Screening	What It Checks For	When and How Often
Height and weight	General health; obesity	Periodically*
Blood pressure	High blood pressure and general health	Periodically*
For young women only:		
Papanicolaou (Pap) test	Cervical cancer	Every one to three years for sexually active females or beginning at age 18
Chlamydia screen	Chlamydia, a sexually transmitted disease	Routine screenings recommended for all sexually active females*
Rubella serology or vaccination history	Determines if rubella vaccine was given or if you've had German measles	Recommended for all females of child-bearing age

*   *Discuss frequency with your doctor.*

Screenings—Ages 25 to 64 Years

Screening	What It Checks For	When and How Often
Height and weight	General health; obesity	Periodically*
Blood pressure	High blood pressure	Periodically*
Cholesterol	High total cholesterol, and low HDL cholesterol	Periodically* for males between ages 35 and 64; and females between ages 45 and 64
Fecal occult blood test	Colorectal cancer	Annually* beginning at age 50
Sigmoidoscopy	Colorectal cancer	Every three to five years, beginning at age 50
For women only:		
Clinical breast exam	Breast cancer	Annually between ages 50 and 69
Mammogram	Breast cancer	Every one to two years starting at age 40**
Chlamydia screen	Chlamydia, a sexually transmitted disease	Sexually active females*
Papanicolaou (Pap) test	Cervical cancer	Every one to three years for sexually active females who have not had a hysterectomy

*   *Discuss frequency with your doctor.*
** *Effective Jan. 1, 1998, Medicare requires coverage for annual mammograms for all women ages 40 and older.*

Screenings—Ages 65 Years and Older

Screening	What It Checks For	When and How Often
Height and weight	General health; obesity	Periodically*
Blood pressure	High blood pressure	Periodically*
Cholesterol	High total cholesterol, and low HDL cholesterol	Periodically*
Eye exam	Glaucoma and other vision problems	Annually
Hearing test	Hearing difficulties	Periodically*
Fecal occult blood test	Colorectal cancer	Annually* beginning at age 50
Sigmoidoscopy	Colorectal cancer	Every three to five years
For women only:		
Papanicolaou (Pap) test	Cervical cancer	Every one to three years for sexually active females who have not had a hysterectomy
Clinical breast exam	Breast cancer	Annually between ages 65 and 69
Mammogram	Breast cancer	Every one to two years starting at age 40**

* Discuss frequency with your doctor.
** Effective Jan. 1, 1998, Medicare requires coverage for annual mammograms for all women ages 40 and older.

partner to help with hard-to-see places. Look for any unusual changes on your skin, such as scaliness, oozing or bleeding. Pay special attention to moles and freckles.

Think ABCDE, and if you see any of these signs, promptly report them to your doctor:

- Asymmetry—one half of your mole looks different than the other

- Border—the edges are irregular, notched or scalloped

- Color—blue, white or red patches, or a mixed brown or black color, or a change in color

- Diameter—the mole is the size of a pencil eraser or larger, or it has grown noticeably

- Elevation—the mole is raised

■ **Breast self-exam.** Early detection of breast cancer can dramatically increase the chances of recovery. Discuss with your doctor how often to do breast self-exams. He or she also can teach you the proper technique.

Talk with your doctor about the difference between the natural, healthy texture of your breasts and possible warning signs.

See your doctor if you notice any:

- Lumps
- Swelling
- Dimpling
- Redness
- Discharge

The best time to do a breast self-exam is during the week following your menstrual period.

■ **Testicular self-exam.** Males between ages 15 and 35 are most vulnerable to testicular cancer. With early detection, it's very curable. Talk with your doctor about the value of testicular self-exams.

The best time is after a warm bath or shower when your scrotum is relaxed. While standing, gently roll each testicle between your thumbs (on top) and your index and middle fingers (underneath). If you find any lumps or notice other changes, see your doctor.

Home health tests. Knowing your health status is easier with the convenience of home health tests and devices. Perhaps your doctor wants you to monitor your blood glucose levels or blood pressure. The results you collect can help your doctor develop the best possible treatment plan for you.

There also are home tests for pregnancy, high cholesterol, colon cancer, HIV and other health concerns. Some test kits require you to mail the test to a lab. You may be able to call for anonymous results. Many of these tests are available at your local pharmacy and are relatively inexpensive. They can be useful, but keep these tips in mind:

- Don't rely on a home health test to replace your doctor's diagnosis. Inaccurate results may be possible.
- Be sure to use a test that's approved by the Food and Drug Administration.
- Read all instructions carefully. Follow each step. Dispose of test materials as instructed. Don't use a test past its expiration date.
- If the kit contains chemicals, keep it out of the reach of children.

Home health tests offer a great opportunity to take an active part in your health care. But remember—they won't be of any value if you don't share the information with your doctor. He or she can determine if the results are accurate. From there you can work together to develop a plan for making the most of your health.

Medications

4

You may use them occasionally when you're sick, or every day to manage an ongoing health condition. They may be prescription or over-the-counter. In any case, medications can play an important role in helping you feel better and stay healthy.

For the sake of your health, it's critical to understand the medications you take. If not used properly, they can be ineffective—or even dangerous. Talk with your doctor about your medication history; ask lots of questions; and use and store your medications safely for best results.

If you're pregnant, or think you may be, check with your doctor before taking any prescription or over-the-counter medications, vitamins or supplements.

Work With Your Doctor

Tell your doctor about:

- Any known allergies to medications or side effects you've experienced
- Existing health conditions, including if you're pregnant, or may be pregnant
- All the medications you're taking—including over-the-counter drugs, vitamins and herbal supplements

Ask your doctor:

- What's the name of the medicine and what does it do?
- Is a generic version of this medicine appropriate for you?
- How often—and for how long—should you take it?

- What happens if you don't take it?

- What are the possible side effects?

- Do you need to take it with food or on an empty stomach?

- Is it safe to drink alcohol while taking this medication?

- What should you do if you miss a dose?

- What signs indicate you need to call the doctor back?

- Will a refill be needed? If so, will that require a return doctor visit?

Take Advantage of Your Pharmacy

- Ask your pharmacist any questions you may have about your prescription. He or she also can help you choose over-the-counter medicines.

- Check the prescription label before leaving. Make sure it's your prescription, and that you can read and understand the directions. Ask for more information, if needed.

- If you need to crush or split pills to help swallow them, ask your pharmacist if this is safe for your specific medication.

- Ask if your pharmacy has a computerized service that allows them—and your doctor—to keep track of all your medications. This can help prevent interactions.

Use and Store Medication Safely

- Take the prescribed amount of medication—no more, no less.

- Spread out the dosages appropriately. For instance, if a medication is supposed to be taken twice a day, take each dose 12 hours apart—not, for example, at lunch, then at dinner.

- Finish all your medications if your doctor tells you to do so—even if your symptoms have gone away.

- Don't ever share your prescription medications. They can be dangerous to someone else.

- Give children medication and dosages intended for them. If no children's dosage is listed on the package, don't guess. Ask your doctor or pharmacist.

- Take your medication in a well-lit room. Make sure you've grabbed the right medicine. It's easy to make a mistake late at night or when you don't feel well.

- Beware of potential interactions. Alcohol, other medicines, vitamins and herbal supplements—and even some foods—can interact with your medication. Ask your doctor or pharmacist about this.

- If you take several medications, make a chart to keep track of when you need to take each (see Page 348).

- Keep medications in their original containers.

38

- Don't use medicine past its expiration date. Throw out prescription medications you no longer use. Dispose of them by flushing the contents down the toilet.

- Keep medicines locked up and away from children—including those medications you may have in your purse or briefcase.

- Teach your children and grandchildren about medication safety.

Over-the-Counter Medications

Over-the-counter, or OTC, medications can help relieve minor symptoms. They can be helpful for nasal congestion, fever, headache and more. Follow these tips to make the most of these convenient self-care tools:

- Choose a product designed for the symptoms you have. Don't over-medicate with ingredients you don't really need.

- Read and follow all instructions and warnings carefully.

- Aren't sure about your symptoms? See your doctor for an accurate diagnosis. Also, call your doctor if you've tried self-care but your symptoms haven't improved.

- Pregnant women should talk with their doctors before taking any over-the-counter medication.

Pain Relievers

Aspirin reduces pain, inflammation and fever. It's one of several nonsteroidal anti-inflammatory drugs, or NSAIDS. While aspirin is effective for some illnesses or conditions, it also has some well-known side effects. For some people, prolonged use of aspirin can lead to gastrointestinal upset or ulcers. Reduce potential stomach irritation by using aspirin labeled "enteric coated," and taking it with food or milk. Aspirin increases the risk of bleeding in general.

As with all medication, check with your doctor before using aspirin.

> Don't give aspirin to anyone younger than age 19! It's linked to Reye's syndrome, a rare but sometimes fatal condition (see Page 361).

Acetaminophen relieves pain and reduces fever. Some people find it as effective as ibuprofen in relieving the pain of osteoarthritis. In general, it's considered safer than aspirin for people with various health concerns, and for children. Acetaminophen seldom causes stomach problems, and it doesn't cause bleeding.

Ibuprofen and naproxen sodium also are NSAIDs. For some people, these pain relievers/fever reducers can be easier on the stomach than aspirin. However, they sometimes can cause ulceration. Be sure to take these medications with food or milk. These two NSAIDs don't interfere with blood clotting in the same way as aspirin, but they can cause bleeding in some people, including some older adults.

Cold and Allergy Remedies

Decongestants relieve nasal congestion by constricting blood vessels. For this reason, these medications may not be right for people with high blood pressure, heart disease, diabetes, glaucoma and many other conditions. Read the warning labels carefully. Prolonged use of decongestants can cause a "rebound" effect—particularly nasal decongestant sprays. They can leave you even more congested.

Antihistamines are effective in controlling allergy symptoms such as sneezing and runny nose. They sometimes are included in cold remedies to help dry congested nasal passages. Over-the-counter antihistamines should be used sparingly. They can cause drowsiness and may become less effective over time.

A note about decongestants and antihistamines: These medications—alone or in combination—are particularly hazardous for older men with benign prostatic hyperplasia (see Page 300).

Cough Medications

Some coughs are productive, generating mucus and helping to clear your lungs. Others are dry and unproductive. Typically, it's best not to suppress a productive cough unless it's keeping you from sleeping.

Expectorants help loosen mucus, making it easier to cough up. These products aren't designed to stop your cough. They're intended to help clear your lungs.

Cough suppressants, or antitussives, help relieve a dry, unproductive cough. Be aware that these medicines can cause drowsiness. If you have asthma, bronchitis or emphysema, talk with your doctor before using these products.

Heartburn Relief

Antacids neutralize stomach acid. They also help relieve heartburn caused by gastroesophageal reflux disease (GERD). Most antacids contain aluminum, calcium carbonate, magnesium or sodium. Liquid and tablet forms seem equally effective.

Sodium-based antacids can increase fluid retention and raise blood pressure. Avoid this type if you have heart or kidney disease, or high blood pressure. Aluminum-based antacids can interfere with the absorption of medications. If you're taking any medications, check with your doctor before using antacids. Taking large doses of antacids containing calcium carbonate can cause "acid rebound," resulting in even more stomach acid.

Other OTC Remedies

Antidiarrheals commonly work by absorbing many times their weight in water. This makes stools firmer and slower to pass. These products generally take two to three days to work. Be sure to drink lots of water when taking these medications, or constipation may result.

Some antidiarrheals work by interrupting nerve messages within the intestines, reducing the frequency of bowel movements. This type, including certain strengths of loperamide, work more quickly. Drowsiness is a possible side effect.

Laxatives help relieve constipation. Bulk-forming laxatives contain nondigestible fibers that absorb water in the intestines. This makes stools softer and easier to pass.

Stool softeners encourage fluids to be absorbed into the stool, making elimination easier. Stool softeners are slow and gentle. Other stimulant laxatives are very fast acting. They cause water to quickly flush out the stool.

Use laxatives sparingly. If you use them too frequently, your bowels may become dependent on them. Instead, be sure to drink plenty of water, eat fiber-rich foods and exercise regularly.

Antifungal medications help treat infections, such as vaginal yeast infections, oral thrush, athlete's foot and ringworm. Antifungals are available as creams, ointments, powders, sprays, lozenges and tablets. Ask your doctor or pharmacist which is right for your situation.

From Medicine Cabinet to Medicine Center

It used to be that the bathroom medicine cabinet was where we often stored remedies for our family's minor illnesses. But, the bathroom's heat and humidity can damage the effectiveness of medications. Instead, choose a cool, dry spot for your home "medicine center" and keep it well stocked. Be sure it's out of the reach of children. Choose a storage place that can be locked.

This list will give you ideas for your home medicine center. You may have many of these items in your first-aid kit, too (see Page 2). Keep your kit intact for emergencies and use your medicine center for routine self-care.

- Antacid
- Antidiarrheal medication
- Antihistamine
- Antiseptic cream
- Bandages—assorted sizes and shapes
- Cough medication
- Cold medication
- Decongestant
- Eyeglass prescription
- Gauze pads
- Hydrocortisone cream or calamine lotion
- Pain relievers/fever reducers such as acetaminophen, ibuprofen, naproxen sodium and aspirin
- Petroleum jelly
- Rubbing alcohol
- Saline nose drops
- Saline solution
- Scissors
- Sore throat lozenges
- Sunscreen
- Syrup of ipecac
- Thermometer
- Tweezers

Also, be sure to keep an ample supply of important prescriptions that are used daily for ongoing conditions. Store them in the same secure place.

Working With Your Doctor

Developing a comfortable and open relationship with your doctor is key to your well-being. Your doctor can be much more than someone you see only when you're sick or injured. Through prevention and education, he or she can help you achieve long-term good health. Think of your doctor as someone who can provide comfort and peace of mind.

Take a proactive approach to making the most of your relationship with your doctor. There are many ways to do this—knowing how to choose a doctor, planning the questions you'll ask at your appointments, and understanding your health plan.

Finding a Doctor

At some point, we all need to choose a doctor—whether due to moving, changing jobs and health plans, or developing a new health concern. These tips can help as you begin your search:

- First, check your health plan's provider list to be sure you choose a doctor who accepts your insurance or health coverage plan. These lists sometimes give information on doctors' credentials, specialties, and which languages they can accommodate.
- Ask family, friends and co-workers about doctors they recommend.

- Check with local doctor-referral services such as through hospitals or medical associations. These resources also may have credential information.

- Consider what's most important to you. Do you want a family practitioner, or separate doctors for yourself and your children? Which location is most convenient—close to home or work? Do members of your family have special needs?

Making the Choice

Depending on your needs and where you live, you may find there are several doctors or practices from which to choose. Call those you're interested in. Ask each one the same questions to help you make a decision.

- Are they taking new patients?

- Do they accept your health insurance or other coverage plan?

- What are their days and hours?

- How many doctors are in the practice? What are their specialties?

- Which hospital is the doctor associated with?

- How do they schedule "sick" visits and routine "well" visits?

- How do they handle urgent appointments? Do they have 24-hour, on-call coverage?

- What services do they have? For instance, is phone advice available? Do they have a physician's assistant

or nurse practitioner? Do they have X-ray equipment onsite?

- How are co-payments or other fees handled?

Schedule a "Get Acquainted" Appointment

It's ideal to meet with the doctor you're considering. Admittedly, this may be a luxury of time not everyone can afford. But, if you can fit this into your busy schedule, a meeting can help you decide if this is the doctor for you. Some doctors charge a fee for this visit, so be sure to ask when you call.

Bring a notepad and some prepared questions about issues important to you. Tell the doctor what you're looking for in a physician. Let him or her know about any special health concerns. As he or she answers your questions, you can begin to determine if this is going to be a good match. Trust your instincts. They're probably right.

Use this list of things to notice, and questions to ask to get started:

- Does the office seem clean and organized? Is there enough staff? Are they friendly and helpful?

- How long has the doctor been practicing? How long has he or she been at this office?

- What treatments does he or she usually recommend for any ongoing health concerns you or your family members may have?

- Does the doctor or a staff member always follow up with patients?
- What is the doctor's philosophy on preventive health?
- Is the doctor carefully listening to your questions, giving you time to talk?
- Is he or she answering in a clear, understandable manner?
- Is the doctor's communication style a good match for you?
- Would you feel comfortable with this doctor?

Make the Most of Your Appointments

Being an active participant in your health care will benefit you in the long run. You'll feel confident and your doctor will be able to serve you better.

Come prepared. Arrive in plenty of time to fill out any paperwork so that you don't feel rushed. Bring your health insurance card and any other information you'll need to provide.

Share information. Your doctor can choose the most appropriate and effective care only if he or she knows as much about you as possible. Share information about past and ongoing medical conditions and treatments; symptoms or other concerns you have now; all prescription and over-the-counter medicines, vitamins, supplements and herbal remedies you're taking; drug allergies or intolerances you may have; any complementary therapies you're using; and lifestyle habits such as whether you smoke or how much you exercise. Jot these things down ahead of time to help you remember everything and feel more relaxed.

Ask questions. It's not uncommon to leave the doctor's office and then think of questions you wish you'd asked. Use the list on the following page to help you prepare your questions ahead of time. Leave room on your list to take notes.

Follow your doctor's instructions. Your doctor's treatment or prevention plan can be effective only if you follow his or her instructions closely. Take medications as prescribed. Make any healthy lifestyle changes recommended. Keep your follow-up appointments as needed.

Communicate your preferences and concerns. Be actively involved in the development of your treatment plan. If you prefer a specific approach, or you're worried about something, let your doctor know. Don't be afraid to say that you may want a second opinion, if that's the case. Your doctor should understand that it's important for you to have as much information as possible.

You and Your Health Plan

Knowing what your health plan covers can save time, confusion and even disappointment. For instance, if you're having a planned surgery, do you need to follow preauthorization or other special procedures? What tests or screenings are covered? Are you covered when traveling outside the United States?

Read through your covered benefits carefully. If you have any questions, call your plan representative so that you feel knowledgeable about your coverage.

Keep good records. Review your statements to make sure they're correct. If you have a question about your statement or how a claim was handled, call your health plan right away to resolve it. Have your insurance card and your records handy.

Questions to Ask Your Doctor

- What is the diagnosis?

- Are any tests required?

- What are the benefits and side effects of the recommended treatment or medication?

- What are the possible health consequences if I don't follow your recommended course of action?

- Are generic medications appropriate for my situation?

- What should I know about my medication, including side effects?

- What should I do if I forget to take a dose of medicine?

- Are there self-care measures that I can do at home?

- Are there alternative or complementary treatments that would be helpful (if you're interested)?

- What should I do if my symptoms get worse?

- Do I need to come back for a follow up? If yes, when?

Symptoms

No matter how well we take care of ourselves, injuries and illnesses can be an inevitable part of life. The symptoms they bring can be worrisome—especially when you don't know what to do. Understanding when a symptom is minor or potentially serious can help you take charge of your health.

The pages that follow describe a wide range of symptoms and possible causes. Each symptom provides an easy-to-follow decision chart. Using this tool can help you determine the course of action that's right for you. You also will find information specifically geared toward children's health.

This chapter can help you:

- Decide on the appropriate level of care for your situation
- Recognize emergency situations
- Learn how to care for minor symptoms at home
- Develop questions to ask your doctor and make the most of your next visit
- Know when your child's symptoms require special care

The most important thing is to be proactive about your and your family's health. When in doubt about any symptoms you may have, be sure to call your nurse information service or doctor to learn more.

ABDOMINAL CRAMPING

Cramping or pain in the abdominal area

Causes

Appendicitis. You may have pain near your belly button, that shifts to your lower right abdomen. The pain may be severe. It may get worse when you move, take deep breaths, cough or sneeze. You also may have nausea, vomiting, constipation, diarrhea or low-grade fever. You may not be able to pass gas. In appendicitis, your appendix becomes inflamed, and may burst, causing infection and even death. Seek emergency help immediately. Don't take enemas or laxatives—this can make the condition worse. Also, avoid pain relievers. They may mask symptoms that your doctor needs to know about.

Irritable bowel syndrome (IBS) (See Page 262). You may have abdominal cramping and stomach pain, diarrhea, constipation or bloating. The cause of IBS is unknown, but stress, dairy products, and high-fat or gas-producing foods may make it worse. Your doctor may prescribe medication to help control symptoms.

Gastroenteritis. Along with abdominal cramping you may have diarrhea, fever, headache, nausea or vomiting. Gastroenteritis most often is caused by viral infections or food poisoning (see Page 90). See your doctor and try self-care.

Female reproductive concerns. You may have abdominal cramping and pain. You are or might be pregnant. You also may have vaginal bleeding. This may indicate a miscarriage or an ectopic pregnancy (see Page 234)—see your doctor immediately. In women who aren't pregnant, recurrent cramping or pain other than ordinary menstrual cramps may indicate endometriosis. See your doctor for a diagnosis. If you have pain and cramping in your lower abdomen and pelvis; heavy vaginal discharge with an unpleasant odor; irregular menstrual bleeding; or pain during intercourse, you may have pelvic inflammatory disease (see Page 312) or another health condition. See your doctor.

Other causes may include menstrual cramps (see Page 316).

Self-Care

- If you have gastroenteritis, drink plenty of water or other clear fluids to prevent dehydration. Get plenty of rest. Try bland foods or the BRAT diet— bananas, rice, applesauce and toast.

- Try acetaminophen, ibuprofen or naproxen sodium to help ease menstrual cramps. Also, try placing a heating pad on your abdomen.

Prevention

- If you have IBS, eat a low-fat, high-fiber diet. Avoid substances that may trigger IBS. Cabbage, caffeine, alcohol and dairy products may cause flare-ups in some people.

- Follow safe food-handling procedures. Keep hot foods hot, and cold foods cold.

- Use latex condoms or practice abstinence to help prevent sexually transmitted diseases.

SEEK EMERGENCY HELP

▶ You have a lump or mass in your abdomen that pulsates. You also feel confused or faint.

▶ The pain is severe and you're pregnant or you think you might be.

▶ The pain is constant, localized or rapidly getting more intense.

▶ You've had pain near your belly button that may have moved to your lower right abdomen; nausea or vomiting; and a fever.

▶ The pain has lasted more than two hours; repeated vomiting hasn't relieved the pain; or your abdomen is swollen and tender.

▶ You had a hard blow to the abdomen, followed by pain, inability to urinate, or vomiting.

▶ You have excessive thirst, or fast breathing or heartbeat.

▶ You have a fever and you've been using tampons.

CALL YOUR NURSE INFORMATION SERVICE OR DOCTOR

▶ You have bloody or painful urination.

▶ You've tried self-care but the mild abdominal pain hasn't improved. You may have no other symptoms. Or, you may have diarrhea that's lasted more than 24 hours.

TRY SELF-CARE

▶ You have relatively mild pain but no other symptoms except possibly diarrhea for less than 24 hours.

YOUR CHILD'S SYMPTOMS

Seek emergency help if your child screams with pain at the slightest movement or touch, or if he has blood in his stool along with abdominal pain.

Call your nurse information service or doctor if your baby stops eating and seems to have abdominal pain.

Abdominal pain and your child. If your infant age 2 weeks to 4 months cries for a long time for no apparent reason, he may have colic. This is especially true if he stops crying after passing gas or having a bowel movement. Babies with colic typically have excellent appetites.

If your baby has colic, try these tips to soothe him:

- Give him a warm bath.
- Hold him close. Gently rub his back or abdomen.
- Rock with him in a rocking chair.
- Take him for a car ride.
- Play soothing music or sounds of nature.

! *Don't give aspirin to anyone younger than age 19! It's linked to Reye's syndrome, a rare but sometimes fatal condition.*

49

ACNE OR PIMPLE

Blackheads; whiteheads; clusters of red, inflamed cysts; or thick, painless lumps below the skin surface on the face or other areas

Causes

Tiny sebaceous glands all over your body produce a skin lubricant called sebum. Puberty, menstruation, pregnancy, other shifts in hormone balance, hereditary factors or certain medications may trigger the production of too much sebum. In addition, sloughed-off skin cells can block the sebum follicles. This plugs your skin's pores and produces whiteheads. Skin pigments, not dirt, turn them into blackheads. Normal skin bacteria can cause infection and pus. Pimples result when whiteheads rupture the follicle wall and allow sebum, dead cells and bacteria to invade the skin.

In many cases, acne can cause a great deal of embarrassment. It sometimes can lead to lower self-confidence—especially among adolescents and teen-agers. Fortunately, acne is harmless and typically clears up after adolescence. Antibiotics, drying preparations or medications such as oral isotretinoin often are prescribed.

Rosacea. Your skin may be red, as though you are blushing or have a sunburn. You also may have small, red, solid or pus-filled pimples. Rosacea is a skin condition that most often occurs in adults between ages 30 and 60. It often is called adult acne or acne rosacea. It's very different from acne, however. Using acne medications actually may make your symptoms worse. Rosacea can be treated with prescription medications and self-care. Talk with your doctor.

Self-Care

- For mild cases of acne, use benzoyl peroxide preparations.
- Wash your skin gently with a warm, clean washcloth and soap to remove skin oil. Steam may help open clogged pores. Avoid scrubbing and using abrasive soaps.
- Bathe or shower after exercising or sweating.
- Shampoo often. If needed, use a dandruff shampoo.
- Shield face from hairsprays and gels.
- Avoid stress—it may aggravate inflammation.

Prevention

- Keep skin clear by gently washing twice daily.
- Don't use oil-based makeup.
- Avoid cortisone preparations.

- Don't pick or squeeze pimples.
- Minimize sun exposure and avoid tanning bed use.
- Don't touch your face a lot. This may encourage inflammation.

SEE YOUR DOCTOR

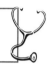

▶ **You have large, painful cysts.**

CALL YOUR NURSE INFORMATION SERVICE OR DOCTOR

▶ **You have pimples or blackheads on your face, neck, chest or back, and you're beginning puberty.**

▶ **You've tried self-care but your acne hasn't improved.**

TRY SELF-CARE

▶ **You have pimples but no other symptoms.**

YOUR CHILD'S SYMPTOMS

Acne and your child.
Approximately one-third of all infants develop "baby acne" on their faces about three weeks after birth. This possibly is caused by the mother's hormones which are passed to the baby before birth. This acne looks like small whiteheads and isn't inflamed. It usually disappears within a few weeks. However, it may last for months. Simply wash your baby's face with mild soap and water. Don't use any other treatment.

ANKLE PAIN OR SWELLING

Painful, swollen or bruised ankle

Causes

Injury. Your ankle may be tender, swollen and discolored. You may have strained or sprained it. If your ankle is deformed or if you can't bear weight on it, seek emergency help.

Achilles' tendinitis. Your tendons may have become inflamed from overuse, causing your ankle to swell slowly over a period of weeks. Call your nurse information service or doctor.

Fluid or circulation problem. Your ankles may have been swollen for more than a day, with no other symptoms. If you've been sitting for a long time, such as on a long trip, fluid may pool in your feet and ankles. It should go away within two days, especially with leg elevation. You may have insufficient valves in the veins in your legs. This is known as varicose veins.

Other causes may include a history of deep venous thrombosis (see Page 164).

Self-Care

- If you have a sprain or strain, try the PRICE remedy—protect, rest, ice, compression and elevation. Protect your ankle from further injury. Rest it for a day or so. Wrap crushed ice in a thin towel and apply for 15 to 20 minutes, three to four times a day. Use an elastic wrap or bandage. Whenever possible, keep your ankle elevated above the level of your heart to help reduce swelling.
- Try an over-the-counter pain reliever such as acetaminophen, ibuprofen, naproxen sodium or aspirin.
- Ease Achilles' tendinitis by inserting a lift or pad in your shoe heel.
- After the pain and swelling lessen, gently rotate and bend your ankle several times a day to keep it flexible.
- Ask your doctor about surgical support stockings to help reduce chronic swelling.
- Exercise regularly. Walking or jogging will strengthen your muscles. It also can help support tissues around your ankle, and improve circulation.

Prevention

- Stretch before and after exercising. Wear shoes that fit well and are appropriate for the activity.
- Balance-related exercises can help strengthen the muscles around your ankle.
- Wear comfortable shoes—avoid those that are tight or have high heels.

- Use cushioned inner soles if you're on your feet a lot.
- Place arch supports in shoes that need them. This can help keep your feet from rolling inward.

SEEK EMERGENCY HELP

▶ Your ankle looks deformed or bent the wrong way. The pain is so severe you can't move it or put weight on it.

▶ After an injury, your ankle swells up immediately and turns blue.

▶ One ankle is swollen, red and hot, and you have a fever.

▶ One ankle or the calf of one leg is swollen or tender, or you have a history of blood clots.

▶ Your foot suddenly is pale, blue or gray and feels cold.

SEE YOUR DOCTOR

▶ One or both ankles recently became swollen, and you're short of breath, or have heart, kidney or liver disease.

▶ There's been no improvement more than three days after an injury to your ankle.

▶ You've tried self-care but the pain or swelling hasn't improved.

CALL YOUR NURSE INFORMATION SERVICE OR DOCTOR

▶ The ankle pain is still too severe to walk 24 hours after the injury.

▶ Your ankle has gradually become painful and stiff over months or years.

▶ Your ankle has been hurting for more than four days for no apparent reason.

▶ Both ankles have been mildly swollen for months, without pain.

TRY SELF-CARE

▶ You have pain in one ankle following an injury.

YOUR CHILD'S SYMPTOMS

! *Don't give aspirin to anyone younger than age 19! It's linked to Reye's syndrome, a rare but sometimes fatal condition.*

APPETITE LOSS

Not hungry; food is unappealing

Causes

Aging. If you're age 60 or older, you may feel hungry less often. With age, one's metabolism slows down and muscle mass decreases. You don't need as many calories as you once did. So, your appetite decreases to compensate. Your senses of taste and smell also may diminish, making food less appealing. Report any unintentional weight loss to your doctor. It may indicate an underlying health problem.

Anorexia nervosa (see Page 333). You may eat very little. Perhaps you've lost a great deal of weight but you still think you're fat. If you're female, you may have stopped having menstrual periods. Anorexia nervosa is a disease that often affects women and adolescent girls. It may cause them to virtually deny the need to eat. While not as common, men also can suffer from this disorder, so possible symptoms should not be ignored. Anorexia nervosa can be a life-threatening disorder if not effectively treated. Talk with your doctor.

Other causes may include depression (see Page 332), gastritis (see Page 298), hepatitis (see Page 156), illness, kidney disease, certain medications, pancreatic and some other cancers, peptic ulcer disease (see Page 298), recent surgery, or zinc deficiency.

Self-Care

Self-care isn't appropriate for anorexia nervosa.

If you're taking medication and you haven't been hungry lately, talk with your doctor.

- If zinc deficiency is causing a loss of appetite because of diminished sense of taste, over-the-counter supplements may help. Talk with your doctor.

- Eat small, frequent, appetizing meals. Eating your favorite foods is a good way to stimulate your appetite and get the calories you need.

Prevention

- Exercising regularly can increase your appetite.
- If you have a diminished sense of smell or taste, try using herbs and spices to add more flavor to your foods.

CALL YOUR NURSE INFORMATION SERVICE OR DOCTOR

▶ You've been experiencing loss of appetite for more than two weeks.

▶ You've had loss of appetite with severe fatigue; decreased taste sensitivity; persistent pain anywhere on your body; fever; or weight loss.

▶ You have a fever; swollen glands; whitish bowel movements or dark urine; frequent urination; pain when swallowing; or a rash.

▶ You're feeling blue or hopeless, and have lost interest in pleasurable activities.

▶ You're underweight according to height and weight charts. Yet, you still limit food intake because you feel you need to lose more weight.

▶ You've tried self-care but your appetite hasn't improved after two weeks.

TRY SELF-CARE

▶ You have appetite loss but no other symptoms.

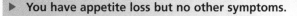

YOUR CHILD'S SYMPTOMS

Call your nurse information service or doctor if your child seems fatigued or sickly, or is failing to grow at the expected rate.

Appetite loss and your child. Changes in a child's appetite are normal. Children's appetites are affected by their energy requirements. They may have larger appetites during growth spurts. As long as your child is growing normally and doesn't seem tired or sickly, don't worry. Don't force her to eat. Remember that your young child's stomach is small. She can be satisfied with small portions.

Children sometimes go through phases in which they'll eat only one or two types of food. There's little danger that this will lead to malnutrition. Usually, it's best to ignore it. Boredom or curiosity eventually will stimulate your child to accept more foods. But don't give her unhealthy foods simply because she prefers them.

Toddlers sometimes suck on bottles not just to quench their thirst, but as a way to deal with boredom, frustration or fatigue. When they fill up on too much liquid, they may refuse to eat solid foods. Limit the amount of liquid your child gets from a bottle or spout cup to 24 ounces a day. If she's really thirsty, she'll take sips from an open cup.

BACKACHE

Pain or stiffness in the upper, middle or lower back

Causes

Injury. You may have injured your back. Perhaps you were lifting something heavy or working in the garden. If the pain isn't severe, try self-care.

Osteoarthritis (see Page 255). You may have pain and stiffness in your joints, including your knee, hip, hands, feet or spine. It may be worse when you move. Osteoarthritis is common but treatable. Talk with your doctor.

Other causes may include cancer (see Page 264), depression (see Page 332), herniated disk (see Page 184), viral or bacterial infection, inflammation, obesity, osteoporosis with compression (see Page 294), poor posture, or pregnancy (see Page 321).

Self-Care

- For a muscle injury, make a cold pack by wrapping ice in a thin towel. Apply for 15 to 20 minutes. Sometimes alternating cold and heat or applying heat alone may be more effective. Repeat three to four times a day.

- Avoid complete bed rest. Gentle activity can help you recover.

- When in bed, take the pressure off of your lower back by lying on your side.

Bend your knees and place a small pillow between them. Or, lie on your back with a pillow under your knees. Get up slowly. Roll onto your side, swing your legs to the floor and push off the bed with your arms.

- Try an over-the-counter pain reliever such as acetaminophen, ibuprofen, naproxen sodium or aspirin.

Prevention

- Lift objects properly (see illustration).

- Stand up straight. Ask your nurse information service or doctor for exercises to increase your flexibility and strengthen your abdominal muscles.

- Sleep on a firm mattress.

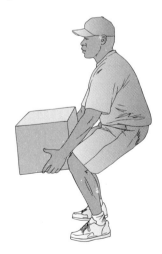

Prevent back problems by lifting from your knees.

SEEK EMERGENCY HELP

▶ The pain started in your chest and moved to your upper back. You're also dizzy, sweating or having difficulty breathing. You even may have an uneven pulse, nausea or vomiting, or anxiety.

▶ You have sudden loss of bowel or bladder control; lack of mobility; numbness; or tingling or weakness in your arms, legs, hands or feet.

▶ You have numbness or tingling in a saddle pattern— that is, if you were riding a horse, the area of your body that would be touching the saddle.

▶ You have severe backache accompanied by a tearing sensation.

SEE YOUR DOCTOR

▶ You feel pain or burning when you urinate.

▶ You have pain often on one side or the other, or in your lower back just above your waist. You also feel sick, or have a fever, or blood in your urine.

▶ You have a history of back injury or surgery, and the pain is persistent or severe.

CALL YOUR NURSE INFORMATION SERVICE OR DOCTOR

▶ You have severe pain across your whole upper back. It started suddenly, for no apparent reason.

▶ You're pregnant.

▶ You've tried self-care but your backache hasn't improved.

TRY SELF-CARE

▶ The pain started after you lifted something or moved awkwardly, but you have no other symptoms.

YOUR CHILD'S SYMPTOMS

Seek emergency help if your child complains of back pain after an injury, and has difficulty moving his arms and legs.

Call your nurse information service or doctor if your child complains of any back pain. Backaches are unusual in children.

! *Don't give aspirin to anyone younger than age 19! It's linked to Reye's syndrome, a rare but sometimes fatal condition.*

BED-WETTING

Involuntary urination during sleep, more often than once a month

About Bed-Wetting

Bed-wetting is quite common in children up until age 7 years. It's not your child's fault. He or she doesn't do it deliberately. Most children are embarrassed and ashamed of wetting their beds. They would gladly stop if they could. Therefore, they need support and encouragement, not punishment.

Causes

In the great majority of cases, the causes of bed-wetting in children aren't known. Bed-wetting may be related to sleeping patterns. It's especially common in children who are heavy sleepers.

Sometimes, bed-wetting may be caused by a urinary tract infection (see Page 230) or, rarely, diabetes (see Page 281).

Self-Care

- Be supportive. Avoid showing disgust or disappointment. Don't scold.
- Buy disposable, absorbent underpants for your child to wear to bed.
- Remain calm and comforting as you change your child's bedsheets or underpants.
- Your doctor may suggest that you try a reward system to help motivate your child to stop bed-wetting. This often involves keeping track of his or her progress. A small reward is offered when a goal is reached. Let your child create a colorful chart and mark off dry days. This can help build confidence.

Note that these reward systems are most helpful after ages 5 to 6 years. However, they're effective only if the child indeed is motivated.

Prevention

- Make sure your child urinates before going to bed at night.
- Limit fluid intake for two hours before bedtime.

CALL YOUR NURSE INFORMATION SERVICE OR DOCTOR

- ▶ You have dribbling urine, a weak urinary stream, painful urination, difficulty urinating, blood in the urine, or fever.

- ▶ You have lower back or abdominal pain, excessive thirst or hunger, fatigue or weight loss.

- ▶ Your child, previously dry at night, begins to bed-wet.

- ▶ Your child experiences bed-wetting after age 5 years.

TRY SELF-CARE

- ▶ Your child wets the bed but has no other symptoms.

BITE, ANIMAL OR HUMAN

Bite by an animal or person; wound may be deep, or superficial—affecting only the top layer of skin

About Bites

Bites often can be treated like other cuts or puncture wounds. Some bites are more serious, however. If the bite is from a cat, or on your face, hands, legs or feet, see your doctor. People who have diabetes or peripheral vascular disease should seek emergency help for bites on the face or lower extremities. Any bite can be dangerous, including presenting the possibility of tetanus. Call your doctor regardless of your tetanus status.

Causes

Animal. If you've been bitten by an animal, you may have been infected with rabies. Rabies is a viral disease that attacks the central nervous system. It is extremely serious—even fatal. If you've been bitten by a wild animal, seek emergency help. Report the bite to the local health authority or animal control agency. Do so even if the animal doesn't show the classic signs of active rabies—foaming at the mouth or acting aggressively. You may need to get a rabies vaccine or anti-rabies serum. If you've been bitten by someone's pet, it's less likely that you've been infected

with rabies. Ask the owner if the animal has had its required immunizations. All animal bites should be reported to the appropriate authorities.

Human. Bites from people also can cause infection. Bites by children are less likely to become infected than bites by adults. If the bite was from a person who may have hepatitis B (see Page 156) or HIV (see Page 284), or if the bite is the result of abuse, seek emergency help.

Self-Care

Note: Self-care alone isn't sufficient. These tips should be used in addition to your doctor's recommendations.

- Rinse the bite wound by running it under cold water. Wash it thoroughly with soap and water, or saline solution, and rinse again. Remove any foreign material with tweezers soaked in rubbing alcohol. However, if the material is deeply embedded, see your doctor.

- For the next four to five days, clean the wound with warm, soapy water three to four times a day. Watch for signs of infection—increased redness, swelling, pain or tenderness.

60

- If necessary, cover the wound with a loose, sterile bandage. Change the dressing often.

Prevention

- Avoid animals that act strangely, attack for no reason, drool or foam at the mouth. They may have rabies.
- Teach your children how to stay safe around animals.

SEEK EMERGENCY HELP

▶ You have extensive bleeding; loss of consciousness; or the bite is on your face, scalp, genitals, hand or foot, or near a joint.

▶ You have multiple bites, and some of them are deep or wide.

▶ You can't move the affected area; you have a foreign object in the wound; a bleeding disorder; a prosthetic valve or joint; or you're immunocompromised.

▶ The bite is from an HIV- or hepatitis B-positive person.

▶ The bite is from a wild or potentially rabid animal.

▶ The bite is from abuse.

SEE YOUR DOCTOR

▶ The bite is from a human or a cat, and it broke the skin.

▶ There is numbness or tingling at the site of the bite.

▶ You have a fever or chills.

▶ You've tried self-care but now see signs of infection such as redness, warmth or swelling.

CALL YOUR DOCTOR

▶ The bite was from a pet that doesn't have a current rabies vaccine, or you don't know its rabies status.

▶ The bite broke the skin.

BLEEDING

Blood flowing from a cut or wound that won't stop even when pressure is applied; bleeding heavily from a minor injury

Causes

Injury. You may have cut yourself or have a scrape. Depending on the injury, you may be bleeding quite a bit. If you feel faint or can't stop the bleeding after several minutes, seek emergency help.

Von Willebrand's disease. You may bruise easily, have frequent nosebleeds and bleed heavily from cuts, or during menstrual periods. You may have blood in your urine or stool. Von Willebrand's disease is caused by the lack of a clotting factor in the blood. See your doctor.

Thrombocytopenia. You may have nosebleeds and your cuts may bleed for a long time. Your menstrual periods may be heavy. You may get a rash of tiny bright- and dark-red spots wherever your skin is irritated—and sometimes even where it's not. This illness may result from medication or a recent viral infection. It's sometimes associated with leukemia or Hodgkin's disease, and is caused by a low level of platelets in the blood. Talk with your doctor.

Other causes may include hemophilia.

Self-Care

To stop the flow of blood:

- Press down firmly and directly over the wound for several minutes, using a clean cloth or gauze pad. Don't use a tourniquet.

- Wrap an adhesive bandage, or clean cloth, firmly but not tightly around the wound.

- Elevate the limb or body part that's bleeding.

- If blood oozes through, add another bandage on top. Don't remove the original bandage—the bleeding may start again.

- When the bleeding has completely stopped, cleanse the wound with soap and water, or saline solution. If the wound is gaping open, see your doctor.

- Styptic pencils can help stop bleeding from nicks.

- For nosebleeds, sit up straight and lean your head slightly forward. Don't tilt your head back—this can cause blood to flow down your throat. Pinch your nose just above your nostrils. Hold it firmly shut for 10 minutes and breathe through your mouth. If your nosebleed is caused by a minor trauma or injury, apply ice wrapped in a thin towel directly to your nose for 30 minutes. After the bleeding has stopped, avoid strenuous activity for six to eight hours.

Prevention

■ If you're prone to bleeding, don't take aspirin, ibuprofen or naproxen sodium. Instead, use acetaminophen for pain or headaches. Talk with your doctor about other medications you're taking.

SEEK EMERGENCY HELP

▶ You've bled so much that you feel faint.

▶ You have numbness or paralysis in your fingers or toes. You also have uncontrolled bleeding despite applying steady pressure.

SEE YOUR DOCTOR

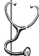

▶ You bleed easily and uncontrollably from minor injuries. Or, you have frequent nosebleeds, unexplained bruises and red rashes.

▶ The bleeding stopped 24 hours ago but now the wound is oozing pus, red and swollen. You also have a fever.

CALL YOUR NURSE INFORMATION SERVICE OR DOCTOR

▶ Your last tetanus shot was more than five years ago or you're unsure of your tetanus status.

TRY SELF-CARE

▶ The bleeding is moderate, from a cut or wound that's narrow and shallow.

BLISTER

A bump on the skin that's tender to the touch and contains fluid

Causes

Friction. Perhaps you've been wearing shoes that don't fit well. Maybe you've been raking leaves and now you have a blister. Most blisters are caused by friction—something rubbing against your skin. Self-care is often all that's necessary.

Herpes simplex. You may have had a tingling or burning sensation before watery blisters appeared on your genitals or your lips, inside your mouth or on other body parts. The blisters fill with pus. They become large, painful sores that crust or dry before healing. Although the rash may clear, herpes simplex virus is contagious and never leaves your system once you've been infected. With a few precautions, you can live an active, healthy life. Work with your doctor. Prescription medication can help prevent outbreaks.

Medication. You may have started taking a medication recently. Now you notice blisters forming on your body. Sensitivity or allergy to medication, including antibiotics, diuretics and pain relievers, can cause blisters. Call your doctor.

Other causes may include burns, chemicals, chickenpox (see Page 191), plants such as poison ivy (see Page 190) or rash.

Self-Care

- If the blister is intact, leave it alone. If needed, cushion it with a bandage.

- If the blister is on your foot, cushion it with nonmedicated callus or corn pads. Wear shoes that fit well. If you have diabetes, see your doctor.

- If your blister is open, wash the area thoroughly with soap and water. Fold the skin back over it to protect the sore area. Cover it with a bandage.

- For herpes:
  - Use your prescription medication immediately to shorten outbreaks.
  - Wash the infected area twice a day with soap and water. Take a warm bath if you can tolerate it.
  - Wear loose, cotton clothing.
  - Avoid stress.
  - Try an over-the-counter pain reliever such as acetaminophen, ibuprofen, naproxen sodium or aspirin.

Prevention

- Try to protect your skin from friction.

- Wear shoes that fit well. Break in new shoes or boots gradually.

- Keep your feet dry. Change your socks if they get wet or sweaty.

- Wear heavy gloves for activities such as gardening.
- Avoid sexual contact with anyone who has sores on the genitals, anus, mouth, lips or tongue, or who complains of genital tingling or irritation.
- Use a latex condom or practice abstinence to prevent sexually transmitted diseases.
- If you've had herpes, talk with your doctor about preventive medications.

SEEK EMERGENCY HELP

▶ The blister is on the mucous membrane of your eye.

▶ Blisters appear and you're very sick. You're weak, can't eat and feel there's something terribly wrong.

SEE YOUR DOCTOR

▶ The blister is on your nose or upper half of your face.

▶ The blister is pus-filled, red, hot or painful.

▶ You're pregnant or you recently gave birth and you have a blister with no known cause.

CALL YOUR NURSE INFORMATION SERVICE OR DOCTOR

▶ The blister appeared for no apparent reason.

▶ You have diabetes.

▶ You have a large blister, or widespread, small blisters.

▶ You have painful blisters around your mouth or genitals.

▶ You've recently started taking a new medication—or one you've taken previously with no problem.

▶ You've tried self-care but the blister hasn't improved after two to three days.

TRY SELF-CARE

▶ You have a blister but no other symptoms.

! *Don't give aspirin to anyone younger than age 19! It's linked to Reye's syndrome, a rare but sometimes fatal condition.*

BREAST PAIN

Pain, swelling and tenderness in one or both breasts

Causes

Premenstrual syndrome (see Page 316). Your breasts may feel full and painfully tender. Wearing a bra that provides good support, and using self-care may help. Regular breast self-exams can help you become familiar with the texture of your breasts (see Page 35). The best time to do a breast self-exam is during the week after your period.

Mastitis. You may be breast-feeding, and your nipples are dry and slightly cracked. Bacteria may have produced an infection, making part of your breast swollen, red, painful or tender, and hot. Drain the infected breast by nursing more frequently on that side or by using a breast pump. Use warm compresses to massage the tender area while nursing or pumping. If you have a fever, you also may need antibiotics. See your doctor.

Milk production. Breast discomfort is very common a few days after child-birth. This usually is the result of breast engorgement, or swelling, when milk is produced. You can help relieve the pain by breast-feeding. Warm showers and compresses also can help.

Fibrocystic breasts. Your breasts may be tender or lumpy, especially the week before menstruation. You may have several distinct, round lumps that move freely inside your breast tissue. If you find a new or different lump, see your doctor. The pain can be severe. Talk with your doctor about pain relief.

Self-Care

- If the pain occurs before your period, try non-impact exercises such as walking, swimming or biking. Wear a bra that provides good support, not just while exercising, but at all times—even in bed. Ibuprofen or a cool compress may help.

- For mastitis, in addition to your doctor's recommended treatment, acetaminophen may relieve discomfort. But, be sure to check with your doctor before taking any medication.

Prevention

- To avoid sore or cracked nipples during breast-feeding, make sure your nipple is positioned far back in your infant's mouth. Proper positioning and latch-on usually will fix this problem. Letting your nipples air-dry after nursing also can help.

CALL YOUR NURSE INFORMATION SERVICE OR DOCTOR

▶ You could be pregnant.

▶ You have a lump or discharge from your nipple; or the shape or appearance of your breast has changed.

▶ The pain is severe.

▶ You're taking hormone replacement therapy.

▶ You're breast-feeding and have sore or painful nipples; a painful, red, breast lump; fever; or chills.

▶ You're male and have noticed a breast lump or enlargement.

▶ You've tried self-care but your breasts are painful and tender after your period has ended.

TRY SELF-CARE

▶ You have breast pain but no other symptoms.

▶ Your breasts are painful and tender, and your period is due within one week.

BREATH, BAD

Breath has an offensive odor

Causes

Poor dental hygiene. You may notice that your breath has an unpleasant odor, although you have no other symptoms. Perhaps you sometimes forget to brush your teeth twice a day, or often rush through the task. Not brushing or flossing well enough is the most common cause of bad breath. The odor is caused by bacteria that live on decaying food particles lodged between your teeth. Fortunately, self-care can correct this problem, but you also should visit your dentist twice a year for professional cleanings.

Dry mouth. You may have bad breath, and your mouth often feels parched. Saliva has enzymes that help minimize the bacterial contamination in your mouth. When your mouth lacks saliva, bacteria multiply, producing bad breath. Dry mouth causes the "morning breath" that many adults experience when they wake up. Certain medications, including antihistamines and some antidepressants, also can cause dry mouth. Talk with your doctor or dentist.

Tooth decay. You may have bad breath along with tooth pain—especially after eating sweet or sour foods. You also may have tooth sensitivity to heat and cold, and an unpleasant taste in your mouth. Tooth decay may be the cause. See your dentist.

Sinus infection. You may have a sore throat, swollen lymph nodes in your neck, fever, stuffy nose, yellowish-green nasal discharge and a mucus-producing cough. The discharge can drain into the back of your throat causing bad breath. Call your nurse information service or doctor.

Other causes may include diabetes (see Page 281), gastritis (see Page 298), gastroesophageal reflux disease (GERD) (see Page 144), gum disease (see Page 130), liver or kidney diseases, ulcers (see Page 298) or Vincent's infection (see Page 130). Some of these are serious illnesses, of which bad breath is just one symptom.

Self-Care

- To avoid bad breath from dry mouth, stay well hydrated. Drink plenty of water each day.

- Practice good oral hygiene. Floss, and brush your teeth at least twice a day—in the morning and at night before bed. Use fluoride toothpaste and a soft toothbrush. Hard bristles can irritate your gums and wear away tooth enamel. Gently brush along the gum line, one section of your teeth at a time. Brush for at least three minutes. Time yourself to make sure that you're brushing thoroughly. Rinse well.

- Don't forget to brush your tongue. Bacteria and plaque on your tongue can be significant sources of bad breath. Brush as far back on the tongue as you can. Gently brush the insides of your cheeks, too.

- Avoid using mouthwash with a high alcohol content. It can irritate your mouth, which may make the problem worse.

Prevention

- Remember to brush at least twice a day, including your gums, tongue and the insides of your cheeks. Floss every day and stay well hydrated.

- Replace your toothbrush every three months.

- Avoid foods that cause bad breath. Onions and garlic are the biggest offenders.

- See your dentist twice a year.

CALL YOUR NURSE INFORMATION SERVICE, DOCTOR OR DENTIST

▶ You have red, swollen or bleeding gums.

▶ You have pain in one or more teeth when you eat sweet or sour foods. Your teeth are sensitive to heat or cold.

▶ You've had a sore throat or sinus pain, and fever for more than three days.

▶ You have persistent bad breath—for more than two weeks—despite good oral hygiene.

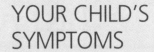

YOUR CHILD'S SYMPTOMS

Call your nurse information service or doctor if your child has bad breath and unusual nasal discharge.

Bad breath and your child. Upper respiratory tract infections can cause bad breath in children because they breathe through their mouths. If your child's breath has a foul odor, check for other signs of upper respiratory tract infection, such as throat pain.

A foreign object lodged in a nostril can cause bad breath in a young child. This may be the cause especially if you notice yellowish-green drainage from only one side of the nose.

BREATHING DIFFICULTY

Feeling breathless or having trouble breathing

Causes

If you're having difficulty breathing and don't know why, don't try to diagnose yourself. Seek emergency help.

Acute respiratory illness. Your breathing is labored or noisy, and you cough and have chills, fever and a sore throat.

Asthma (see Page 258). There may be times when you wheeze or have severe difficulty breathing. Your symptoms may be worse when exposed to triggers such as pollen or smoke. In some cases, an asthma attack can be life-threatening. Asthma is treatable, and people who have this condition can live active lives. See your doctor.

Chronic respiratory disease. You may be a current or former smoker. Perhaps you've had trouble breathing for some time and it's getting worse. You may have a habitual cough with gray or yellowish-green sputum, or get winded easily. These symptoms could signal chronic bronchitis or emphysema (see Page 270) or lung cancer. See your doctor.

Hyperventilation. You may be under stress. You may start breathing faster, your mouth or hands tingle, and you may feel panicky. Although this isn't dangerous, it can be frightening. Breathing exercises can help you stay calm and regain control. Call your nurse information service or doctor.

Anaphylaxis (see Page 15). You may have been stung by a bee. Perhaps you've eaten something to which you're severely allergic. You may feel lightheaded, and have difficulty breathing. You even may lose consciousness. Anaphylaxis is a severe and potentially life-threatening allergic reaction. Seek emergency help immediately. If you have severe allergies, talk with your doctor about prescription medication for emergency situations.

Other causes may include bronchitis.

Self-Care

- For hyperventilation, ask your nurse information service or doctor about breathing techniques and exercises that can help you relax in stressful situations.
- Quit smoking (see Page 25).

Prevention

- Don't smoke.

■ Exercise at least 30 minutes a day, five times a week. Swimming is a good choice if you have asthma. Talk with your doctor about exercises that are right for you.

SEEK EMERGENCY HELP

▶ You have difficulty breathing. You also may have chest pain, or blueness around your lips. Or, you have sharp pain that seems to take your breath away, or gets worse when you breathe in.

▶ You're wheezing constantly. Or, it's so hard to breathe, you can say only a couple of words between breaths.

▶ You have shortness of breath and your tongue is becoming swollen at the back of your throat.

▶ You recently had surgery or were treated for a fracture of a long bone.

SEE YOUR DOCTOR

▶ Lately you find it more difficult to breathe.

▶ You cough up discolored sputum, or work in a place where you inhale fumes or dust.

▶ Your ankles recently have become swollen or puffy. Pressing them with your finger leaves a dent.

▶ You have a fever, and you're coughing up yellowish-green or rust-colored sputum.

▶ You become breathless easily, even while resting or sleeping. You have trouble breathing when lying down.

CALL YOUR NURSE INFORMATION SERVICE OR DOCTOR

▶ You have a cough and chills, fever, sore throat or aching muscles.

▶ Your symptoms are mild but haven't improved.

YOUR CHILD'S SYMPTOMS

Seek emergency help if your child has any of the following: wheezing or breathing loudly enough to be heard 10 feet away; grunting or making a noise like a barking seal when coughing; high fever with a cough; drooling or refusing to swallow food or saliva because it hurts; flaring nostrils and rapid breathing; or your child can't lie down and rest because he's working so hard to breathe.

Breathing difficulty and your child. If your child has asthma and it's well managed, he should be able to participate fully in life. Encourage him to stay active, especially in sports such as swimming. You may help cut down on the number of attacks by identifying and eliminating triggers. Don't expose him to secondhand smoke or burning fires in the fireplace. Work closely with your doctor to tailor medication to your child's needs.

Parents often worry about their newborn's noisy breathing. If your infant is eating and sleeping well, some noisy breathing probably is normal. This may include grunts and snorts.

BRUISE

Discolored area on the skin; blue, purple or black at first, gradually fading to yellow

Causes

Bruises occur when blood vessels break under your skin and the blood seeps into the surrounding area. The discolored area is the blood that's visible under your skin. As the healing process continues, the leaked red blood cells break down and the bruise fades.

Injury. Perhaps you fell down or bumped yourself, and now the area is black, blue or purple. Bruising is a normal reaction to an injury. The size and shape of the bruise depend on the force of the blow; the part of your body that's injured; and how easily you bruise. If you injure an area where your skin is thin, such as your eye, the bruise and accompanying swelling are likely to be worse. Women generally bruise more easily than men. And, everyone bruises more easily after they reach middle age, or if they use aspirin on a regular basis. Bruises are especially common in older adults on the back of the hands and may appear without any injury. Bruises almost always can be treated with self-care.

Bleeding disorders. In addition to bruising easily, you may notice groups of small, pinpoint-sized red specks under your skin. You also may have frequent nosebleeds, prolonged menstrual periods and dark stools. Your gums may bleed when you brush your teeth. You may experience fatigue. See your doctor.

Blood disease. You may bruise easily, and you may have frequent nosebleeds. You may have minor bleeding in your mouth or just under your skin that looks like tiny, red pinpoints. You also may have itching, dizziness, night sweats, fatigue, headache or blurred vision. See your doctor.

Self-Care

- If injury is the cause, apply ice right away. This will help minimize black-and-blue marks. Wrap crushed ice in a thin towel and apply for 15 to 20 minutes, three to four times a day.

- If the bruise is large and on your arm or leg, raise the limb above the level of your heart for 24 hours. This will keep blood from pooling and help minimize the bruise.

- Don't rub or massage the area. This will make your bruise worse.

Prevention

- Make sure you're getting enough vitamin C. Citrus fruits are good sources.

- If you bruise easily, use acetaminophen when needed. Don't use aspirin, ibuprofen or naproxen sodium.

- Wear appropriate protective gear—such as elbow pads, knee pads and helmets—when playing sports or doing other activities that may cause bruises.

- Prevent falls by removing hazards such as toys and loose rugs from the floor. Install rails along stairways and in the bathroom.

- Talk with your doctor if you think your sense of balance is impaired.

SEEK EMERGENCY HELP

▶ Your arm or leg is cold, numb or misshapen. You're in severe pain or can't bear weight on your arm or leg.

▶ You have a large bruise that's rapidly getting bigger.

▶ Your bruises are due to abuse.

CALL YOUR NURSE INFORMATION SERVICE OR DOCTOR

▶ You bruise often. The bruises take longer than one week to disappear.

▶ In addition to bruising easily, you have bleeding from your nose or gums, or have heavy menstrual periods.

▶ You have a rash anywhere on your body that looks like a group of red pinpricks, particularly on your lower legs.

▶ You've tried self-care for a bruise that developed after injuring yourself but it hasn't faded after one to two weeks, or it has become hot.

TRY SELF-CARE

▶ You developed a bruise after a minor injury.

BURN

Red, blistered, blackened or white skin due to a scald, or exposure to fire, chemicals or too much sun

About Burns

Burns can be caused by hot liquids, steam, electric shock, chemicals, flames and sun exposure. Children and older adults are at greater risk for complications and should seek emergency help.

First-degree burn. Only the outer layer of skin is burned. Skin is red and tender but not blistering. First-degree burns usually can be treated with self-care.

Second-degree burn. You have a severe burn or scald. The burn may be painful and swollen. It may have blisters and a weepy, watery surface. See your doctor. Self-care can help your burn feel better and heal within one week.

Third-degree burn. Your burn is severe, deep and possibly exposes underlying flesh. Your skin may be charred or whitened. If your nerves have been burned, you may feel pain around the edges of the burn, but not right on it. Seek emergency help.

Self-Care

- Third-degree burns: Seek emergency help—self-care isn't appropriate.
- Second-degree burns: Place small burns under cold running water for at least 10 to 15 minutes. Wash gently with soap and rinse. Apply antibiotic ointment. Lightly cover with a bandage. Don't break any blisters.
- First-degree burns: Wash with cold running water for at least two to three minutes. Cover with a clean, dry gauze or cloth bandage. Don't use cotton, or apply any ointment or medication. Don't use local anesthetic sprays or creams—they can delay healing. Try an over-the-counter pain reliever such as acetaminophen, ibuprofen, naproxen sodium or aspirin.
- All burns: Remove or cut away any clothes that might stick to the burn. After immediate first aid, elevate the burned body part, if possible. Keep dressings clean. Watch for any signs of infection, including redness or swelling. New skin may be dry and may crack—try moisturizing cream.
- You may need a tetanus shot if your skin is broken, and your last tetanus shot was more than five years ago or you're unsure of your tetanus status.

Prevention

- Don't smoke—especially not in bed.

- Take safety measures to prevent fires in your home.
- Install smoke alarms (see Page 29).
- Follow safety procedures when using chemicals.
- Avoid prolonged exposure to the sun. Always wear sunscreen when outdoors—at least SPF 15 with both UVA and UVB protection.

SEEK EMERGENCY HELP

▶ The burn covers an extensive area; your skin is broken; severely blistered or charred; or you're in severe pain.

▶ You have singed nasal hairs, soot or sputum in your mouth or nose, or a new onset of hoarseness. Or, you may have inhaled toxic vapors released in a house fire.

▶ The burn goes all the way around your neck, chest, arm, leg, head or fingers.

▶ You have a burn that is red, tender and blistered on your face, hands, feet, groin, genitals, or knee, elbow or other joint.

▶ You have difficulty breathing; severe wheezing; irregular pulse; rapid or irregular heartbeat; drowsiness or faintness; or bleeding that won't stop.

▶ Your eye is burned.

▶ You have an electrical, chemical or radiation burn.

CALL YOUR NURSE INFORMATION SERVICE OR DOCTOR

▶ It's been 24 hours since the burn was treated, and you feel numbness, tingling or loss of sensation in the area.

▶ You're still in pain 48 hours after medical treatment or self-care.

TRY SELF-CARE

▶ You have a minor burn but no other symptoms.

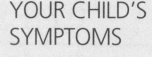

YOUR CHILD'S SYMPTOMS

Seek emergency help if your child has been burned. Children are at high risk of complications from burns.

! *Don't give aspirin to anyone younger than age 19! It's linked to Reye's syndrome, a rare but sometimes fatal condition.*

CHEST PAIN

Pain in the chest that may be crushing, squeezing, burning, dull and pressing, or sharp and stabbing

Causes

If you're having a new onset of chest pain, don't try to diagnose yourself. Seek emergency help.

Heart attack. The blood supply to your heart is partially blocked, causing part of your heart muscle to die. You may have severe, crushing pain in the center of your chest that may spread to your arm, shoulder or jaw. Other symptoms include sweating, shortness of breath, and nausea or vomiting. You may feel faint, dizzy or very anxious. Women often experience different symptoms than men—sometimes causing them to delay seeking help.

When a heart attack occurs, you might not experience all of these symptoms. If you notice one or more of these signs in yourself or another person, seek emergency help immediately (see Page 10).

Angina. Part of your heart isn't getting enough oxygen. You may feel a squeezing pressure, heaviness or mild ache in your chest. The pain typically occurs when you're active and decreases when you rest. This usually is seen in men ages 40 or older, postmenopausal women, and people who smoke, or have high blood pressure (see Page 287), diabetes (see Page 281), high cholesterol, or family history of coronary heart disease (see Page 278) before age 55.

Other causes may include gastro-esophageal reflux disease (GERD) (see Page 144), respiratory infection, or sprain or strain of the chest muscle.

Self-Care

Apply these self-care measures only if a doctor has diagnosed the cause of your chest pain. Don't diagnose yourself.

- If you think you're having a heart attack, call for emergency help. If you have no aspirin allergies, chew and swallow one aspirin of any dose (see Page 10).

- To relieve angina, try resting in a chair. If you've been diagnosed with angina, follow your doctor's instructions about taking your medication. Discuss with your doctor, in advance, what to do if your medication doesn't relieve the pain.

- If you have an infection, your chest pain may not go away until the infection is treated. Cough medicine may help—as long as you're not coughing up mucus. A cool-mist vaporizer or humidifier will moisten the air and may provide relief. Be sure to clean it daily or as instructed by the manufacturer.

Prevention

- Make heart-healthy lifestyle choices (see Page 17). Exercise regularly. Eat a balanced, low-fat diet. And, don't smoke.

- If you have high blood pressure or diabetes, manage your health condition closely.

SEEK EMERGENCY HELP

▶ You have pain in your arms, neck or jaw; difficulty breathing; dizziness or faintness; sweating; uneven pulse; nausea or vomiting; or anxiety and nervousness.

▶ You sense that you're about to die.

▶ You've taken your prescribed angina medication but have no relief from symptoms.

▶ You have chest pain after recent use of cocaine.

▶ You have a recent chest or rib injury.

▶ You feel a squeezing or heavy sensation, or a mild ache that gets better when you rest.

▶ You have sudden shortness of breath and chest pain that get worse when you take a deep breath.

▶ You've had a recent illness or injury that's kept you in bed a long time. The pain gets worse when you take a deep breath.

CALL YOUR NURSE INFORMATION SERVICE OR DOCTOR

▶ You have a cough or fever, and you're coughing up sputum.

▶ You've tried self-care but your chest pain hasn't improved.

TRY SELF-CARE

▶ Your chest is tender to touch.

▶ You have a burning sensation that gets worse when you bend or lie down, especially within an hour of a meal.

YOUR CHILD'S SYMPTOMS

Seek emergency help if your child has chest pain or light-headedness occurring only with exercise; or if she injures her chest while playing, and the pain or breathing difficulty lasts more than a few minutes.

Chest pain and your child. Chest pain in children is unlikely to be due to heart problems, unless the child is known to have a heart disorder.

In early adolescence, sharp chest pain, lasting only a few seconds and occurring at rest, is common and usually of no concern. This type of chest pain typically gets worse with moving the chest wall, such as with deep breathing. It often is located where the rib and breastbone come together.

! *Don't give aspirin to anyone younger than age 19! It's linked to Reye's syndrome, a rare but sometimes fatal condition.*

CONFUSION OR FORGETFULNESS

Not knowing who or where one is, or what day it is; difficulty remembering things—suddenly or over a long period of time

About Confusion or Forgetfulness

Sudden onset. Profound confusion or forgetfulness that comes on suddenly may indicate a serious medical problem. Seek emergency help.

Common causes of sudden confusion or forgetfulness may include head trauma (see Page 9); hypothermia (see Page 8); heatstroke (see Page 12); low blood sugar (see Page 112); shock (see Page 15); stroke (see Page 16); high fever; or alcohol or illegal drugs.

Delirium is a state of acute mental confusion. This can be common in some hospitalized older adults.

Gradual onset or dementia. Confusion and forgetfulness may come on gradually— over months or years. Though dementia can be common in older adults, it's not a normal sign of aging. It also shouldn't be mistaken for occasional forgetfulness. Symptoms may include asking the same questions repeatedly; becoming lost in familiar places; and getting disoriented about time, people and places. The person may become unconcerned about

cleanliness and appearance. He or she may be unable to remember what just happened. Talk with your loved one's doctor.

Common causes of dementia may include Alzheimer's disease (see Page 252); or poor blood flow to the brain, as in vascular disease and advanced stages of Parkinson's disease (see Page 296). Alzheimer's disease accounts for approximately half of all cases. Multi-infarct dementia, also called vascular dementia, is caused by strokes.

Other causes may include alcohol or substance abuse (see Page 328); encephalitis; fever; kidney, liver or lung disease; infectious diseases; certain medications; metabolic diseases; psychiatric disorders; toxins; or vasculitis.

Self-Care and Caregiving

Seek emergency help for sudden onset of symptoms. Don't leave a confused person alone.

■ If the person has diabetes, is confused and has low blood sugar, this is an emergency situation. He or she needs a quickly absorbed sugar product immediately. Make sure you know what snacks the doctor recommends in case of sudden low blood sugar.

Prevention

- Dementia often can't be prevented. Staying healthy can help you avoid diseases that may contribute to dementia. Eat well and exercise regularly.
- Don't smoke.
- Seek help for alcohol or substance abuse.
- Take up hobbies and interests that stimulate both your mind and your body.

SEEK EMERGENCY HELP

▶ Your confusion started suddenly, following a recent head injury.

▶ You have difficulty speaking; dizziness; blurred vision; numbness or tingling; or weakness in your limbs.

▶ You have a headache, vomiting and drowsiness.

SEE YOUR DOCTOR

▶ You gradually became confused or forgetful.

▶ You have a fever.

▶ You have a loss of bladder control; change in personality; poor personal hygiene; or are forgetful of recent events.

▶ Before the confusion began, you were drinking alcohol or taking a new prescription medication.

▶ You have diabetes, or heart or lung disease.

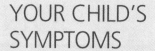

YOUR CHILD'S SYMPTOMS

Seek emergency help if your child is talking gibberish; acting agitated or dazed; or seeing or hearing things that aren't there. Get help immediately if he won't bend his head forward or drink anything.

See your doctor if your child has a fever and is confused.

! *Don't give aspirin to anyone younger than age 19! It's linked to Reye's syndrome, a rare but sometimes fatal condition.*

CONSTIPATION

Infrequent bowel movements—two or fewer per week;
hard stools that are difficult or uncomfortable to pass

Causes

Insufficient fluid and fiber intake. Not getting enough fluid and fiber in your diet is by far the most common cause of constipation. Fiber is the undigestible bulk found in some foods. It acts like a sponge in the intestines, drawing in water and making the stool softer. It also keeps your bowel movements regular. Add fiber to your diet with whole grains, fruits and vegetables. Be sure to drink plenty of water each day.

Inactivity. Perhaps your job requires you to sit all day. Or, you rarely exercise. Physical activity helps stimulate muscle contractions inside the bowel.

Change in dietary pattern. You may have been traveling. Perhaps you've been skipping lunch or breakfast. Regularly scheduled meals help your body regulate its bowel movements.

Bowel obstruction. You may have constipation along with abdominal pain; unexplained weight loss; rectal bleeding; or diarrhea. This may be caused by a blockage in your intestines possibly due to colorectal cancer, a hernia (see Page 144) or inflammatory bowel disease (IBD) (see Page 261). See your doctor.

Other causes may include irritable bowel syndrome (IBS) (see Page 262), certain medications, neurological disorders, pregnancy (see Page 321), rectal pain or thyroid conditions (see Page 308).

Self-Care and Prevention

Try a few of the following tips in combination for the best results:

- Set aside a regular time each day for bowel movements. The best time is often within one hour after breakfast. Don't hurry. Sit for at least five to 10 minutes, whether or not you actually have a bowel movement.

- Try drinking a cup of hot decaffeinated coffee or tea, or water in the morning.

- Include fruits, vegetables, beans, and bran or other whole-grain cereals in your diet.

- Drink plenty of water each day. Avoid too much caffeine or alcohol, which can dehydrate you.

- Increase your physical activity. Brisk walking, jogging and aerobic exercise can help stimulate bowel movements.

- Add an over-the-counter fiber supplement to your diet. Be sure to take it with enough fluid, or you may become more constipated than before.

- If you're pregnant, be sure to talk with your doctor before making any changes to your diet or usual activity.

SEEK EMERGENCY HELP

► You have severe abdominal pain for more than two hours, or severe pain when you touch your abdomen.

► You have a prior history of abdominal surgery, along with nausea and vomiting.

CALL YOUR NURSE INFORMATION SERVICE OR DOCTOR

► Your stools have become unusually narrow. You have abdominal cramping, gassiness or vomiting. You've lost weight without trying.

► You have pain or discomfort around your anal area.

► You've recently begun taking a new medication.

► You've had constipation for more than two weeks. You know that neither travel nor change in diet or activity is the cause.

► You're pregnant or think you might be.

► You've tried self-care but your symptoms haven't improved after two weeks.

TRY SELF-CARE

► You have constipation but no other symptoms.

YOUR CHILD'S SYMPTOMS

See your doctor if your child is experiencing a long period of constipation or "stool holding." This can lead to a condition in which she doesn't know that she's soiling her pants. Don't put off talking with your doctor.

Constipation and your child. Children, like adults, don't need to have a bowel movement every day—or even every other day. Don't suspect constipation unless your child has difficulty or pain when trying to have a bowel movement; complains of discomfort in her anal area; or passes large, hard, dry stools fewer than three times a week.

Children who have just started toilet training, or who recently have been toilet trained, sometimes hold their stools, resisting the urge to have a bowel movement. If you think your child is doing this, be reassuring. Let your child know that it's fine to wear diapers for bowel movements and "big-girl pants" the rest of the time. Let her give up diapers at her own pace.

CORN OR CALLUS

Corn—a small bump of thickened skin on top of a toe joint
Callus—a thickened, hard, rough, yellowish patch of skin

About Corns and Calluses

Corns and calluses are very much alike. Their difference is in location and size. Corns are small and round. They form on the bony area on top of toe joints or between toes. Calluses are larger and flatter. They can appear on any part of the body that's repeatedly subjected to pressure and friction—the balls or heels of your feet, the palms of your hands, or your knees.

Corns and calluses are your body's way of protecting itself against constant pressure or repeated friction. Both are very common, and they usually disappear when the pressure or friction is removed. Corns and calluses rarely cause serious problems.

Self-Care

If you have diabetes (see Page 281) or circulatory problems, don't use self-care for corns and calluses. Talk with your doctor.

- If your corn or callus isn't causing discomfort, no action is needed.
- Wear comfortable shoes that fit well— with plenty of room around your toes. Your feet tend to swell in hot weather, during pregnancy and as you get older.

Don't assume that your shoe size is the same now as it was in the past. Have your feet measured each time you buy new shoes.

- Soak the affected area in warm, soapy water every day for at least five minutes. Then, use a pumice stone, callus file or rough towel to gently rub away the outer layer of thickened skin.
- Take care when using over-the-counter, acid-based corn and callus removers. They may cause infection. If you decide to use one, follow the package directions carefully.
- Don't use ointments that contain salicylic acid.
- Apply a doughnut-shaped piece of felt or moleskin around the corn or callus to help relieve any pressure.

Prevention

- Wear comfortable shoes that fit well.
- Wear work gloves when doing heavy manual work.

CALL YOUR NURSE INFORMATION SERVICE OR DOCTOR

▶ You have diabetes or any other circulatory problem.

▶ You have signs of infection on or near your corn or callus—such as redness, swelling, pus or warmth.

▶ You've tried self-care but your symptoms haven't improved after two to three weeks.

TRY SELF-CARE

▶ You have a corn or callus but no other symptoms.

COUGH

The body's reflex to an irritation in the sinuses, throat, breathing tubes or lungs; a productive cough brings up mucus; a non-productive cough is dry and hacking

Causes

Respiratory infection. You may have a productive cough and fever. You may be extremely tired and your muscles may ache. Coughing up white mucus is usually a sign of a viral infection. Self-care can help relieve these symptoms. Green or rust-colored mucus is often a sign of a bacterial infection, which may require an antibiotic. See your doctor.

Cigarette smoking. Your cough may be nonproductive, or productive and gagging. It may be worse when you wake up or after smoking. Talk with your doctor about effective ways to quit smoking (see Page 25).

Other causes may include allergies (see Page 303), asthma (see Page 258), bronchiectasis, certain blood pressure medications, chronic bronchitis or emphysema (see Page 270), gastro-esophageal reflux disease (GERD) (see Page 144) or tuberculosis.

Self-Care

- If your cough is productive, don't suppress it, except at night to get some sleep. Take a hot shower, or use a cool-mist vaporizer or humidifier. Clean it daily or as instructed by the manufacturer.

- Try an over-the-counter cough expectorant that contains guaifenesin. Don't use guaifenesin if you have a persistent or chronic cough with a lot of mucus, or an asthma-related cough. Drink plenty of liquids.

- If your cough is nonproductive, try throat lozenges, or an over-the-counter cough suppressant. Look for the ingredient dextromethorphan. Don't use dextromethorphan without your doctor's permission if you're taking a monoamine oxidase inhibitor (MAOI).

- For postnasal drip, try over-the-counter decongestants or antihistamines to help dry up the mucus.

Prevention

- Don't smoke. Avoid exposure to secondhand smoke.

SEEK EMERGENCY HELP

▶ Your sharp cough developed without warning and you're gasping, panting or wheezing.

▶ You have a new onset of coughing, and trauma to the chest within the past 48 hours.

▶ You have a cough and shaking chills—not just shivering.

▶ You have a cough and fever of 104° F or higher.

▶ You're coughing up blood—more than just blood-tinged sputum.

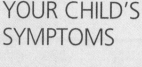

SEE YOUR DOCTOR

▶ You have a new cough and fever, and you're either immunocompromised or age 65 or older, or you've just had surgery.

▶ You cough when you exercise.

CALL YOUR NURSE INFORMATION SERVICE OR DOCTOR

▶ You've had a fever for more than four days.

▶ Your cough has lasted more than a month, or you're coughing up sputum that's thick, green, yellowish-green or dark red, and foul-smelling.

▶ You have a sharp pain in your chest when you cough or breathe.

▶ You've tried self-care but your symptoms haven't improved after seven days.

▶ You've tried self-care but you've had a cough and runny nose, sneezing and a sore throat for more than 10 days.

TRY SELF-CARE

▶ You're coughing up yellow or white sputum.

▶ You have a cough and runny nose, sneezing and a sore throat.

YOUR CHILD'S SYMPTOMS

Seek emergency help if your child suddenly starts coughing sharply and doesn't have a cold; or if you suspect he may have food or some other small object lodged in his windpipe. (See Page 6 for the Heimlich maneuver.)

Call your doctor if your child develops a cough that sounds like a seal's bark, is accompanied by hoarseness, and is worse at night. This may be croup, an inflammation of the air passages. Croup is common in children.

Call your nurse information service or doctor if a child age 3 months or younger develops a cough. Although congestion is common, a persistent cough is unusual in very young infants.

Try self-care to help ease the symptoms of croup. Expose your child to humid air. Take him into the bathroom and close the door. Stand with your child outside the bathtub and turn the shower on hot—full blast so he can inhale the steam in the room. Or, take a walk in the cold night air, or use a cool-mist vaporizer or humidifier near his bed.

! *Don't give aspirin to anyone younger than age 19! It's linked to Reye's syndrome, a rare but sometimes fatal condition.*

CUT

Skin or flesh that has been sliced open

About Cuts

Most cuts heal with self-care. However, some are severe and require medical attention. If the cut has affected a muscle, tendon, ligament, nerve or joint, or is wide or deep, see your doctor. You may need a tetanus shot if your skin is broken and your last tetanus shot was more than five years ago or you're unsure of your tetanus status.

A deep cut caused by a sharp, pointed object is considered a puncture wound (see Page 246).

Self-Care

■ Rinse the cut by running it under cold water. Wash it thoroughly with soap and water or saline solution, and rinse again. Remove dirt, glass or any other foreign material with tweezers soaked in rubbing alcohol. However, if the material is deeply embedded, see your doctor.

■ If the cut is bleeding, apply a pressure bandage, or hold a gauze pad tightly against it. Close a small gaping cut with a butterfly bandage. If the wound is more than 1/8 inch deep and doesn't stay closed with a bandage, you may need stitches. See your doctor.

■ If the cut is painful but without signs of infection—redness, swelling or pus—try acetaminophen, ibuprofen, naproxen sodium or aspirin.

■ Don't pick at scabs as the cuts heal.

Prevention

■ Take care when using sharp tools or knives. Store them safely, not jumbled together in a drawer. Never leave sharp kitchen utensils, such as knives, in a sink full of water.

■ Wear heavy gloves when doing construction or repair work.

■ For general safety tips, see Page 28.

SEEK EMERGENCY HELP

▶ The cut is spurting blood or bleeding uncontrollably despite applying firm pressure for several minutes.

▶ You've been stuck by a needle already used on someone else.

▶ The cut is severe and it's on your outer-ear cartilage, the palm of your hand, or over a joint.

▶ The cut is on your arm or leg, and you're numb or weak in that limb. Or, you have paralysis in your fingers or toes.

▶ You have a large or deep cut on your face, chest, neck stomach or back.

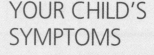

SEE YOUR DOCTOR

▶ The cut is dirty, and your last tetanus shot was more than five years ago or you're unsure of your tetanus status.

▶ The cut is gaping, or jagged, with flaps of skin or tissue at the edges.

▶ You have increasing tenderness or pain, swelling and redness, pus, red streaks or unexplained fever.

▶ There's an object in the wound.

▶ The cut is on your face or feet, and you have diabetes or peripheral vascular disease.

CALL YOUR NURSE INFORMATION SERVICE OR DOCTOR

▶ You have a cut that's not necessarily large or dirty, and your last tetanus shot was more than five years ago or you're unsure of your tetanus status.

TRY SELF-CARE

▶ You have a minor cut but no other symptoms.

YOUR CHILD'S SYMPTOMS

Call your doctor if your child has a cut that's more than shallow. This is especially important if the cut is on his head or hand.

! *Don't give aspirin to anyone younger than age 19! It's linked to Reye's syndrome, a rare but sometimes fatal condition.*

DANDRUFF

Scalp sheds white flakes

Causes

Seborrheic dermatitis. You may have very small flakes on your shoulders, but no other symptoms. Or you may have heavy scaling and dandruff flakes around your eyebrows or nose; behind your ears; in the center of your breastbone; or under your arms. There may be redness, crusting and oozing. The cause of seborrheic dermatitis isn't known. It may be due to a type of fungal infection. It's associated with excessive oiliness often made worse by physical or emotional stress; extremely hot, humid weather; or very dry, cold air. Self-care usually helps.

Psoriasis. You may have started with dandruff. But, now you have plaques—patches of raised, red bumps covered with white, flaking scales—on your scalp, knees, elbows or buttocks. The patches may be itchy or painful. You also may have loosened, discolored nails, and joint pain and stiffness. Call your nurse information service or doctor.

Fungal infection. You may have itchy, flaking, red or grayish patches on your scalp. You also may have some hair loss. Fungal infections are caused by microscopic organisms. Flare-ups can range from mild to severe. Over-the-counter or prescription medication may help.

Other causes may include certain medications. Some shampoos and other hair products, such as dyes, may cause allergic dermatitis.

Self-Care

- Shampoo with a prescription or over-the-counter dandruff shampoo containing sulfur, salicylic acid, selenium, tar or antifungal medication. Follow instructions carefully. Be sure to rinse thoroughly. A conditioner also may help.

Prevention

- Use dandruff shampoo occasionally, between uses of regular shampoo. Try alternating regular shampoos, too. Switch every few days.
- Don't overuse styling products such as hairspray, mousse or gel.
- Avoid exposing the scalp to excessive heat—such as prolonged hair drying.

CALL YOUR NURSE INFORMATION SERVICE OR DOCTOR

▶ You have unusually large flakes along your hairline, elbows, knees or genitals.

▶ You have scaly patches of dandruff that ooze, form crusts or leak pus.

▶ You've tried self-care but your symptoms haven't improved after three weeks.

TRY SELF-CARE

▶ You have flaky dandruff but no other symptoms.

YOUR CHILD'S SYMPTOMS

Dandruff and your child. If your baby has greasy, scaly, yellow-brown patches on the top of her head, she probably has cradle cap. This is a very common condition, and it can be stubborn to remove.

Apply baby oil a few minutes before you give her a shampoo. Use a baby's brush to gently work the shampoo onto the affected areas of her scalp. Be careful not to rub too hard. Gently use your fingernail or a fine-toothed comb to remove any remaining scales.

Never use petroleum jelly— it's too difficult to wash out. For stubborn cases of cradle cap, just try to remove a little each day.

DIARRHEA

Unusually watery, frequent bowel movements; may be preceded by gas and abdominal cramping

Causes

Food poisoning. You may have eaten spoiled food. Symptoms such as headache, nausea, vomiting and diarrhea can occur two hours to two days after eating contaminated food. Call your nurse information service or doctor.

Diet. Sorbitol and fructose-sweetened foods can cause diarrhea. Too much alcohol and laxative-type foods such as apple or grape juice can cause diarrhea, too. Try self-care.

Food allergies. You may have abdominal cramping, diarrhea, nausea, vomiting, itching, sneezing and hives. Reactions usually develop within one hour. Common food allergies include shellfish such as shrimp and lobster, peanuts and tree nuts. Food allergies often are confused with food intolerance, indigestion or other conditions. True food allergies can be life-threatening. If you have symptoms, seek emergency help.

Infection. You may have had several episodes of diarrhea, and you feel sick. You also may be vomiting. This is a common sign of an intestinal tract infection—caused by viruses, bacteria or parasites picked up in food or drinking water. Diarrhea is the body's way of getting rid of the infection. It's usually best to let diarrhea run its course. Try self-care. Certain intestinal tract infections require antibiotics. Talk with your doctor.

Other causes may include Crohn's disease (see Page 261), irritable bowel syndrome (IBS) (see Page 262), lactose intolerance (see Page 122), certain medications or ulcerative colitis (see Page 261).

Self-Care

- For the first 24 to 48 hours of diarrhea, drink plenty of clear liquids to prevent dehydration (see Page 220).

- When you're ready to eat solid foods, try the BRAT diet—bananas, rice, applesauce and toast.

- Avoid caffeine, dairy products, alcohol and highly seasoned foods while the diarrhea lasts and for the first few days after it stops.

- If you think you may have lactose intolerance, see your doctor for a diagnosis. Lactose-free dairy products and lactase-replacement products are available.

- Use over-the-counter antidiarrheal medication only if you don't have a fever, severe abdominal pain or blood in your stool.

Prevention

- Wash your hands often, especially before eating, before and after preparing food, and after using the bathroom. Use soap and warm running water.

- To prevent food-associated gastrointestinal infection, follow safe food-handling procedures. Keep hot foods hot, and cold foods cold.

- Avoid foods, spices or other triggers that may cause diarrhea.

SEEK EMERGENCY HELP

▶ You have large amounts of bloody diarrhea.

▶ You have a very low or absent urine flow, dry lips and mouth, rapid pulse, and dizziness when standing up.

SEE YOUR DOCTOR

▶ You have black stools, or watery stools and abdominal cramping after 24 hours of consuming nothing but clear liquids.

▶ You have a fever, rectal urgency, or blood in your stools.

CALL YOUR NURSE INFORMATION SERVICE OR DOCTOR

▶ You've had diarrhea for more than three days.

▶ You've started taking a new medication.

▶ You recently traveled to a foreign country.

▶ You've tried self-care but your symptoms haven't improved after three days.

TRY SELF-CARE

▶ You have diarrhea but no other symptoms.

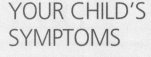
Seek emergency help if your child is eating poorly and is drowsy and unresponsive. He also may have bloody or tarry stools; sunken eyes; dry skin or drowsiness; and may not be able to urinate. Abdominal pain and vomiting along with diarrhea require emergency care.

Call your nurse information service or doctor if your child's diarrhea lasts more than three or four days, or if you see blood in the stool.

Diarrhea and your child. Short-term diarrhea may not have a serious cause. It shouldn't be a health risk as long as your child drinks plenty of fluids while the diarrhea lasts. Many children develop diarrhea from drinking juice—especially apple juice—or milk. See Page 220 for information about dehydration.

Breast-fed babies normally have frequent, yellow, liquid stools. So, it may be difficult to tell if they have diarrhea—which is watery, and clear or green tinged.

"Toddler's diarrhea" may be the cause if your child's stools are foul-smelling and runny, and the diarrhea lasts for several days. If your child remains active, seems healthy, doesn't have a fever and stays well hydrated, you don't need to be concerned.

DIZZINESS

Feeling off-balance, whirling or falling; the room may seem to be spinning

Causes

Vertigo. You may get dizzy when you lean forward or backward; move your head; or look up or down. Dizziness also may occur when you turn your head quickly; roll over in bed; or after vigorous exercise. Your symptoms may last only a few seconds. Often there's no apparent reason for vertigo. It sometimes can be related to head trauma (see Page 9) or stroke (see Page 16). If you become dizzy when you stand up suddenly, your blood probably has pooled in your lower legs, temporarily depriving your brain of oxygen. Vertigo usually is harmless, unless it happens often and you have other symptoms.

Labyrinthitis. You may have intense vertigo with nausea or vomiting. Your eyes may move jerkily. You may have ringing in your ears. Your symptoms may have started abruptly and lasted for several hours or even days. Your inner ear may be inflamed from a viral infection, disrupting your balance mechanism. See your doctor.

Other causes may include allergies (see Page 303), arrhythmia, cardiovascular disease, dehydration (see Page 220), hyperventilation (see Page 70), low blood pressure, certain medications, Ménière's disease (see Page 98), motion sickness or sinusitis (see Page 303).

Self-Care

Dizziness can have many causes. It may be a symptom of a serious health problem. If you have unexplained dizziness, don't diagnose yourself. See your doctor.

- Move slowly, sit very still and look straight ahead for a few minutes. Or, lie down until the dizziness goes away.

- For motion sickness, talk with your doctor about over-the-counter medications before traveling.

Prevention

- Avoid stress and tension. Try some relaxation techniques. If you're hyperventilating, use breathing exercises to help calm yourself.

- Don't sit up or stand up suddenly. Avoid getting out of bed quickly, especially if you're an older adult.

- Cool down after strenuous exercise—walk slowly or stretch your muscles.

- Ask your doctor about exercises to reduce dizziness caused by head movement.

SEEK EMERGENCY HELP

▶ You have difficulty speaking; blurred vision; numbness or tingling on one side of your body or face; weakness or paralysis.

▶ You have chest pain or shortness of breath, or lose consciousness.

▶ You've had a head trauma in the past 72 hours.

▶ You have sudden dizziness after exposure to possible allergens such as medicine, food or an insect sting.

▶ You have sudden difficulty walking straight.

CALL YOUR NURSE INFORMATION SERVICE OR DOCTOR

Always report any dizziness symptoms to your doctor.

▶ You feel fatigued, nauseated—especially in the morning—or you recently have missed a menstrual period.

▶ You have a noise in your ear, an ear infection, or nausea or vomiting. You recently started a new prescription or over-the-counter medication.

▶ You're recovering from the flu, a cold or other upper respiratory infection.

▶ You're having a panic or anxiety attack—unexplained fear, rapid heartbeat, perspiration, dry mouth or shortness of breath.

▶ You're dizzy after quickly getting up from sitting or lying down, or other sudden change in position.

▶ You have a history of high blood pressure. Or, you're taking high blood pressure medication.

TRY SELF-CARE

▶ You have nausea or vomiting, and your dizziness occurred while traveling in a car, plane, train or boat.

YOUR CHILD'S SYMPTOMS

Try self-care if your child is dizzy. Have her lie down with her legs propped up above head level.

DROWSINESS

Sleepiness; difficulty keeping eyes open, or concentrating

Causes

Inadequate sleep. The most common cause of drowsiness is lack of sleep. Most people need eight to nine hours of un-interrupted sleep each night. Getting less than this amount can lead to drowsiness throughout the day. Sleep is essential to good health.

Irregular sleep pattern. You may be working the late shift. Maybe stress or personal worries are keeping you awake at night. Perhaps you're not going to bed and waking up at the same time every day. You may have disturbed your natural sleep/wake cycle.

Sleep apnea. You may snore loudly, and feel tired during the day. You may wake up with a headache. Sleep apnea occurs when the muscles in the back of your throat relax, causing your airway to nar-row or close. Then, your brain awakens you to reopen your airway. Therefore, sleep is interrupted constantly. You may be at higher risk if you're overweight, age 40 or older, or male. Sleep apnea can be treated. See your doctor.

Other causes may include alcohol or drugs, central nervous system disease, depression (see Page 332), liver or kid-ney failure or certain medications.

Self-Care

- Get at least eight to nine hours of uninterrupted sleep in every 24-hour period.

- Try to go to bed and wake up at the same time every day.

- If your schedule allows, try taking a nap in the middle of the afternoon. A 45-minute nap helps many people feel more alert. But, some find that it has the opposite effect. Don't nap if you have trouble sleeping at night.

- Exercise. You're most likely to feel drowsy during periods when you're not physically active. Taking a walk—preferably in the sun—at the first sign of drowsiness may help.

- Don't drive when feeling drowsy.

Prevention

- Get at least eight to nine hours of uninterrupted sleep in every 24-hour period. Teens need at least nine to 10 hours of sleep.

- Limit your intake of coffee, tea, soft drinks and other caffeinated products such as chocolate and some over-the-counter medications.

- Exercise regularly. But avoid exercising four to six hours before going to bed. You may have trouble sleeping.

- Eat a balanced diet—insufficient vitamins and minerals may affect your alertness.

SEEK EMERGENCY HELP

▶ You have confusion.

▶ You have a headache, fever, nausea or vomiting.

CALL YOUR NURSE INFORMATION SERVICE OR DOCTOR

▶ Your drowsiness makes you less alert and puts you or others in physical danger—such as when driving.

▶ You've had episodes of drowsiness for one week or more even though you're getting eight to nine hours of sleep a night.

▶ You snore excessively, or your sleep often is interrupted.

▶ You often fall asleep in inappropriate places. Or, sleep overtakes you so suddenly that you can't prevent it.

TRY SELF-CARE

▶ You have drowsiness but no other symptoms.

EAR, OBJECT IN

Foreign object in the ear; may include ear pain or hearing loss

About Objects in the Ear

A surprising variety of objects can end up in ears—especially children's ears. Marbles, tiny toys, bits of paper, cotton swabs, jewelry, seeds and earplugs are a few possibilities. It also isn't unusual for insects to fly into ears.

The ear's structure prevents most objects from penetrating the middle and inner ear, but it's possible for an object to scratch or tear the eardrum. You're most likely to perforate your eardrum as you attempt to remove objects. If you or your child has an object lodged in the ear, follow these self-care tips and warnings.

Self-Care

If there's a foreign object in your ear, make only one attempt to remove it—but only if it's a blunt object. Never try to remove anything that has sharp edges.

- Work with gravity by tilting your head to the affected side. Gently jiggle your earlobe or shake your head toward the ground to try to dislodge the object. Don't strike your head.

- Cotton swabs are meant for cleaning the outside of your ears only. Don't use cotton swabs to try to remove the object from your ear canal. You may risk pushing the object farther into your ear.

- Don't try to grasp the object with tweezers—you may push it farther in.

If the foreign object is an insect:

- Lie down on your side with the affected ear up.

- If you have no history of ear injury and don't have ear tubes, fill the ear canal, drop by drop, with room temperature oil. You can use mineral oil, baby oil, cooking oil or olive oil. Very gently, pull the earlobe upward and backward to open the canal.

- The insect will drown and float to the top. Blot it away with a tissue. Then lie on your side to drain the remaining oil.

Don't use this technique unless you're certain that the object is an insect. Another foreign object might expand as it absorbs the oil, making it more difficult to remove.

Don't put oil in your ear if you have a history of eardrum injury, such as perforation, or if you have tubes in your ears.

Prevention

- Never insert any object into your ear.

CALL YOUR NURSE INFORMATION SERVICE OR DOCTOR

▶ You have a complete loss of hearing, dizziness, severe pain, or bleeding from your ear.

▶ Something has entered your ear, but isn't visible in the outer ear canal.

▶ You've tried self-care but can't remove the object after one attempt.

TRY SELF-CARE

▶ The object is visible in your outer ear, and you can grasp it without entering the ear canal.

▶ The foreign object is an insect.

EAR, RINGING IN

A buzzing, ringing or hissing noise in the ear; also called tinnitus

Causes

Loud noise. You may work in a loud environment. Perhaps you frequently listen to loud music on a headset. You may hear sounds in your ear when no sound is present. You also may have hearing loss. Loud noise can damage the sensitive hair inside your ear. Try to minimize your exposure to loud noise, and wear ear protection as needed.

Barotrauma. Your symptoms may have begun after you took an airplane trip or went deep-sea diving. This might be the case, especially if you started out with a cold or stuffy nose. You also may be dizzy and feel like your ears are plugged. Symptoms of barotrauma usually clear up on their own. If they don't go away after several days of decongestant therapy, you may need antibiotics. See your doctor.

Ménière's disease. You may have tinnitus, dizziness, fluctuating hearing loss and pressure in your ear. This condition is due to an increase of fluid in the part of the inner ear most involved in balance. It usually affects one ear, then both. See your doctor.

Other causes may include aging, aspirin, certain medications or nerve damage.

Self-Care

- For minor symptoms, try relaxation or biofeedback techniques. Listen to white noise. In a quiet setting, turn on a fan, soft music or low-volume radio static to help mask the noise of tinnitus.

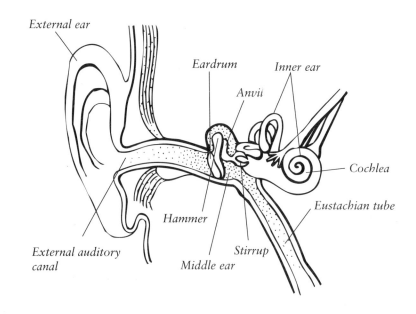

External ear

Eardrum

Inner ear

Anvil

Cochlea

Eustachian tube

Hammer

Stirrup

External auditory canal

Middle ear

- For mild symptoms of barotrauma, try taking a decongestant three to four times a day. Carefully follow package directions. Blow gently through your nose while holding your nostrils closed.

Prevention

- Wear ear protection when exposed to loud noises.
- Avoid air travel when you have a cold. If you must travel, taking a decongestant before your flight may help. Chew gum or suck on hard candy, especially during takeoff and landing.
- If using aspirin, caffeine or alcohol, do so in moderation. Avoid nicotine products.
- Have your hearing checked regularly.

CALL YOUR NURSE INFORMATION SERVICE OR DOCTOR

▶ You have a sudden loss of hearing or severe pain in your ears, forehead or cheekbones.

▶ You've been taking aspirin or arthritis medication containing salicylates.

▶ You have a sudden earache, partial hearing loss, and slight bleeding or discharge from your ear.

▶ You've tried self-care but your symptoms haven't improved after two to three days.

TRY SELF-CARE

▶ You have ringing in your ears after air travel.

YOUR CHILD'S SYMPTOMS

! *Don't give aspirin to anyone younger than age 19! It's linked to Reye's syndrome, a rare but sometimes fatal condition.*

EARACHE

Pain in one or both ears that's dull and throbbing, or sharp and stabbing; may range from mild to severe

Causes

Infection. You may have severe ear pain that may be accompanied by fever. You also may have a sticky yellow, green or bloody discharge. Although ear infections can occur in adults, they're most common in infants and children. Ear infections may need to be treated with antibiotics. See your doctor.

Swimmer's ear, or inflammation of the ear canal. Your earache may have started after swimming. Swimmer's ear is an infection that requires antibiotic drops. Discomfort can be relieved by drying up the water that has entered your ear. See your doctor.

Cerumen wax blockage. Everyone's ear canals make some wax. It's the body's way of protecting the ear. But excessive wax buildup can block the canal. This can cause painful pressure on your ear's sensitive lining tissue. Blockages should be removed by a doctor.

Other causes may include a foreign object in the ear, temporomandibular joint disorders (see Page 158) or trauma.

Self-Care

If your pain is caused by a bacterial infection, you may need an antibiotic. See your doctor.

To relieve discomfort:

- Try an over-the-counter pain reliever, such as acetaminophen, ibuprofen, naproxen sodium or aspirin.

Prevention

- Shake your head after swimming or showering to remove trapped water. If you often have swimmer's ear, try using a solution of equal parts rubbing alcohol and white vinegar, or over-the-counter eardrops each time your ear canal gets wet. Don't remove earwax before swimming—it protects the ear canal from moisture.

- Avoid air travel when you have a cold. Use a decongestant before take-off. Yawn, chew gum or suck on hard candy during takeoff and landing.

- If you tend to have excessive wax buildup, talk with your doctor about using an over-the-counter eardrop solution and ear irrigation kit.
- Never insert objects into your ear—including cotton swabs.

CALL YOUR NURSE INFORMATION SERVICE OR DOCTOR

▶ Your earache worsens when you pull on your earlobe.

▶ You have a fever, and there's a sticky yellow, green or bloody discharge coming from your ear.

▶ You have pain in your teeth or jaw.

▶ Your earache began after a plane trip or deep-sea diving, and it hasn't improved after one week.

▶ You have a cold and the pain has lasted more than two days, gotten worse or you have a fever.

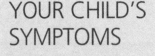

TRY SELF-CARE

▶ The earache began after a plane trip or deep-sea diving, and your ears feel plugged.

▶ You have a cold.

YOUR CHILD'S SYMPTOMS

Call your nurse information service or doctor if your child is extremely irritable, especially when lying down. He may or may not tug at his ear.

Earaches and your child. Ear infections are common in babies and young children. They usually are a complication of an upper respiratory infection. They can be very painful. Since babies can't express their discomfort in words, they may repeatedly tug at one or both ears. But remember, children normally play with parts of their bodies, including their ears. So watch for other symptoms.

If your child has an ear infection, he also may have a fever and cry constantly despite being comforted. He may be particularly irritable when lying down. He also may not be eating well and may be unresponsive to loud noises or to the sound of your voice.

To prevent earaches, hold your baby with his head elevated while breast- or bottle-feeding.

! *Don't give aspirin to anyone younger than age 19! It's linked to Reye's syndrome, a rare but sometimes fatal condition.*

ELBOW PAIN

Pain and possible swelling, tenderness, redness or bruising in the elbow

Causes

Fracture or dislocation. You may have fallen, or injured your elbow. It may be swollen, bruised or bleeding. It also may look twisted or deformed. You may find that it's also painful, tender, hard to move or stiff within a half hour after the injury. Your elbow may be dislocated or broken, or you may have chipped a bone or torn soft tissue around your elbow. See your doctor.

Bursitis. You may have swelling around your elbow. It's painful, especially when you press on it. You also may have a fever. See your doctor. He or she may want to drain the fluid to be sure there's no infection. Your doctor also may recommend a compression wrap and an anti-inflammatory medication such as ibuprofen, naproxen sodium or aspirin. Try to avoid placing direct pressure on the affected area.

Compression injury. You may have pain in your elbow. You also may have numbness and tingling in your fourth and fifth fingers. Perhaps you've been repeatedly leaning your elbow on a hard surface, such as a desk or the handlebars of a bicycle. You may have damaged your ulnar nerve, which passes under your elbow at a spot commonly referred to as the funny bone. Call your nurse information service or doctor. Try not to lean on your elbow, and use a protective pad when you do.

Tennis elbow. Perhaps you've been playing tennis or using a screwdriver or wrench. You may have pain in the outer part of your elbow and upper forearm after repeatedly rolling or twisting your forearm. Try self-care and prevention measures.

Self-Care

If the pain is caused by trauma with no dislocation or fracture:

- For the first 48 hours, use the PRICE remedy—protect, rest, ice, compression and elevation. Protect your elbow from further injury. Rest it, using a sling if needed. Avoid stress or strain on the joint. Wrap crushed ice in a thin towel and apply for 15 to 20 minutes, three to four times a day. Whenever possible, keep your elbow elevated above the level of your heart to help reduce swelling.

- Try an over-the-counter, anti-inflammatory pain reliever such as ibuprofen, naproxen sodium or aspirin.

- After 48 hours, begin carefully moving your elbow through its range of motion every hour or so. Ask your nurse information service or doctor about elbow exercises.

Prevention

- Ask your nurse information service or doctor about exercises that will strengthen your forearm, upper arm and shoulder.

- Use proper equipment, posture and movement for repetitive motion activities such as typing, using tools, or playing golf, tennis or baseball.

- For tennis elbow, ask an instructor to make sure your grip is correct. Reduce your hours of play, and warm up before playing. Apply ice afterward and use a tennis-elbow strap.

SEE YOUR DOCTOR

▶ **Your elbow is red or swollen, you have a fever and you feel sick.**

▶ **Your hand is numb or weak.**

CALL YOUR NURSE INFORMATION SERVICE OR DOCTOR

▶ **The pain started after falling on or injuring your elbow.**

▶ **The pain gets worse when you use your elbow and better when you don't, or it's stiff in the morning.**

▶ **Your elbow's normal range of motion is impaired.**

TRY SELF-CARE

▶ **You have pain in your elbow and outer forearm, and you play tennis, golf or baseball, or do plumbing or carpentry work.**

YOUR CHILD'S SYMPTOMS

See your doctor if your young child's arm is dislocated—which can happen if she's pulled by her arm. Also see your doctor if your child's elbow is red or hot, or if the pain lasts or feels worse the following day. She also may have a fever. She might avoid using her elbow and keep her arm flexed.

Elbow pain and your child. Most elbow injuries or sprains in children are effectively cared for with ice, and perhaps an elastic bandage or sling to rest the arm.

! *Don't give aspirin to anyone younger than age 19! It's linked to Reye's syndrome, a rare but sometimes fatal condition.*

EYE, ITCHY OR RED

Itchy or red eyes

Causes

Allergies (see Page 303). You may have been exposed to an allergen. Common allergens include air pollution, smoke, perfume, pollen or cosmetics. Your eyes may be itchy, red and swollen. You also may be sneezing or have a runny nose. Try to avoid things that irritate your eyes.

Keratitis. Your eyes may be inflamed and painful, but you have no other symptoms. Perhaps you've been wearing your hard contact lenses longer than recommended, or you've been over-exposed to sunlight. Your corneas may be injured. See your doctor.

Blepharitis. Your eyes may be red and itchy. The edges of your eyelids may be inflamed and scaly. This condition often accompanies dandruff. If self-care doesn't work or your symptoms are severe, call your doctor. You may require a prescription ointment.

Dry eye. Your eyes may be red and dry, and you have few or no tears. The white of your eye is red, and your eye feels hot and gritty. Dry eye sometimes accompanies rheumatoid arthritis (see Page 256). It occurs more often in women than men and is a frequent complaint during menopause. Some medications also can cause dry eye. Call your nurse information service or doctor. Self-care measures may help.

Other causes may include conjunctivitis (see Page 108).

Self-Care

- If conjunctivitis is the cause, see Page 108.

- For keratitis, try an over-the-counter pain reliever such as acetaminophen, ibuprofen, naproxen sodium or aspirin. Don't wear contact lenses until you talk with your doctor.

- For blepharitis, wash away the scales twice a day with warm water or baby shampoo.

- For dry eye, relieve the discomfort with over-the-counter artificial tears.

- If a painless red patch on the white of your eye appears suddenly, leave it alone. It usually is harmless and will clear up on its own.

- To relieve redness, apply a cool compress with a clean cloth.

Prevention

- To avoid the spread of infection, wash your hands often. Don't share wash-cloths or towels. Launder them often. Never share eye makeup.

- Replace eye makeup every three months or after an eye infection.
- To prevent keratitis, carefully follow instructions for contact lens cleaning and use. Don't exceed recommended time limits for wearing contact lenses.
- Wear sunglasses to protect your eyes from bright light and ultraviolet rays.
- Avoid possible allergens, including perfumed tissues, cosmetics and detergents.

SEEK EMERGENCY HELP

▶ You have extreme eye pain, light sensitivity or a yellowish-green discharge that hasn't responded to self-care after 24 hours.

SEE YOUR DOCTOR

▶ Your eyes are inflamed and painful, and you wear contact lenses, or have been in strong sunlight.

CALL YOUR NURSE INFORMATION SERVICE OR DOCTOR

▶ Your eyes are red, dry and gritty.

▶ You've tried self-care but your symptoms haven't improved after two days.

TRY SELF-CARE

▶ You have redness and scaliness around the edges of one or both eyelids.

! *Don't give aspirin to anyone younger than age 19! It's linked to Reye's syndrome, a rare but sometimes fatal condition.*

EYE, OBJECT IN

Foreign object in the eye

About Objects in the Eye

Most specks that may enter your eye are harmless and can be taken care of when you blink or when your eye fills with tears. If you think an object may have penetrated your eye, don't try to remove it—seek emergency help. If your eye is obviously injured, you have sudden severe pain or trouble seeing, or you develop a fever, you may have an injury that poses a serious threat to your sight. Seek emergency help.

Self-Care

Never try to remove an object that's stuck or embedded in your eye. Instead, cover both eyes with a sterile or clean cloth. Seek emergency help.

It's important to cover both eyes. If the unaffected eye is open, the pupils in both eyes will change in reaction to light exposure. This may worsen your eye pain. If you can't close your eye, cover it with a small paper cup. Don't put pressure on your eye.

To remove an object on the surface of your eye or under your eyelid:

- Don't rub or apply pressure—this can damage your eye.
- Wash your hands. Then gently pull your lower eyelid down. If the object is there, remove it with the tip of a moistened cotton swab or the corner of a clean cloth. Be careful not to scratch the cornea.
- If the object isn't visible, grasp the eyelashes of the upper eyelid and pull out and down until the upper lid over-laps the lower. Wait a moment until your tears wash the object out.

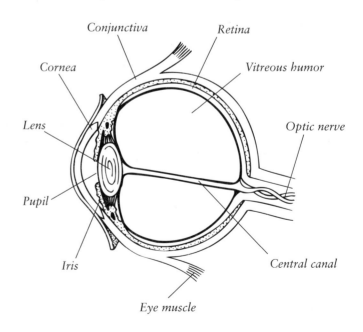

Conjunctiva *Retina*
Cornea *Vitreous humor*
Lens *Optic nerve*
Pupil
Iris *Central canal*
Eye muscle

- If the object is still there, wash the eye using an over-the-counter, eye-irrigating solution, or open your eye under running water.

- For lingering pain or discomfort after an object is removed, call your nurse information service or doctor.

Prevention

- Always wear eye protection when doing carpentry, metalwork, heavy yard maintenance or any activity involving loose dirt, wood splinters, sawdust, metal, glass or any other particles.

SEEK EMERGENCY HELP

- ▶ Something exploded or flew into your eye.

- ▶ Something seems to be stuck in your eye.

- ▶ You can see blood in your eye, or you're having trouble with your vision.

CALL YOUR NURSE INFORMATION SERVICE OR DOCTOR

- ▶ You still can see the object even though you've washed your eye.

- ▶ The object is trapped under your eyelid.

- ▶ You've tried self-care but your condition hasn't improved.

TRY SELF-CARE

- ▶ You have a scratchy feeling that hurts and makes you blink.

EYE DISCHARGE

Clear or yellowish discharge; eyes may be swollen, itchy and red, and possibly so crusty they're difficult to open upon waking

Causes

Viral conjunctivitis. Your eyes may be itchy, red and swollen. They also may be producing a clear, watery discharge. Conjunctivitis, or pinkeye, that's caused by a virus usually is less severe and bothersome than bacterial conjunctivitis. Viral conjunctivitis may be a complication of a cold or the flu. It can take several days to clear up. Because it's caused by a virus, antibiotics won't help. Call your nurse information service or doctor.

Bacterial conjunctivitis. Your eyes may be itchy, red and swollen, with a thick, whitish or yellowish discharge. They may be stuck shut when you wake up. Conjunctivitis, or pinkeye, is an inflammation of the membrane that covers the white of the eye and the inner surface of the eyelids. Bacterial conjunctivitis can cause ulceration of the cornea, and must be treated with antibiotic eye drops. Untreated pinkeye can permanently impair vision. It's highly contagious and commonly caused by sharing eye makeup. See your doctor.

Allergic reaction. You may have been exposed to an airborne irritant to which you're allergic. Now your eyes are watery, red, swollen and itchy. Allergens include pollen, dust, mold spores, animal dander—tiny flakes of hair, feathers or skin—cosmetics and contact lens solution. If possible, avoid the allergen that's bothering you. Otherwise, try self-care.

Self-Care

For conjunctivitis:

- Conjunctivitis is extremely contagious. Wash your hands. Don't share washcloths or towels.

- If your eyes are crusted shut when you wake up, loosen the crusts with a warm, clean washcloth. Don't use this washcloth again until it's laundered.

- Apply a washcloth soaked in warm water to your closed eyes for five minutes, three to four times a day.

- Throw out any eye makeup you were using when the infection started.

- Don't wear eye makeup or contact lenses while you have an eye infection.

- Don't wear a patch over your eye. It may allow an infection to spread.

- To relieve the itching and irritation of viral conjunctivitis, try over-the-counter eye drops.

If allergens are the cause:

- Use antihistamines and eye drops for relief.

Prevention

- Don't share eye makeup, eye drops or contact lens supplies with others.
- Keep your contact lenses clean. Don't exceed recommended time limits for wearing contact lenses. Remove them as soon as you feel eye pain.
- Replace eye makeup every three months.

SEE YOUR DOCTOR

- ▶ Your vision is affected, your eye area is swollen and you have severe eye pain, sensitivity to light, or a fever.
- ▶ The discharge resembles pus, or is yellowish-green.

CALL YOUR NURSE INFORMATION SERVICE OR DOCTOR

- ▶ You've tried self-care but your symptoms haven't improved after two to three days.

TRY SELF-CARE

- ▶ You have eye discharge but no other symptoms.

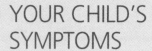

YOUR CHILD'S SYMPTOMS

See your doctor if your child's eyes become swollen.

Call your nurse information service or doctor if your child has allergic conjunctivitis. This condition feels itchy. It's in both eyes but has no discharge. Prescription medicines can help.

Viral conjunctivitis is non-itchy and often accompanies a cold. Your child's eyes may be watery, but without discharge. This usually clears up on its own.

Eye discharge and your child. Bacterial conjunctivitis, or pinkeye, is common in children because it's so contagious. They tend to rub their eyes with dirty hands, which is another contributing factor. Call your nurse information service or doctor.

EYE PAIN

Throbbing or sharp pain, or scratchiness in one or both eyes

Causes

Eye pain can have many causes and may be a symptom of a serious problem. If you have eye pain, don't try to diagnose yourself. See your doctor.

Eyestrain. Your eyes may feel tired and you may have a headache. If your vision is blurred at close distance or your ability to focus on objects at close range has been getting worse, you may need corrective lenses.

Injury. You may have sudden pain in your eye, decreased vision, or redness after being struck in the eye. Many eye injuries can be avoided. Take preventive measures while playing sports or participating in other potentially hazardous activities. Wear eye protection when appropriate.

Sty. You have a small, red painful bump on your upper or lower eyelid. It may feel as if there's something in your eye. Your eyes may be watering excessively. A sty is caused by a bacterial infection of an eyelash follicle. Try self-care.

Uveitis. Your eyes may be red, painful and sensitive to light. You may have blurred or decreased vision. The cause of uveitis often is unknown, but many cases are related to an autoimmune disorder or an infection. Uveitis can be treated. See your doctor.

Corneal ulcer or infection. You may have severe eye pain, blurred vision, excess tears, light sensitivity and difficulty keeping your eyelids open without severe pain. See your doctor.

Other causes may include chemical or flash burns, chalazion, acute closed-angle glaucoma (see Page 267), migraines (see Page 290), object in the eye, optic neuritis or sinusitis (see Page 303).

Self-Care

- Rest your eyes.
- Wear sunglasses to protect your eyes from bright light and ultraviolet rays.
- Use cool or warm compresses—whichever give more relief—for one hour, several times a day.
- Place a pillow or foam wedge under the mattress to elevate the head of the bed.
- Try artificial tears to relieve dryness or irritation.

For sties:

- Apply a warm, clean washcloth to the area for 10 minutes, three to four times a day.

■ Never squeeze a sty. This may spread the infection and cause other sties to develop.

Prevention

■ Wear protective eye gear while playing sports or doing work, as needed.

■ Keep your contact lenses clean. Don't exceed recommended time limits for wearing contact lenses. Remove them as soon as you feel eye pain.

■ Be careful. Makeup brushes, fingernails and sprays can scratch or irritate your cornea.

■ Wear sunglasses to protect your eyes from bright light and ultraviolet rays.

■ Get regular eye exams, including screenings for glaucoma.

SEEK EMERGENCY HELP

▶ You have pain behind your eye. You also have light sensitivity, lethargy, severe headache, confusion or worsening of pain when you bend over.

SEE YOUR DOCTOR

▶ You have severe pain in one eye, blurred vision and sensitivity to light.

▶ You have pain behind your eye, along with tenderness in the temple on that side of your head.

CALL YOUR NURSE INFORMATION SERVICE OR DOCTOR

▶ Your eye is red, and it feels gritty and sticky.

▶ You've tried self-care but your eye pain hasn't improved.

TRY SELF-CARE

▶ You have eye pain but no other symptoms.

FAINTNESS

Brief loss of consciousness

Causes

Postural hypotension. You may feel dizzy or faint when you sit up or stand up quickly. This is due to a sudden drop in blood pressure. It has many causes and is common in older adults, especially following a meal. Try to move slowly when changing position. If it happens often, talk with your doctor.

Anemia. You may feel faint or have fainted. Perhaps you've been feeling tired and weak, and looking pale. You may have shortness of breath, rapid heartbeat when you exert yourself, weight loss or appetite loss. You also may have a sore, red tongue or bleeding gums. Call your nurse information service or doctor.

Vasovagal syncope. You may feel faint, or have fainted at the sight of blood. Or, perhaps something else made you fearful or anxious. The vagus nerve slows the heart rate. When this nerve becomes stimulated—typically from unpleasant emotional or physical stimuli—the heart rate can slow enough, and blood pressure can fall enough, to cause fainting. Symptoms may include nausea, weakness and sweating. Don't diagnose yourself. Call your nurse information service or doctor.

Low blood sugar. You may feel faint, hungry, anxious and irritable. Perhaps you're perspiring and trembling. You also may have palpitations, confusion and loss of coordination. Quickly eating or drinking some sugar or carbohydrates may relieve the faintness, but you should call your nurse information service or doctor.

Other causes may include dehydration (see Page 220), heart disturbances, heat exposure (see Page 11), certain medications or neurological disorders.

Self-Care and Caregiving

- Check to see if the person who has fainted is breathing and has signs of circulation—normal breathing, coughing or movement in response to stimulation. If not, seek emergency help and perform CPR if you've been trained in it (see Page 3).

- Raise the person's legs above his or her head, loosen clothing and make the person comfortable.

- Don't sit up or stand immediately upon regaining consciousness. Weakness after fainting is common.

- If you have diabetes and haven't eaten for six hours, try hard candy, dried fruit or orange juice. Ask your doctor for other snack ideas.

- If you're pregnant, avoid standing for prolonged periods. Move around to stimulate circulation.

- If you have low blood sugar that's been diagnosed, carry glucose tablets, sugar or candy to eat when you feel faint. Drinking fruit juice also can help.

- Drink plenty of liquids, especially in hot weather. Dehydration can trigger or aggravate faintness. Avoid alcohol.

Prevention

- Don't sit up or stand suddenly.
- Stay hydrated by drinking plenty of fluids.
- Eat three meals a day.

SEEK EMERGENCY HELP

▶ You have an injury from a fall; head or chest pain; difficulty breathing; numbness; weakness; or rapid heartbeat.

▶ You've been out in the sun or in an overheated environment. You have a headache, dizziness, weakness or dry skin.

▶ You have heart disease, and your heartbeat changed noticeably before you fainted.

▶ You have diabetes, and you're insulin dependent.

▶ You faint upon exertion.

SEE YOUR DOCTOR

▶ You're pregnant.

▶ The cause of fainting is unknown.

▶ You have diabetes, and you haven't eaten in more than six hours or you've exercised more than usual.

TRY SELF-CARE

▶ You feel faint when you suddenly stand up after sitting or lying down, or you're recovering from an illness.

▶ Your faintness was triggered by some very specific, upsetting event.

YOUR CHILD'S SYMPTOMS

Seek emergency help if your child suddenly fell to the ground, and his face or limbs twitched while he was unconscious (see Page 14).

113

FATIGUE

Tired or lacking energy

Causes

Lifestyle. If you're not getting enough rest, nor practicing healthy habits, you may experience fatigue. Perhaps you stay up very late at night and tend to oversleep in the morning. You may eat an unbalanced diet, get very little exercise, smoke, drink excessively or work long hours. Stress and anxiety also can drain your energy. You may need to make lifestyle changes to combat your fatigue (see Page 17).

Infection. You may have profound fatigue, low-grade fever and swollen glands in your neck. You could have mononucleosis (see Page 126) or viral hepatitis (see Page 156). If your fatigue has lasted for at least six months, you may have chronic fatigue syndrome. If you also have achy joints, a headache and possibly may have been exposed to ticks, you may have Lyme disease (see Page 192). Call your nurse information service or doctor.

Anemia. You may feel faint and a little breathless, look pale, or have heart palpitations. Anemia may be the cause, especially if you're a woman who has heavy menstrual periods. You also may have anemia if you eat a diet low in iron or have suffered blood loss. Call your nurse information service or doctor.

Hypothyroidism (see Page 308). Perhaps you're middle-aged, feel tired all the time and have difficulty keeping warm. You may gain weight, your hair may be thinning, and your skin may be dry. If so, you may have an underactive thyroid gland. This condition is treatable. See your doctor.

Depression (see Page 332). You may have fatigue accompanied by sadness, loss of appetite and loss of pleasure in activities. You may be unable to concentrate, or have trouble sleeping. Depression is treatable. If these symptoms last longer than two weeks, talk with your doctor. He or she also can determine if there is an underlying health problem causing your symptoms.

Other causes may include alcohol, chronic illnesses, certain medications, rheumatoid arthritis (see Page 256) or sleep disorders.

Self-Care

- Get at least eight to nine hours of uninterrupted sleep in every 24-hour period. Teens need at least nine to 10 hours of sleep.
- Start a program of moderate, regular exercise. Check with your doctor first if you've been inactive for a while.

- Reduce your activity if you've been working out excessively.

- If you've been diagnosed with iron-deficiency anemia, iron supplements will help. Ask your doctor about dietary changes or treatment.

- Eat a healthy, balanced diet and drink plenty of water.

- Learn some relaxation and stress-relieving techniques.

Prevention

- Regulate your sleep, eat a balanced diet and stay hydrated by drinking plenty of water each day. Avoid stimulant medications, caffeine and alcohol.

SEEK EMERGENCY HELP

▶ You have any combination of faintness, paleness, breathlessness or palpitations.

CALL YOUR NURSE INFORMATION SERVICE OR DOCTOR

▶ You've been too tired to function normally for more than two weeks, without any apparent cause, such as overwork.

▶ You have swelling in your neck, armpit or groin, or sore throat, headache or fever.

▶ You have constant discomfort or heaviness in the left part of your abdomen.

▶ You're more sensitive to cold than usual, and you're losing hair, gaining weight or suffering from dry skin.

TRY SELF-CARE

▶ You have fatigue but no other symptoms.

FEVER

Adult temperature higher than 99.5° F, taken orally; feeling hot and sweaty, or hot and chilled

Causes

Viral and bacterial infections. Your fever is lower than 103° F. You also may have a mild sore throat, aches and pains, headache, runny nose or sneezing. You may have a common cold or the flu. Self-care can help. However, if you become short of breath, even while you're at rest, or if you cough up discolored sputum, you may have pneumonia or bronchitis. See your doctor.

Kidney, urinary tract or female reproductive infection. You may have a sudden fever of 102° F or higher. You also may have shaking chills and burning, frequent urination. And, if you're female, you may have bloody or yellow vaginal discharge. Your lower back may hurt, and you may feel nauseated. Fever right after childbirth, or pain in your lower abdomen with foul-smelling or heavy vaginal discharge, may signal a serious infection.

Other causes may include excessive exposure to heat or sunlight (see Page 11).

Self-Care

- Try an over-the-counter fever reducer such as acetaminophen, ibuprofen, naproxen sodium or aspirin.

- Sponge bathe with tepid water. Bath water that's about 70° F may lower fever. Cold water may cause shivering which can raise your body temperature. Dress in thin, loose clothing. Use light sheets or blankets.

- Drink plenty of fluids—including water, juice, decaffeinated tea, broth and sports drinks—to replace lost nutrients and prevent dehydration.

Prevention

- Exposure to viruses and bacteria is very common, so prevention is difficult. Hand washing can help prevent the spread of infection.

- Avoid overexposure to heat and sun.

SEEK EMERGENCY HELP

▶ The person with a fever is having convulsions—the body stiffens, eyes roll and limbs thrash. He or she also may feel confused, behave strangely or have difficulty breathing.

▶ You have a stiff neck, severe headache, confusion or drowsiness.

▶ Your skin is very dry. Your fever is higher than 104° F.

▶ Your infant younger than age 1 month appears sick.

SEE YOUR DOCTOR

▶ Your fever has returned for no apparent reason.

▶ You've been sweating heavily for several consecutive nights.

▶ Your fever has lasted more than three days. You feel faint and your eyes are sensitive to light.

▶ You have chills, back pain, or frequent or burning urination.

▶ You've had a severe sore throat for three or more days, rash, earache or cough with discolored sputum.

▶ Your infant younger than age 3 months has a rectal temperature higher than 100.4° F.

CALL YOUR NURSE INFORMATION SERVICE OR DOCTOR

▶ You've recently traveled abroad—especially in a tropical country.

▶ You've had a DPT or MMR shot, or taken immunosuppressant medication.

▶ You've tried self-care but your symptoms haven't improved.

TRY SELF-CARE

▶ You have a fever but no other symptoms.

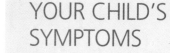

YOUR CHILD'S SYMPTOMS

Seek emergency help if your child has difficulty breathing, true difficulty swallowing liquids, or pain when touching her chin to chest.

Call your nurse information service or doctor if your child has swollen glands, headache, sore throat that makes it uncomfortable to eat or drink, diarrhea, vomiting, earache, runny ear discharge or rash in addition to fever.

Fever seizures, or febrile seizures, and your child. These seizures are fairly common between ages 6 months and 5 years. They usually last one to five minutes and are typically harmless. Report all fever seizures to your doctor. Follow these steps immediately:

■ Make sure she can breathe. Clear food or vomit from her mouth. Gently move her head until her neck is arched, with her chin slightly tipped up in a "rose-sniffing" position. Turn her head to the side.

■ Try sponging or bathing her for 20 to 30 minutes. Use lukewarm water. Check her temperature every half hour until it drops below 102° F. Avoid warm blankets. Rectal suppositories of acetaminophen can be given.

! *Don't give aspirin to anyone younger than age 19! It's linked to Reye's syndrome, a rare but sometimes fatal condition.*

FINGER PAIN OR INJURY

Pain in the finger

Causes

Injury. You may have injured your finger in any number of ways. You even may have pierced your finger with a fishing hook (see illustration). If your injury seems serious, see your doctor.

Tendinitis. Your fingers may be painful and tender, more so at night. You may have trouble moving your fingers and may have muscle spasms in your hand. Tendinitis can develop after a sudden physical trauma or prolonged repetitive movement. Most commonly, it affects the shoulders, elbows, wrists, ankles and fingers.

Tenosynovitis (repetitive strain disorder). You may have trouble straightening your finger, and then it suddenly may snap straight. This sometimes is called "trigger finger." It happens when the membrane covering the tendon becomes inflamed and narrowed. Repetitive movement or infection may be the cause. Call your nurse information service or doctor.

Severed tendon. You may have cut your finger severely across an area where tendons run lengthwise from your wrist to your fingertips. You may not be able to move one or more fingers. Seek emergency help.

Self-Care

- To treat an injury, try the PRICE remedy—protect, rest, ice, compression and elevation. Protect your finger from further injury. Rest the affected area for a day or so. Wrap crushed ice in a thin towel and apply for 15 to 20 minutes, three to four times a day. Use an elastic wrap or bandage. Whenever possible, keep your finger elevated above the level of your heart to help reduce swelling.

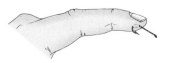 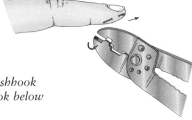

To remove a fishhook, use a wire-cutting tool. Push the fishhook through so that you can see the pointed barb. Cut the hook below the barb. Pull the hook out backward.

- Try an over-the-counter pain reliever such as acetaminophen, ibuprofen, naproxen sodium or aspirin.

- For painful joints, apply a moist-heat pad, or warm, moist towel for 15 to 20 minutes, three to four times a day.

Prevention

- Avoid repetitive strain by varying activities or taking frequent breaks.

SEEK EMERGENCY HELP

▶ You have a protruding bone, misshapen finger, severe pain, or loss of sensation or function following an injury.

▶ Your injured finger shows signs of impaired circulation— pale, blue or gray, and feels cold.

▶ You can't remove a ring from an injured finger due to swelling.

CALL YOUR NURSE INFORMATION SERVICE OR DOCTOR

▶ You have heavy bleeding under your fingernail, or a loose or missing nail.

▶ You have numbness or tingling in your fingers and severe pain when your hand is still.

▶ Your fingers hurt after exposure to the cold, and they look white.

▶ You can't straighten your fingers.

▶ Your finger has been smashed.

▶ The pain began after engaging in physical activity, such as sports.

▶ You've tried self-care but your symptoms haven't improved after two weeks.

TRY SELF-CARE

▶ You have finger pain but none of the symptoms or situations listed above.

YOUR CHILD'S SYMPTOMS

! *Don't give aspirin to anyone younger than age 19! It's linked to Reye's syndrome, a rare but sometimes fatal condition.*

119

FOOT PAIN OR ITCH

Pain, itching, swelling or irritation in one or both feet

Causes

Athlete's foot. Your feet sting, itch and burn, especially between and underneath your third, fourth and fifth toes. Your skin may be red, cracked, scaly and peeling. Athlete's foot is a fungal infection. It's mildly contagious and transmitted by contact—often in public showers, locker rooms and swimming areas, or by sharing towels or footwear. It's not serious, but it can be very uncomfortable.

Morton's neuroma. You may have burning pain and cramping above your third and fourth toes. Morton's neuroma usually is a result of wearing tight shoes.

Calcaneal spur. You have an overgrowth of the heel bone. This places pressure on other structures in the heel and may result in irritation. This may be associated with plantar fasciitis—pain in the sole of the foot often caused by overuse (see Page 146).

Plantar warts. You have small lumps that have one or more little black dots in the center. These may appear on the bottom of one or both feet. They are contagious and may cause pain (see Page 240). Call your nurse information service or doctor.

Other causes may include bunions (see Page 224), contact dermatitis (see Page 190), dyshidrosis or stress fractures.

Self-Care

- If you have diabetes, or impaired circulation, be sure to talk with your doctor about any foot problems you might have.

- If you have athlete's foot, wear clean, cotton socks. Keep your feet dry and air them out as often as possible. Only wear shoes that let your feet breathe. Avoid plastic shoes or shoes that are lined with plastic. Use an over-the-counter antifungal powder during the day when you wear shoes and socks. Apply antifungal creams at night.

- If you have Morton's neuroma, wear wider and flatter shoes. Massage your feet for relief.

- Use orthotic-type arch supports and heel cushions.

- Do foot exercises and try an ice massage after standing for long periods.

Prevention

- Many foot problems are caused by wearing shoes that are too small. Your feet may grow during pregnancy or as you age. Have your feet measured each time you buy shoes.

- Elevate your feet whenever possible, especially during hot weather. Limit your intake of salt.

- To prevent athlete's foot, keep your feet as clean and dry as possible.

- If you're treating a plantar wart or athlete's foot, wear slippers, shower sandals or socks to prevent the spread of infection.

SEEK EMERGENCY HELP

▶ **Your foot shows signs of impaired circulation—pale, blue or gray, and feels cold.**

SEE YOUR DOCTOR

▶ **You have diabetes and two or more of these symptoms: redness, warmth or swelling of the feet, oozing, red streaks or fever.**

▶ **You have persistent numbness or tingling in your foot.**

CALL YOUR NURSE INFORMATION SERVICE OR DOCTOR

▶ **You have a wart on the bottom of your foot.**

▶ **You have abnormalities or lesions on your feet that won't go away.**

TRY SELF-CARE

▶ **Your feet are burning, itchy, red, scaly and cracking, especially between your toes.**

▶ **You have sharp or burning pain in the ball—or bottom front—of your foot and it shoots into your toes.**

YOUR CHILD'S SYMPTOMS

Foot pain or itch and your child. Young children might not be able to tell you when their shoes are too tight. Be sure to have your child's feet measured at least three times a year.

If your child has an itchy, red rash on the bottom of both feet, he may be allergic to material in his shoes. Have him wear different shoes and walk barefoot when at home.

121

GAS OR FLATULENCE

Uncomfortable fullness in the abdomen; rumbling stomach; burping or frequently expelling gas

Causes

Gas-producing food. You may have gas after eating high-fiber foods. These include beans, bran, fibrous vegetables, and beverages containing yeast—such as beer—or carbonation.

Lactose intolerance. You may have gas or flatulence after eating ice cream or other dairy products. You also may have abdominal cramping, bloating or diarrhea. Lactase is an enzyme that helps digest lactose—the main sugar in dairy products. Many adults don't have lactase. This makes it very difficult, if not impossible, for them to digest dairy products. Try self-care. Also, call your nurse information service or doctor for tips on getting enough calcium.

Other causes may include altered intestinal motility; eating too fast; gastrointestinal infections—especially giardiasis, a parasitic infection; certain medications or swallowing air.

Self-Care and Prevention

■ Eat slowly and try not to gulp air as you swallow.

■ Eat fewer gas-producing foods. These include apples, beans, bran, broccoli, cabbage, cauliflower, nuts, onions, peaches, pears, popcorn, prunes and soybeans.

■ Reduce your intake of beer and carbonated drinks.

■ Don't chew gum.

For lactose intolerance:

■ Try lactose-free dairy products. Or, try lactase replacement products. These are available at grocery stores and pharmacies.

CALL YOUR NURSE INFORMATION SERVICE OR DOCTOR

▶ You taste bitter fluid when you belch. Or, you have pale, greasy, foul-smelling bowel movements. You also may have trouble gaining weight.

▶ You have cramps in your lower abdomen that are relieved by a bowel movement. You suffer alternately from constipation and diarrhea.

TRY SELF-CARE

▶ You've been eating high-fiber foods, such as beans, cabbage or bran, or drinking beer or carbonated beverages.

GENITAL SORE

Bump, blister, wart or rash on the penis or vagina, or in the genital area

Causes

The most common causes of genital sores are sexually transmitted diseases (see Page 311).

Herpes simplex. You may have had a tingling or burning sensation before watery blisters appeared in your genital area, on your lips, inside your mouth or on other body areas. The blisters fill with pus and become large, painful sores that crust or dry before healing. Although the rash may clear, herpes simplex virus is contagious and never leaves your system once you've been infected. With a few precautions, you can live an active, healthy life. Work with your doctor—prescription medication can help prevent outbreaks.

Genital warts. You may have small, flat, flesh-colored bumps or a cluster of tiny, cauliflower-like bumps in your genital or anal area. You also may have itching, burning, tenderness or pain. Genital and anal warts result from sexual transmission of human papillomavirus (HPV). See your doctor.

Syphilis. You may have a hard, red, painless, ulcer-like sore on your genitals, or possibly around your mouth or anus.

This sore is a chancre—pronounced "shanker." It may heal after one to five weeks. But, if syphilis goes untreated, the disease will progress. Sometimes there may be other symptoms, such as swollen lymph nodes, but the chancre usually is the telltale sign. See your doctor for a diagnosis. Any sexual partners in recent months should be informed.

Self-Care

It's important to see your doctor if you think you may have a sexually transmitted disease. Early diagnosis is key. There are treatments that may help speed your recovery and prevent complications, as well as prevent the spread of infection to others. These tips may help ease some of the discomfort.

For herpes:

- Using your prescription medication immediately can shorten the length of an outbreak.
- Wash the infected area twice daily with soap and water. Take a warm bath if you can tolerate it.
- Wear loose, cotton clothing.
- Avoid stress.

124

- Try an over-the-counter pain reliever such as acetaminophen, ibuprofen, naproxen sodium or aspirin.
- Avoid sexual contact until after you've been treated. Use prevention techniques at all times.

Prevention

- Always use a latex condom during all sexual contact, or practice abstinence to help prevent sexually transmitted diseases.
- Avoid sexual contact with anyone who has sores on the genitals, anus, lips or tongue, or who complains of genital tingling or irritation.

SEE YOUR DOCTOR

▶ You have a sore that interferes with urination.

CALL YOUR NURSE INFORMATION SERVICE OR DOCTOR

▶ You have pain when urinating, watery vaginal discharge or swelling of your penis.

▶ You have a fever, headache and swelling in your groin.

▶ You have a hard, red sore; an ulcer; or soft, fleshy growths on or around your genitals.

YOUR CHILD'S SYMPTOMS

! *Don't give aspirin to anyone younger than age 19! It's linked to Reye's syndrome, a rare but sometimes fatal condition.*

GLANDS, SWOLLEN

Lumpy swelling often just below, in front of or behind the ears; down both sides or on the back of the neck; or in the armpit or groin

Causes

Infection. Your glands may be swollen or mildly tender in two or more places. You may have a fever and generally feel sick. Many viruses and bacteria can cause swollen glands. Scalp infections may cause swelling in the back of your neck. Some foot infections can cause swollen glands in your groin. Certain sexually transmitted diseases also can cause groin swelling. Call your nurse information service or doctor.

Mononucleosis. Your neck, groin and armpit glands may be swollen, and you also may have a high fever, severe sore throat, trouble swallowing and fatigue. In mononucleosis, the spleen—located in your upper left side, below your ribs—may become enlarged. See your doctor.

Sore throat or tonsillitis. You may have a sore throat and difficulty eating solid food. The glands may be swollen on the sides of your neck. Self-care may provide some relief, but see your doctor if your symptoms are severe.

Other causes may include an abscessed tooth, chronic fatigue syndrome, connective tissue disease such as lupus, HIV infection (see Page 284), leukemia, lymphoma or mumps.

Self-Care

Self-care alone isn't sufficient for persistent swollen glands. See your doctor.

■ If you feel uncomfortable, apply a warm compress—a washcloth soaked in warm water, for example—as often as needed.

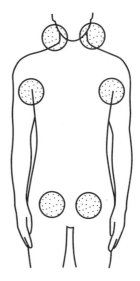

Glands are located throughout the body, including in the neck, armpits and groin.

- Try an over-the counter pain reliever such as acetaminophen, ibuprofen, naproxen sodium or aspirin. Tenderness or soreness usually goes away in a couple of days. But, swelling may last longer.

- If you have mononucleosis, avoid sports or activities in which your spleen might be hit. It may be enlarged and could rupture.

Prevention

- Exposure to viruses and bacteria is very common, so prevention is difficult. Hand washing can help prevent the spread of infection.

- Certain conditions such as mumps are preventable by immunization. Make sure you and your children are immunized (see Page 31).

CALL YOUR NURSE INFORMATION SERVICE OR DOCTOR

▶ Your glands are red, tender, painful or warm to the touch, or the swelling has become worse.

▶ You have a large, hard gland, fever, trouble swallowing or chronic sore throat.

▶ The swelling is in your groin or behind your ear.

▶ You have a swollen gland, and sore throat or earache.

▶ You've tried self-care but your symptoms haven't improved after two weeks.

TRY SELF-CARE

▶ You have swollen glands but no other symptoms.

YOUR CHILD'S SYMPTOMS

Call your nurse information service or doctor if your child has had a fever for more than three days or if she's refusing to drink.

Swollen glands and your child. Use warm compresses and have your child drink plenty of cold liquids. Don't force her to eat solid foods if it hurts to swallow, or if she isn't hungry.

! *Don't give aspirin to anyone younger than age 19! It's linked to Reye's syndrome, a rare but sometimes fatal condition.*

GROIN ITCH

Itching, redness and scaling in the groin area

Causes

Jock itch. Your groin may itch after frequent workouts or in other situations that may cause constant moisture in your groin area. You may have an itchy, red, scaly rash on your groin. The fungus that causes jock itch thrives in warm, moist, dark places. Self-care and prevention usually are effective.

Pubic lice, or "crabs." These lice can be passed from one person to another by sexual contact or contact with infested bed linens or towels. Pubic lice look like little pieces of sand attached at the base of pubic hair.

Scabies. You may have small, red blisters that itch severely. The itching may be worse at night or after a hot bath. Scabies is caused by tiny mites that burrow into your skin. Areas typically affected are wrists, armpits, elbows, ankles, soles of the feet, around the breasts and genitals and on the buttocks. You may see tiny tracks that look like burrows. Blisters appear about two weeks after the mite has dug under your skin. Mites and eggs caught under your fingernails after scratching may be transmitted to other parts of your body. You can catch scabies from close physical contact with an infected person or from contaminated bedding or clothing. Over-the-counter and prescription treatments are available. Family members without symptoms also should be treated.

Medication. You've recently started taking a new medication and have itching in your groin area. Certain prescription and over-the-counter medications can cause itching as a side effect. Call your nurse information service or doctor.

Other causes may include contact dermatitis (see Page 190) possibly due to elastic on underwear, skin rashes associated with being overweight, or urinary incontinence.

Self-Care

- Wash your groin gently and blot dry with a towel, which should be laundered afterward.
- Try an over-the-counter antifungal remedy.
- Sleep naked or in loose-fitting shorts.
- For pubic lice and scabies, try using a 5 percent permethrin cream, available over-the-counter. Follow the instructions on the package exactly. Don't use this cream on your face. A second application after seven to 10 days may be necessary. Clothing and bedding should be washed in hot water.

- If you're pregnant, talk with your doctor before using any treatment.

Prevention

- Keep your groin area clean and dry.

- Launder athletic supporters frequently.

- Don't leave damp clothes in your locker or gym bag.

- Wear absorbent, loose, cotton underwear, including under your supporter during sports.

- Change clothes as soon as possible after sweating.

CALL YOUR NURSE INFORMATION SERVICE OR DOCTOR

- ▶ The itching is severe or spreading from your groin to other parts of your body.

- ▶ You recently had close contact with someone who has scabies or pubic lice.

- ▶ You've tried self-care but your symptoms haven't improved after two weeks.

TRY SELF-CARE

- ▶ The symptoms are mild and limited to your groin area.

GUMS, BLEEDING

Gums bleed easily

Causes

Gingivitis. Your gums may be red, soft, shiny and swollen. They may bleed easily, even from gentle brushing. Gingivitis can be prevented with proper dental hygiene. If not treated, it can lead to serious gum and jawbone disease.

Periodontal disease. You may have untreated gingivitis. Your gums may bleed easily. Plaque, a sticky deposit of debris and bacteria, may collect in pockets between your swollen gums and teeth. You may have an unpleasant taste in your mouth and bad breath. Your gums may pull back from the base of your teeth, exposing areas that are sensitive to hot, cold or sweet foods or drinks. Sometimes an abscess may form deep inside one of your gum-line pockets. The bone around the base of your teeth may be affected, and one or more of your teeth may be loose. This is a serious condition. See your dentist.

Thrombocytopenia or leukemia. If your gums bleed easily, and you also have nosebleeds, fatigue, weakness and a tendency to bruise easily, you may have a blood condition called thrombocytopenia. Or, you may have another blood disorder characterized by low platelets. If you have these symptoms—abdominal pain and swelling, nausea, fever, night sweats, and decreased appetite or weight loss—you may have a type of leukemia. See your doctor.

Vincent's infection or "trench mouth." You may have red, swollen, painful, bleeding gums with a grayish film. It may hurt to swallow. And, you may have bad breath and a bad taste in your mouth. You also may salivate excessively. This is a noncontagious infection associated with poor dental hygiene, physical or emotional stress, poor nutrition or heavy smoking. It must be treated, and the irritating causes such as smoking or eating spicy foods must be eliminated. See your doctor or dentist.

Self-Care and Prevention

- Brush your teeth thoroughly with a fluoride toothpaste at least twice a day and after each meal, if possible. Use dental floss at least once a day.

- Watch your diet. Avoid foods with a lot of sugar, especially foods that stick to your teeth. Eat high-fiber foods such as green vegetables and apples. Finish your meals with a little bit of cheese to counteract acidity.

- Get plenty of vitamins A and C every day. Cantaloupe, broccoli, spinach, liver, fortified dairy products, oranges, grapefruit, tomatoes, potatoes and green peppers are good sources.

- See your dentist twice a year to have your teeth cleaned professionally.

- Quit smoking (see Page 25).

CALL YOUR NURSE INFORMATION SERVICE, DOCTOR OR DENTIST

- ▶ You have swollen, red gums that bleed easily; teeth exposed at the gum line; or teeth that are loose or separated from each other.

- ▶ You have bad breath or a foul taste in your mouth; pus around your gums or teeth; or tooth pain when you eat or drink.

- ▶ You bruise easily, have fatigue, bone pain, nausea, fever or night sweats.

- ▶ You have bleeding gums, pain when you swallow, and excessive salivation.

HAIR LOSS

Hair that's thinning or falling out at an abnormal rate

Causes

Male pattern baldness. Your hair may have thinned slowly. It may have begun to disappear, starting at the temples or front of your scalp, working back over the crown of your head. Male pattern baldness is an inherited condition. It also may be related to an increased sensitivity to androgen—a male hormone—and isn't reversible.

Alopecia areata. You've quickly lost all your hair in one spot or several patches. But you have no infection, and your scalp is normal. This condition often goes away with no treatment—and new hair covers the bald spots within six to nine months. However, you should talk with your doctor.

Ringworm. You have bald patches on your scalp, scaly patches of skin and itching. You also may have blistering and oozing. Remedies applied to the scalp won't get rid of the fungus in the hair shafts. You may need a prescription for an oral antifungal medication. Call your nurse information service or doctor.

Hypothyroidism (see Page 308). Your hair is sparse, coarse and dry, and you may be experiencing other symptoms such as unexplained fatigue, weight gain, muscle pain, cramps, increased sensitivity to cold, constipation and dry skin. These could be signs of an underactive thyroid.

Abnormal androgen level in women. Your hair is becoming thin at the temples or at the crown of your head. But, it's becoming thicker or more noticeable on your face. You also may have abnormally oily skin. Too much male hormone may be genetic or due to menopausal changes or medications—especially birth control pills or hormone replacement therapy. This imbalance usually can be corrected. Rarely, this may be caused by a tumor on the ovaries, or on the adrenal glands which secrete androgen.

Other causes may include childbirth, crash dieting or stress (see Page 334).

Self-Care

- Avoid high-alkaline shampoos.
- Don't towel-dry too vigorously or use a hot hair dryer.
- Comb, don't brush. Don't pull your hair back too tightly in braids or ponytails.
- If you feel self-conscious about your hair loss, you may want to consider wigs, hair transplants or weaves.

- Topical medications tend to be expensive and may be limited in their effectiveness. Ask your doctor if these products are right for you.

Prevention

- Treat your hair gently. Curling irons, hot rollers, lighteners, perms and dyes can damage hair. Even professional styling can be rough on hair.
- When swimming, wear a bathing cap to protect your hair from chlorine.
- Don't share combs and brushes, which can carry bacteria, viruses or parasites.

CALL YOUR NURSE INFORMATION SERVICE OR DOCTOR

- ▶ Your hair is getting thin, and you're taking medication for another condition.
- ▶ You have patchy hair loss.
- ▶ You've tried self-care but your symptoms haven't improved after two to three months.

TRY SELF-CARE

- ▶ Your hair has become thin two to three months after a serious or long illness; major life stress; childbirth; crash dieting; or going off birth control pills.

YOUR CHILD'S SYMPTOMS

See your doctor if ringworm is the cause of your child's hair loss. She'll need a prescription medication. Wash hairbrushes, combs, caps and hair accessories often during treatment. Hair will grow back normally after treatment.

Call your nurse information service or doctor if your child persistently pulls her hair.

Hair loss and your child. Infants often lose their hair, especially if they rub their heads against things. Stronger hair eventually will replace it.

Hair loss also may be caused by tight braids or ponytails, or hair-pulling.

HAND PAIN

Pain, swelling or redness in the hand

Causes

Sprain or strain. You may have injured your hand. You now may have pain or tenderness, and possibly swelling, redness or bruising. If the symptoms are mild, try self-care.

Carpal tunnel syndrome and repetitive motion injuries. You may have pain, numbness and tingling, that often get worse at night, in your wrists and hands. Carpal tunnel syndrome is common among people who do repetitive work or activity with their hands such as keyboarding or assembly-line work. The tendons between the arm and hand become inflamed and swollen, and begin to close in on the major nerve of the wrist. Talk with your doctor.

Arthritis (see Page 255). You may have pain and swelling or stiffness in your hand or in other joints. You also may have limited movement in your wrist. Symptoms of arthritis vary depending on the type. See your doctor.

Tendinitis. Your fingers may be painful and tender, more so at night. You may have trouble moving your fingers and may have muscle spasms in your hand. Tendinitis can develop after a sudden physical trauma or prolonged repetitive movement. Most commonly, it affects the shoulders, elbows, wrists, ankles and fingers. Call your nurse information service or doctor.

Ganglion cyst. You may have a round swelling under the skin of your wrist or the back of your hand. It may be hard or rubbery but not very painful or tender. Ganglion cysts are common and usually need no treatment. If the cyst bothers you, see your doctor.

Other causes may include infectious arthritis, osteomyelitis, rheumatic fever or soft tissue infection.

Self-Care

- If you have tendinitis, or a sprain or strain, try the PRICE remedy—protect, rest, ice, compression and elevation. Protect your hand from further injury. Rest the affected area for a day or so. Wrap crushed ice in a thin towel. Apply for 15 to 20 minutes, three to four times a day. Use an elastic wrap or bandage. Whenever possible, keep your hand elevated above the level of your heart to help reduce swelling.

Prevention

For tendinitis and carpal tunnel syndrome:

- Avoid highly repetitive movement. Take frequent breaks, if possible.
- Use arm and wrist supports appropriate to the activity.

SEEK EMERGENCY HELP

- ▶ The pain immediately followed an injury, or is severe. Or, your hand looks misshapen.
- ▶ You have sudden paralysis or loss of feeling in your hand.
- ▶ Your hand shows signs of impaired circulation—pale, blue or gray, and feels cold.

SEE YOUR DOCTOR

- ▶ You have weakness in your hand or loss of hand function after an injury.

CALL YOUR NURSE INFORMATION SERVICE OR DOCTOR

- ▶ You have numbness or tingling in your hand and the pain is worse at night.
- ▶ Your neck is stiff and painful.
- ▶ Your hands turn white, then blue, then red, especially when they're cold.
- ▶ Your knuckle joints are swollen, and you have hand pain and stiffness that's worse in the morning.

TRY SELF-CARE

- ▶ You have hand pain but none of the symptoms or situations listed above.

YOUR CHILD'S SYMPTOMS

See your doctor if your child has swelling, stiffness and pain in his knuckle joints. Along with these hand pain symptoms, he may have a fever, rash, abdominal pain, weight loss, fatigue, paleness or red eyes.

Call your nurse information service or doctor if your child has joint pain and fever.

HEAD INJURY

Injury to the head, with or without loss of consciousness or other visible symptoms

About Head Injuries

Severe head injuries often result from automobile and motorcycle accidents. Head injuries also occur during sports. In the event of a serious head injury, seek emergency help and follow first-aid techniques (see Page 9).

Concussion. A hard blow to the head creates a sudden movement of the brain within the skull. A concussion often involves loss of consciousness; loss of memory; dizziness; and nausea or vomiting—but not always. Other symptoms may include headache; confusion; sleepiness; trouble concentrating; weakness; seizures; or loss of balance. Seek emergency help.

Intracranial hematoma. A blood vessel ruptures between the skull and the brain. A hematoma—or blood clot—forms, putting pressure on brain tissue. Symptoms such as headache; nausea; vomiting; confusion; loss of strength or feeling; and changes in pupil size may occur. Seek emergency help.

Skull fracture. This is a break in the bone that surrounds and protects the brain. Symptoms include bruising or discoloration behind your ear or around your eyes; blood or clear fluids leaking from your ears or nose; unequal size of pupils; or swelling or depression of your skull. Seek emergency help.

Self-Care

■ The first 24 to 72 hours after a head injury are critical. Symptoms of serious problems may occur during this time. Seek emergency help if you see:

- Noticeable restlessness

- Pupils of unequal size or shape

- Severe headache that lasts longer than four hours after the injury

- Confusion or abnormal behavior

■ Reduce swelling by applying ice. Be aware that the size of the bump isn't an indicator of the severity of the injury.

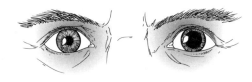

Pupils of newly unequal size indicate emergency treatment is needed.

Prevention

- Motorcycle drivers and passengers, and bicyclists always should wear helmets. Wear protective head gear when playing sports.
- Car drivers and passengers should wear seat restraints. Place children in approved car seats. Never mix driving with alcohol or drugs.

SEEK EMERGENCY HELP

▶ You have severe head or facial bleeding, loss of consciousness, slurred speech or bruising around your eyes or ears.

▶ The head injury occurred while under the influence of drugs or alcohol.

▶ You have a visual problem, bleeding from your eyes, ears or mouth, or fluid draining from your nose or ears.

▶ You have drowsiness or dizziness.

▶ You have a severe headache or one that's progressively getting worse.

▶ You have memory loss; projectile or repeated vomiting; double vision; or loss of strength or sensation in part of your body.

▶ You're having breathing difficulty or seizures, or you feel confused or irritable.

▶ Your pupils are newly unequal in size.

▶ You have a large lump directly behind your ear after an injury.

SEE YOUR DOCTOR

▶ You have severe ear pain or your ears are ringing.

▶ You have a headache that isn't going away.

▶ You've tried self-care but some of your symptoms have gotten worse.

TRY SELF-CARE

▶ You have a mild headache but no other symptoms.

YOUR CHILD'S SYMPTOMS

The symptoms and possible courses of action in the decision chart on this page apply to children, too.

Head injuries and your child. Children often sustain minor head injuries. These symptoms indicate it's probably a minor injury: your child remains conscious even if stunned at first; is easily aroused from sleep even if drowsy—during normal sleep hours after the injury; and both pupils are the same size.

HEADACHE

Head pain that may be constricting, dull, throbbing, pounding, sharp or stabbing; may or may not be accompanied by other symptoms such as nausea or dizziness

Causes

Tension. You may feel a dull, steady pressure around your head or at the back of your neck. You may be contracting the muscles of your head and neck, without even realizing it. Tension headaches are common and tend to run in families. Try self-care.

Migraine (see Page 290). Your head may throb, especially on one side or behind your eyes. You may feel nauseated or be sensitive to light or noise. You may see flashing lights or spots before your eyes. Migraines may be triggered by stress; eating aged cheese or chocolate; drinking red wine; fasting; or changes in your sleep schedule. Call your nurse information service or doctor.

Sinusitis (see Page 303). You may feel pressure in your forehead, behind your nose, or around your eyes or cheeks. You also may be congested or your head may hurt. Sinus headaches tend to feel worse first thing in the morning. Try self-care.

Cluster headaches. You may have intense pain around one eye that may spread to other areas of your face. Your eye may be bloodshot or watery, or your nose may run profusely from one nostril. Cluster headaches generally last from one-half to three hours. You may have multiple headache episodes in one day, recurring over a four- to eight-week period. Talk with your doctor.

Other causes may include alcohol, allergies (see Page 303), consuming something very cold, reactions to monosodium glutamate (MSG) or other substances in foods, or temporomandibular disorders (TMD) (see Page 158).

Self-Care

- Try an over-the-counter pain reliever such as acetaminophen, ibuprofen, naproxen sodium or aspirin as soon as you feel a headache coming on. These can be very effective when taken early. But if you're using them several times a day or for extended periods, call your nurse information service or doctor.

- Tension headaches often can be relieved by massage. Rub the base of your head with your thumbs, starting under your ears and working back and then up to your temples.

- Apply heat to the back of your upper neck.

Prevention

- Look for patterns. Keep track of when and where you get headaches and try to avoid triggers.

- Eat regularly during the day. Avoid foods and beverages that may trigger headaches.

- If you drink alcohol, do so in moderation (see Page 25).

- Keep regular sleeping habits (see Page 27).

SEEK EMERGENCY HELP

▶ Your headache is severe, and it started suddenly, like an explosion in your head.

▶ You have trouble with your vision; difficulty talking or thinking clearly; trouble with coordination; or weakness in your arms and legs.

▶ You have sudden onset of a severe headache, and fever and severe neck pain or stiffness, or dizziness, without a history of migraines.

SEE YOUR DOCTOR

▶ You have a history of high blood pressure.

▶ You have a new, sudden onset of a throbbing headache with nausea or vomiting.

CALL YOUR NURSE INFORMATION SERVICE OR DOCTOR

▶ Your headache has lasted more than three days, and it keeps you from your usual activities.

▶ You have a throbbing headache with nausea or vomiting, and a history of migraines.

TRY SELF-CARE

▶ Your headache feels like a tight band around your head.

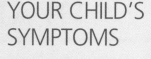
Seek emergency help if your child is age 3 years or younger and her headache isn't the direct result of an injury; or if along with a headache, your child of any age has a stiff neck that hurts more when her head is bent forward.

See your doctor if headaches consistently occur in the morning, or awaken your child from sleep.

Call your nurse information service or doctor if your child is age 3 years or older and has a headache with fever or vomiting without diarrhea, or refuses to drink.

! *Don't give aspirin to anyone younger than age 19! It's linked to Reye's syndrome, a rare but sometimes fatal condition.*

HEARING LOSS

Decreased ability, or inability, to hear some or all sounds; may occur in one or both ears

Causes

Noise. You may have been exposed to loud noises or high-decibel sounds such as machinery, gunshots or very loud music. Noise-induced hearing loss can occur following a short burst of loud sound, such as at a rock concert or fireworks display. Long-term exposure, however, is much more serious. It may damage nerve endings, resulting in decreased hearing.

Aging. You're age 60 or older. It may seem as though people are mumbling a lot lately. You may find yourself asking people to speak a little louder. Those around you may be asking you to turn down the volume on the television and radio. These are all signs of presbycusis, or age-related hearing loss. Talk with your doctor.

Earwax blockage. Your hearing loss may have been gradual, and you may feel as though your ears are blocked. Try self-care.

Other causes may include eighth nerve tumors, eustachian tube dysfunction or Ménière's disease (see Page 98).

Self-Care

- If you have age-related hearing loss, ask your doctor about assistive hearing devices. Don't be embarrassed to ask people to speak clearly and in a normal tone.

- Try an over-the-counter earwax removal kit, with your doctor's approval. Follow directions carefully. Don't use these products if your eardrum is injured or perforated.

- Hearing can be impaired by colds, allergies or plane travel. A decongestant with the ingredient pseudoephedrine may help. But talk with your doctor first if you're pregnant or nursing, if you have heart disease, diabetes or thyroid disease, or if you're taking other medications. If you're taking monoamine oxidase inhibitors (MAOIs), avoid decongestants altogether.

- Try "popping" your ears—pinch your nostrils closed and gently blow out as if blowing your nose.

Prevention

- Avoid exposure to high-decibel sound. If frequent exposure is unavoidable, use well-fitting ear protection.

- If you use portable headphones, keep the volume low.
- Don't put cotton swabs, fingers or any small objects into your ears.
- Blow your nose gently. Don't use too much force.

SEE YOUR DOCTOR

▶ The hearing loss followed an injury or a blow to your head.

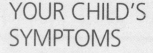

CALL YOUR NURSE INFORMATION SERVICE OR DOCTOR

▶ You have a sticky, yellow discharge from your ear, earache, dizziness, ringing in your ear, or a recent ear or upper respiratory tract infection.

▶ You're taking aspirin or a new medication.

▶ You've tried self-care but your hearing hasn't improved.

TRY SELF-CARE

▶ You feel like your ears are blocked by wax.

▶ You feel like you're talking in an echo chamber, and you've traveled by plane recently.

YOUR CHILD'S SYMPTOMS

Hearing loss and your child. At about age 4 months, a baby begins to respond noticeably to sound by turning toward it. By age 1 year, children usually start speaking. Your child may have hearing loss if he doesn't respond to your voice and is slow in learning to speak.

Children may be born with impaired hearing, or they may develop it as a result of frequent ear or upper respiratory tract infections.

Infants with normal hearing often may ignore sounds. If your infant doesn't respond to sounds that are especially startling, such as a whistle or loud clap—even occasionally—he may have hearing loss.

Many states require newborn hearing screenings. All parents should ask their doctors about this important test.

HEARTBEAT, RAPID

Rapidly beating heart; other symptoms may or may not be present

Causes

A normal adult heart rate is 60 to 100 beats per minute. Most cases of rapid heartbeat are caused by anxiety, smoking, or too much caffeine or alcohol.

Overexertion. You've just done some intense physical activity and now your heart is beating very fast. Physical exertion is a common cause of rapid heartbeat. A heart rate as high as 160 beats per minute isn't unusual with exercise. It generally isn't dangerous if you don't have other symptoms—such as chest pain or faintness—you're in good health and you're age 60 or younger.

Medication. It may feel as if your heart is beating out of your chest. Rapid heartbeat can be a side effect of several over-the-counter and prescription medications—including vitamins or herbal supplements. Examples include appetite suppressants, antihistamines, antidepressants, asthma relievers and decongestants. Call your nurse information service or doctor.

Heart disease (see Page 278). Your heart is beating rapidly. You have shortness of breath, but you haven't had much physical exertion. Rapid heartbeat may occur with any underlying heart abnormality,

as in heart disease. In this case, it's almost always accompanied by other symptoms, such as breathlessness, chest pain, fainting, lightheadedness or fluid retention. See your doctor.

Other causes may include anxiety (see Page 330), stress (see Page 334) or thyroid conditions (see Page 308).

Self-Care

- Make a note of when your rapid heartbeat happens and what you're doing at the time. Record any symptoms and how long they last. Count the number of beats per minute. Give this information to your doctor for a diagnosis.

- Once the cause of your rapid heartbeat is diagnosed, these self-care tips—in addition to any treatment your doctor may prescribe—may help:
  - Limit your intake of caffeine and alcohol.
  - Quit smoking (see Page 25).

Prevention

- Don't smoke.
- Watch your intake of alcohol and caffeinated drinks such as coffee, tea, and cola and some other soft drinks.

■ If you take medication for rapid heartbeat, follow your doctor's instructions. Be sure to keep your medical appointments.

SEEK EMERGENCY HELP

▶ You have chest pain or pain radiating to your arms, shoulders or neck. You also may have shortness of breath, nausea or vomiting.

▶ You have severe breathlessness or lightheadedness.

CALL YOUR NURSE INFORMATION SERVICE OR DOCTOR

▶ You experience skipped beats, extra beats, flip-flops, pounding of your heart or significant changes in your heart rate.

▶ You have a history of panic attacks.

▶ You've tried self-care but your heartbeat is still rapid.

TRY SELF-CARE

▶ You have a rapid heartbeat but no other symptoms.

Rapid heartbeat and your child. Average pulse rates of children vary by age and tend to be a bit higher than those of adults, especially in children ages 8 years and younger. They tend to drop by adolescence. Pulse rates of babies and toddlers differ the most from the pulse rates of older children and adults.

HEARTBURN

Burning pain just below the ribs or breastbone, usually within an hour after a meal; stomach acid backing up into the throat, especially when bending forward or lying down

Causes

Irritation. Heavy meals or eating too fast can cause heartburn. Irritation may be caused by lying down or smoking after a meal; drinking alcohol or coffee—even if it's decaffeinated; taking aspirin; wearing tight clothing; or being overweight. Try self-care.

Gastroesophageal reflux disease (GERD). If you experience heartburn two or more times a week, you may have GERD. Over-the-counter remedies may not provide relief. You may have stomach-acid reflux due to a faulty valve between your stomach and your esophagus. See your doctor.

Pregnancy (see Page 321). Hormonal changes and increased abdominal pressure can produce heartburn. Talk with your doctor.

Hiatal hernia. Heartburn sometimes can be a symptom of a hiatal hernia. Part of the stomach pushes through an opening in the diaphragm—the muscle that separates the abdomen from the chest. Most people with hiatal hernias have few, if any, symptoms. Hiatal hernias usually don't require any treatment. See your doctor if you have persistent heartburn, difficulty swallowing or shortness of breath after eating.

Other causes may include esophageal ulcers, gastritis or peptic ulcers (see Page 298) or certain medications.

Self-Care

- Try a liquid, over-the-counter antacid that doesn't contain calcium. If you're pregnant or have a health condition, call your nurse information service or doctor before taking an antacid, or any other medication.

Prevention

If you frequently have heartburn, you may be able to identify the specific irritating foods. These general tips also may help:

- Improve your posture. Walk and move around. After eating, don't lie down or bend over.

- Place a pillow or foam wedge under the mattress to elevate the head of the bed so gravity can help keep stomach acid down.

- Maintain a healthy weight (see Page 21).

144

- Eat small meals. Don't eat for two to three hours before bedtime. Avoid problem foods.

- Avoid foods that contain air such as whipped cream or carbonated drinks. Don't drink through a straw or from a narrow-necked bottle.

- Avoid tight clothing, especially around your waist.

SEEK EMERGENCY HELP

▶ You're having sudden, severe chest pain. It may get worse if you exert yourself. You're sweating, breathless, nauseated, faint or confused.

▶ You're vomiting, and the vomit is black or red.

CALL YOUR NURSE INFORMATION SERVICE OR DOCTOR

▶ You're having trouble swallowing or you've had the same pain often during the past three days.

▶ The following symptoms get worse at night: belching with an acid aftertaste; difficulty swallowing; or burning discomfort in your chest.

▶ You have moderate pain or discomfort that keeps returning.

▶ You've tried self-care—including eliminating coffee, tea or alcohol from your diet—but the pain persists.

TRY SELF-CARE

▶ You have heartburn but none of the symptoms or situations listed above.

HEEL PAIN

Discomfort in the heel; pain may extend throughout the foot

Causes

Injury. You may have bruised or injured your heel falling or jumping. If your injury isn't severe, try self-care.

Achilles' tendinitis. The Achilles' tendon is one of the strongest tendons in the body. It connects the back of your heel to your calf muscles. It may be inflamed, swollen or tender. You may have strained your calf muscles if they were tight due to lack of stretching. People who run on hard surfaces or wear unsupportive footwear tend to get Achilles' tendinitis. Try self-care.

Bursitis. Fluid-filled sacs called bursae reduce the friction between your tendons and bones. They may become inflamed from poorly-fitting shoes, or from the pressure of landing hard on your heels, such as after a high jump or unexpected fall. The pain may be worse at the end of the day or after standing for a long time. Self-care should help, although you may need a shoe insert to correct improper walking.

Heel spurs. You may have an abnormal bone growth in your heel. Long-term strain—running, jogging or being overweight—sometimes can lead to this. Poorly fitting shoes can aggravate the condition. Talk with your doctor.

Plantar fasciitis. You may have painful inflammation in the sole of your foot, particularly in the tissue that helps support the arch of your foot. Overuse and strain, often caused by being overweight or pregnant, running or playing sports, can cause this. But, you may strain this tissue by moving heavy objects or by wearing unsupportive shoes. Try self-care.

Self-Care

For mild injuries, an inflamed tendon, bursitis, plantar fasciitis or Achilles' tendinitis, try the following:

- Rest your feet as much as possible for one to 12 weeks, depending on the nature and severity of the condition.

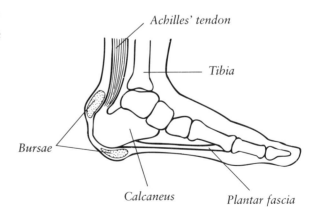

Achilles' tendon

Tibia

Bursae

Calcaneus

Plantar fascia

- Try an over-the-counter pain reliever such as acetaminophen, ibuprofen, naproxen sodium or aspirin.

- Wear shoes that fit well. Use heel pads and arch supports.

- Massage your heels with ice for five minutes after walking, working out or at the end of the day.

Prevention

- Wear comfortable shoes. Use appropriate footwear for exercising. Replace shoes regularly. Running and walking shoes should be replaced every 350 to 500 miles.

- Learn stretching and strengthening exercises for your feet and ankles.

- Maintain a healthy weight (see Page 21).

CALL YOUR NURSE INFORMATION SERVICE OR DOCTOR

▶ The pain began right after an injury or running.

▶ You've tried self-care but the pain hasn't improved.

TRY SELF-CARE

▶ The pain is on the bottom of your foot near the back, or on the back of your heel above the sole.

▶ The pain is in the tendon at the back of your ankle.

▶ The pain is on the bottom of your foot, a little forward from the heel.

YOUR CHILD'S SYMPTOMS

! Don't give aspirin to anyone younger than age 19! It's linked to Reye's syndrome, a rare but sometimes fatal condition.

HIP PAIN

Pain in the upper thigh and lower buttock, or groin area

Causes

Injury. You may have injured your hip in some way. If the pain isn't severe, self-care may help.

Arthritis (see Page 255). You may have pain and swelling or stiffness in your joints. You also may have a limited range of motion. Symptoms of arthritis vary depending on the type. See your doctor.

Pinched nerve. You may have pain in your hip that extends down your leg and is limited to one side. You also may have numbness or tingling in your leg. See your doctor.

Hip fracture. You recently may have fallen, and now you have hip pain. The hipbone—actually the top of the leg bone—can break easily, even after only a slight fall. Older adults and those with osteoporosis (see Page 294) are most at risk. See your doctor.

Bursitis. You may have pain or tenderness in the area of your hip joint. It may spread down your leg to your knee or worsen at night when you lie on it. Bursitis is an inflammation of the bursae, the fluid-filled sacs that cushion the bony part of your hip and reduce friction caused by movement.

Other causes may include avascular necrosis, congenital dislocation, growth-plate slippage or iliotibial band syndrome.

Self-Care

- Avoid activities that aggravate hip pain. But, don't stop exercising entirely. Try gentle stretching and non-weight-bearing exercises.

- Apply a moist-heat pad, or warm, moist towel to your hip for 15 to 20 minutes, three to four times a day. If moist heat isn't available, take a warm bath or shower. Your doctor may recommend ice for bursitis.

- Use an over-the-counter analgesic ointment to soothe pain. Don't use menthol ointment in combination with a heating pad—it can cause serious burns.

- Massage the area around your hip joint.

- Sleep on a firm mattress, preferably on your back. Don't put pillows under your knees or lower back.

- Try an over-the-counter pain reliever such as acetaminophen, ibuprofen, naproxen sodium or aspirin.

Prevention

- Try low-impact exercises, such as swimming, bicycling or walking.
- Wear athletic shoes for any exercise. They increase the stability of the foot.
- Maintain a healthy weight (see Page 21).

SEEK EMERGENCY HELP

▶ The pain began after a fall.

▶ You suddenly can't walk.

SEE YOUR DOCTOR

▶ You're taking oral steroid medication now, or have taken it within the past year, and a persistent hip pain started for no apparent reason.

▶ You have severe pain even when you're not putting any weight on your leg. You also may have a fever, or you can't walk.

▶ The pain started after an injury—even a mild one—and is continuing or getting worse.

CALL YOUR NURSE INFORMATION SERVICE OR DOCTOR

▶ The pain interrupts your sleep, or prevents you from doing your usual activities.

▶ You've tried self-care but your symptoms haven't improved after two weeks.

TRY SELF-CARE

▶ You have hip pain but none of the symptoms or situations listed above.

YOUR CHILD'S SYMPTOMS

See your doctor if your child is limping, or has difficulty moving after an injury. You also should call your doctor if she has redness and heat in the area that hurts. She also may have a fever.

! *Don't give aspirin to anyone younger than age 19! It's linked to Reye's syndrome, a rare but sometimes fatal condition.*

HIVES

Raised, red, itchy ridges or bumps on the skin usually on the face, arms, legs or trunk of the body; less often, they occur on the scalp, hands or feet

Causes

In most cases, hives are an allergic response to something you touched, inhaled or swallowed. Histamine is a chemical your body produces as part of the allergic response. It causes fluid to leak out of blood vessels and collect under your skin as hives. They're more common in allergy-prone people with hay fever, dust allergies or eczema. Some common triggers include:

- Animal dander
- Berries
- Bug bites or stings
- Chocolate
- Dairy products
- Eggs
- Freshwater fish
- Infections
- Nuts
- Pollen
- Pork
- Shellfish
- Wheat products

Certain medications, especially aspirin and aspirin-related drugs, may be triggers.

Hives also can be caused by exposure to cold or heat; pressure; or emotional or physical stress, including exercise. Hives usually are harmless and go away on their own.

In very rare cases, hives may be the first sign of a life-threatening allergic reaction called anaphylaxis (see Page 15). If your symptoms are severe, seek emergency help.

Other causes may include cancer, connective tissue disease, hepatitis (see Page 156) or vasculitis.

Self-Care

- Take cool showers to ease the histamine reaction.
- Wear loose, lightweight clothing.
- Try an over-the-counter antihistamine. Follow package directions. If you're pregnant or breast-feeding, or have a health condition, talk with your doctor before taking any medications.
- Avoid taking aspirin, ibuprofen, naproxen sodium or narcotics—these may aggravate hives.

Prevention

- If you've experienced an outbreak of hives more than once, try to identify the cause.

- Avoid foods and beverages with additives; dusty places; and chemicals that come in contact with your skin such as makeup, cologne, shampoo and soap products.

- Eliminate all possible allergen sources at the same time. Reintroduce them one at a time to identify the cause of your hives.

SEEK EMERGENCY HELP

- ▶ You have wheezing; difficulty breathing; shortness of breath or dizziness; fainting; swollen lips, tongue or throat; or a constricted feeling in your throat or chest.

- ▶ You have large hives that are spreading rapidly.

CALL YOUR NURSE INFORMATION SERVICE OR DOCTOR

- ▶ The hives started after you began taking prescription medication.

- ▶ The hives started after exposure to a possible allergen, such as food or animals.

- ▶ The itching is severe and constant, or you have a fever.

- ▶ You've had hives for more than two days.

TRY SELF-CARE

- ▶ You have one or two hives but no other symptoms.

HOARSENESS OR LOSS OF VOICE

Husky, raspy voice; may be difficult to make any sound at all

Causes

Infection. Your voice may have become hoarse gradually over the past few days. You also may have, or recently had, a cold, sore throat, cough or fever. An upper respiratory tract infection leading to laryngitis is one of the most common causes of hoarseness. You can treat the infection and resulting loss of voice with self-care if the problem is caused by a virus. If you have a bacterial infection, you'll need antibiotics. See your doctor.

Irritant. Respiratory irritants, such as cigarette smoke, can irritate your vocal cords. Cigarette smoke also can cause hoarseness by producing tumors on your vocal cords. Limiting alcohol, quitting smoking (see Page 25) and avoiding exposure to secondhand smoke can help.

Overuse. Excessive talking, singing or shouting can cause laryngitis. You may have overdone it cheering on your favorite team. Or, perhaps you're a teacher or singer, and regular overuse has caught up with you. Self-care, most importantly resting your vocal cords, should help your voice return to normal within one week.

Gastroesophageal reflux disease (GERD). You may have stomach-acid reflux due to a faulty valve between your stomach and your esophagus. This may cause hoarseness or loss of voice. If you experience heartburn two or more times a week, you may have GERD (see Page 144). Over-the-counter remedies may not provide relief. See your doctor.

Other causes may include allergies (see Page 303).

Self-Care

- Speak as little as possible. Avoid talking too loudly or softly. Whispering puts nearly as much stress on your vocal cords as shouting.

- Inhale steam from a hot shower. Or, try a cool-mist vaporizor or humidifier. Clean it daily or as instructed by the manufacturer.

- Stay hydrated by drinking plenty of water each day.

- Try an over-the-counter pain reliever such as acetaminophen, ibuprofen, naproxen sodium or aspirin.

- Avoid gargling. Most mouthwashes contain alcohol, which can cause irritation.

Prevention

- Avoid irritants such as cigarette smoke, chemical fumes and dust.

- Try not to overuse your voice.

SEEK EMERGENCY HELP

▶ You're drooling, and it's very painful to swallow and difficult to breathe.

CALL YOUR NURSE INFORMATION SERVICE OR DOCTOR

▶ You've tried self-care but your symptoms have gotten worse or lasted more than five days.

▶ You've tried self-care but you smoke, and your hoarseness hasn't improved after one week.

TRY SELF-CARE

▶ Your hoarseness started within the past three days, and you also have a cold, cough or sore throat.

▶ You've overused your voice lately.

▶ You smoke, or you've recently been exposed to second-hand smoke or other environmental irritants.

YOUR CHILD'S SYMPTOMS

Seek emergency help if your child has a hoarse cry or inability to make any sound; or if he has a fever and so much trouble breathing that he thrusts his lower jaw out, drools and breathes with his mouth open.

Call your doctor if your child develops a cough that sounds like a seal's bark, is accompanied by hoarseness, and is worse at night. This may be croup, an inflammation of the air passages. Croup is common in children.

Try self-care to help ease the symptoms of croup. Expose your child to humid air. Take him into the bathroom and close the door. Stand with your child outside the bathtub and turn the shower on hot—full blast so he can inhale the steam in the room. Or, take a walk in the cold night air, or use a cool-mist vaporizer or humidifier near his bed.

! *Don't give aspirin to anyone younger than age 19! It's linked to Reye's syndrome, a rare but sometimes fatal condition.*

INSOMNIA

Inability to fall asleep, waking in the night, and inability to get back to sleep; can last for days or months

Causes

Caffeine, alcohol or drug use. You drink coffee, tea or certain soft drinks, or eat chocolate—possibly to excess. Even small amounts of caffeine may make some people restless. Smoking or using over-the-counter decongestants, cold remedies, diet pills or a bronchodilator before bedtime can keep you up as well. Sleeping pills and alcohol may make you feel sleepy, but they can lead to "rebound" insomnia. When this happens, your body becomes dependent on sleeping pills or alcohol in order to sleep. Sleep induced by pills or alcohol also may be shallow and unsatisfying.

Medical concern. You may have chronic pain (see Page 273), especially if you're an older adult and have joint disease. You may have angina (see Page 76) or breathing difficulties. If you snore, sleep fitfully and are sleepy during the day, you may have sleep apnea (see Page 27). Prostate conditions (see Page 300), diabetes (see Page 281) or a urinary tract infection (see Page 230) may be the cause if your sleep is disturbed by the need for frequent urination. If you have allergies (see Page 303) or respiratory ailments, such as chronic obstructive pulmonary disease (COPD) (see Page 270), you may have trouble breathing when lying down, which may keep you awake. Night sweats due to menopause (see Page 317) or other health conditions also can disturb your sleep. Talk with your doctor if any of these medical concerns are preventing you from getting enough sleep.

Other causes may include depression (see Page 332) or certain medications, including some antidepressants and allergy medications.

Self-Care

- Stop struggling to sleep. If you don't fall asleep in 20 minutes, get up and do something to relax. Read a book or a magazine. Use a relaxation technique. Or, listen to soothing music or recorded environmental sounds.
- Don't use alcohol to help you sleep. Try warm milk instead.

Prevention

- Don't use your bedroom for anything not associated with rest, sleep or sex.
- Take a warm (not hot) bath or shower before bed.

- Don't eat for three hours before bed. At dinner, try cereal, bread, fruits and foods rich in the sleep-inducing chemical L-tryptophan—such as milk, turkey or tuna fish.

- Don't smoke—especially right before going to bed.

- Avoid caffeine. Remember that it's found in diet aids, cold and pain medications, coffee, tea, certain soft drinks and chocolate.

- Don't go to bed if you feel wide awake.

- Try getting up at about the same time every day, regardless of your bedtime.

- Make your bedroom dark, cool and comfortable. Use clean sheets and pillowcases. Eliminate, reduce or mask environmental noise.

- Don't exercise too close to bedtime.

- Avoid daytime napping.

CALL YOUR NURSE INFORMATION SERVICE OR DOCTOR

- ▶ You have persistent pain.

- ▶ You have trouble falling asleep, or you fall asleep and then wake up after a few hours.

- ▶ You're a woman age 45 or older and your periods have become irregular.

- ▶ You recently have been experiencing anxiety or depression.

- ▶ You use alcohol, drugs or tobacco.

- ▶ You've been taking sleeping pills regularly for more than a few days.

- ▶ You're awakened by frequent urination.

- ▶ You've tried self-care but your symptoms haven't improved after three weeks.

TRY SELF-CARE

- ▶ Your sleep is disrupted by noise such as a partner's snoring, or extreme temperature.

JAUNDICE

Yellowing of the skin or eyes; itching also may occur

About Jaundice

Jaundice isn't a disease. It's a condition that occurs when your body has too much bilirubin. This substance is formed when old or damaged red blood cells are broken down. Excess bilirubin can be produced for a variety of reasons. Jaundice most commonly is related to liver and gallbladder disorders.

Causes

Bile duct obstruction due to gallstones. In addition to jaundice, you also may have fever, chills, clay-colored stools, or tea- or coffee-colored urine. You also may have severe, steady pain in your upper right abdomen or between your shoulder blades. Gallstones occur when lumps of solid material—usually deposits of cholesterol or calcium salts—form in your gallbladder.

Gallstones often cause no symptoms. But sometimes, they can block the duct between the gallbladder and the small intestine. This can lead to inflammation and infection "upstream" of the blockage. See your doctor. If the pain is severe, seek emergency help.

Hepatitis. You may have flu-like symptoms—including fatigue, headache, loss of appetite, nausea or vomiting, and fever.

As your symptoms get worse, you also may notice a yellowish tint to your skin and the whites of your eyes; brown urine; pale stools; and pain or pressure on your right side, below your ribs. Hepatitis is an inflammation of the liver caused by one of several viruses. Prevention and treatment differ based on the type of virus. See your doctor.

Other causes may include Gilbert's syndrome, hemochromatosis, certain medications, pregnancy-related conditions, Reye's syndrome or sickle cell disease.

Self-Care

Self-care isn't appropriate for jaundice. Symptoms—at any age—need to be evaluated by a health care professional.

Prevention

- Wash your hands frequently, especially before eating and after using the bathroom.
- Practice safer sex (see Page 311).
- Don't share razors or needles. Avoid tattoos, body piercing or acupuncture unless you're sure the professional is certified or licensed, and the equipment is sterile.

- Avoid excess alcohol.

- Avoid any medications not recommended by your doctor—including over-the-counter medications or herbal supplements.

- Stay up-to-date on your immunizations (see Page 31).

- If you think you may have been exposed to hepatitis, call your nurse information service or doctor.

SEEK EMERGENCY HELP

▶ You can't urinate; your mucous membranes are dry; or you feel lethargic.

▶ You have severe abdominal pain or pain between your shoulder blades.

SEE YOUR DOCTOR

▶ You think you may have jaundice and you're pregnant.

▶ You have brown urine or clay-colored stools.

▶ Your abdomen is distended. You also may have nausea.

▶ You have unexplained bruising; or a new onset of severe itching or weight loss.

CALL YOUR NURSE INFORMATION SERVICE OR DOCTOR

▶ You recently were exposed to viral hepatitis.

▶ You have jaundice but none of the symptoms or situations listed above.

YOUR CHILD'S SYMPTOMS

Jaundice and your child. In the first few days of life, more than half of all full-term babies and 80 percent of premature infants who are otherwise healthy can develop jaundice. Normally, the condition develops during the second or third day of life.

Jaundice usually will disappear within one to two weeks, but the condition should be monitored closely by your child's doctor. Jaundice in a child after the first week or two should be evaluated by a doctor.

Carotenemia can occur in children younger than age 2 years who have eaten a lot of yellow and orange vegetables. Your child's skin may appear lemon-yellow in color. The whites of the eyes are unaffected. This is a harmless, temporary condition.

JAW PAIN

Tenderness or severe pain in the area in front of the ear; jaw may be inflamed, swollen or difficult to move

Causes

Temporomandibular disorders (TMD) or TMJ syndrome. Your jaw joint may be inflamed or swollen, and you may have pain in your head, face, teeth, neck or shoulders. It may hurt when you chew, speak or open your mouth wide. You may hear clicking sounds when you open or shut your mouth. You may clench or grind your teeth at night. TMD—often called TMJ, in reference to the temporomandibular joint—occurs when the muscles and ligaments around your jawbone are overused or out of alignment.

Causes of TMD may include trauma to the jaw, tension or stress, or poor alignment of the teeth. Other health conditions, such as rheumatoid arthritis or osteoarthritis (see Page 255), also can affect the temporomandibular joint. Call your nurse information service or doctor.

Dislocated or fractured jaw. An injury to your face may have made your jaw tender, stiff or swollen. You may have difficulty speaking, swallowing or closing your mouth. A dislocated jaw occurs when the mandible, or lower jawbone, is displaced from one or both of the temporomandibular joints. If your jaw is dislocated, don't try to put it back into place yourself. Jaw dislocations and fractures are serious injuries. Seek emergency help.

Heart attack (see Page 10). You may have crushing pain in your chest that radiates to your lower jaw. Seek emergency help.

Other causes may include tension headache (see Page 138) or tooth abscess (see Page 226).

Self-Care

- If trauma is the cause, apply ice packs for the first 48 to 72 hours after an injury—for 15 to 20 minutes, three to four times a day.
- Try an over-the-counter pain reliever such as acetaminophen, ibuprofen, naproxen sodium or aspirin.
- Avoid hard or crunchy foods. Cut food into small pieces.

Prevention

- Avoid extreme jaw movements such as wide yawning.
- Practice relaxation techniques.
- Maintain good posture, which places less stress on your jaw muscles.

- Ask your dentist about a nighttime mouth guard to help reduce pressure on your jaw.

- Wear protective headgear when appropriate—such as for sports or riding a motorcycle.

- See your dentist twice a year.

SEEK EMERGENCY HELP

▶ You have pain in your chest that radiates to your jaw.

▶ You're having difficulty breathing.

▶ You have a jaw injury and are having difficulty speaking, swallowing or closing your mouth.

▶ You have a jaw injury and a jaw deformity or tooth misalignment.

SEE YOUR DOCTOR

▶ You're experiencing signs of infection such as redness, swelling, pain or tenderness, or fever—or you feel sick.

CALL YOUR NURSE INFORMATION SERVICE OR DOCTOR

▶ You have pain or tenderness in your jaw and hear clicking or popping sounds when you open or shut your mouth.

▶ You've had an injury to your jaw and have pain and swelling.

! *Don't give aspirin to anyone younger than age 19! It's linked to Reye's syndrome, a rare but sometimes fatal condition.*

JOINT PAIN

Pain or stiffness in one or more joints

Causes

Injury. You may have pain in one or more of your joints because you've injured yourself in some way. A common cause of injury is overuse. Jogging or hiking, for instance, may cause ankle, knee or other lower extremity pain. Try self-care if your symptoms aren't severe.

Arthritis (see Page 255). You may have pain and swelling or stiffness in your joints. You also may have a limited range of motion. Symptoms of arthritis vary depending on the type. See your doctor.

Gout. You may have pain in the joint at the base of your big toe, or in your foot, ankle, knee, elbow or hand. The pain may have intensified and no position provides relief. Gout is a type of arthritis. There are effective medications for treating gout. Cutting back on rich foods and alcohol also can help. See your doctor.

Infection. You may have pain in your joints, along with swelling that developed rapidly, and a fever. You may need antibiotics if you have a bacterial infection. See your doctor.

Self-Care

- Apply ice as soon as possible to a new injury or to joint pain that has started recently. This will help keep the swelling down. Wrap crushed ice in a thin towel, apply for 15 to 20 minutes, three to four times a day for the first 48 to 72 hours. Remove if the area begins to feel numb.

- Heat may relieve some discomfort in the later stages of a joint injury, or pain you've had for some time. Apply a moist-heat pad, or warm, moist towel for 15 to 20 minutes, three to four times a day. If moist heat isn't available, take a warm bath or shower.

- Rest painful joints. If only one joint is painful, use an elastic bandage or brace to support and rest it. If several joints are involved, sit down, put your feet up and rest for 15 minutes each hour.

- Try an over-the-counter pain reliever such as acetaminophen, ibuprofen, naproxen sodium or aspirin.

Prevention

- Both overuse and underuse can cause joint pain. Exercise regularly. Choose low or moderately intense activities. Swimming and walking in water (about chest-deep) are particularly good choices. Find a balance between rest and exercise.

SEEK EMERGENCY HELP

▶ You've recently injured your joint. You can't move it without severe pain, or it looks misshapen.

SEE YOUR DOCTOR

▶ Your joint is painful, swollen or hot.

▶ You have a fever, weight loss and severe fatigue.

▶ Only one joint is affected and very painful—especially at the base of your big toe, or ankle or knee.

CALL YOUR NURSE INFORMATION SERVICE OR DOCTOR

▶ You've tried self-care but your symptoms haven't improved after three weeks, or progressively have gotten worse.

TRY SELF-CARE

▶ The pain has come on gradually or for no apparent reason, and it isn't severe.

YOUR CHILD'S SYMPTOMS

See your doctor if your child has joint pain. Inflammation of the joint as a result of infection may be the cause of the pain. Your child may need antibiotics.

Call your nurse information service or doctor if the joint pain didn't follow an injury, and your child has a fever and seems ill.

! *Don't give aspirin to anyone younger than age 19! It's linked to Reye's syndrome, a rare but sometimes fatal condition.*

KNEE PAIN

Pain and possible stiffness and swelling in the knee

Causes

Injury. You may have pain and throbbing in your knee, possibly after falling. You also may notice a clicking or grinding sound coming from the joint. Sprains, strains, dislocations and fractures can cause knee pain. See your doctor if the pain is severe.

Arthritis (see Page 255). You may have pain, swelling or stiffness in your knee or other joints. You also may have a limited range of motion. Symptoms of arthritis vary depending on the type. See your doctor.

Gout. You may have pain in the joint at the base of your big toe, or in your foot, ankle, knee, elbow or hand. The pain may have intensified and no position provides relief. Gout is actually a type of arthritis. There are effective medications for treating gout. Cutting back on rich foods and alcohol also can help. See your doctor.

Bursitis. Your knee may be tender, painful or swollen. The twinges of pain can become severe within a few hours, making it difficult to bend your knee. Bursitis is an inflammation of the bursae—fluid-filled sacs around joints. These sacs limit friction and make movement easier. See your doctor.

Other causes may include infection, post-traumatic effusion or "water on the knee," or tendinitis.

Self-Care

- For an injury, try the PRICE remedy— protect, rest, ice, compression and elevation. Protect your knee from further injury. Rest the affected area for a day or so. Wrap crushed ice in a thin towel. Apply for 15 to 20 minutes, three to four times a day. Use an elastic wrap or bandage. Whenever possible, keep your knee elevated above the level of your heart to help reduce swelling.

- Try an over-the-counter pain reliever such as acetaminophen, ibuprofen, naproxen sodium or aspirin.

- If your injury isn't recent or if you've had the pain for a few days, warmth may provide some relief. Apply a moist-heat pad, or warm, moist towel for 15 to 20 minutes, three to four times a day. If moist heat isn't available, take a warm bath or shower.

Prevention

- Avoid overuse of your knees.
- Maintain a healthy weight (see Page 21).

- Use kneepads or a cushion when kneeling. Take frequent breaks. Avoid squatting.
- Exercise regularly. Choose a low-impact activity such as walking or swimming.

SEEK EMERGENCY HELP

▶ **You injured your knee within the past 24 hours. It's now painful, misshapen or unable to bear weight.**

SEE YOUR DOCTOR

▶ **Your knee has swelled up suddenly and rapidly. It's warm to the touch.**

▶ **You have pain or swelling in your calf muscle, below the back of your knee.**

▶ **The pain is accompanied by fever and fatigue, and you feel sick.**

CALL YOUR NURSE INFORMATION SERVICE OR DOCTOR

▶ **You can't move your knee through the normal range of motion.**

▶ **You've tried self-care but the pain is due to overuse and hasn't improved after five days.**

▶ **You've tried self-care but the pain that started gradually hasn't improved after two weeks.**

TRY SELF-CARE

▶ **The pain started due to overuse, such as running or playing sports.**

▶ **The pain started gradually.**

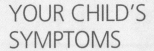

YOUR CHILD'S SYMPTOMS

See your doctor if your child has symptoms of juvenile rheumatoid arthritis (see Page 256)—swollen and painful joints, fever, rash, abdominal pain, weight loss, swollen lymph glands, fatigue and painful, red eyes.

Knee pain and your child. Overuse injuries often center around the lower leg. They're common in children and adolescents, and pass with time. For relief, try the PRICE remedy—protect, rest, ice, compression and elevation.

Growing pains are common in pre-adolescent children. Typically, they complain of calf pain which awakens them from sleep, yet, they have no problem with activity during the day. Calf massage helps. With time, children outgrow this problem.

! *Don't give aspirin to anyone younger than age 19! It's linked to Reye's syndrome, a rare but sometimes fatal condition.*

LEG PAIN OR CRAMP

Pain in the thigh or calf

Causes

Cramp. You may have sudden, severe pain in your calf or foot especially at night or while you're resting. Leg cramps usually aren't serious. In almost all cases, they're caused by strain or overuse. Try self-care.

Injury. Injuries can range from mild, such as a sprain or strain, to severe, such as broken bones. If you can't put weight on your leg, the bone may be broken— seek emergency help. For muscle injuries, try self-care.

Shinsplints. You may feel pain in the front and side of your lower leg during or after exercise. Shinsplints result from repeated stress on the muscles or tendons in your lower leg. This is common in runners. Try self-care.

Intermittent claudication. You may have leg cramping that starts with exercise and stops with rest. This is due to a narrowing of the arteries in your leg. Intermittent claudication is a condition more common in older people and in heavy smokers. Call your nurse information service or doctor.

Deep venous thrombosis. Your calf may be painful and swollen. Deep venous thrombosis is a condition in which a blood clot blocks a vein deep in your leg. If the clot breaks away and lodges in a vital organ, it can be fatal. You may need blood thinners. See your doctor.

Superficial thrombophlebitis. You may have a throbbing or burning pain in your calf. You may notice a red and inflamed vein in your leg. Although this usually isn't serious, you should see your doctor.

Other causes may include cellulitis, degenerative joint disease, fluid or electrolyte imbalance due to diabetes or diarrhea, heat exhaustion (see Page 11), pinched nerve in the lower back, ruptured calf muscle or ruptured disk.

Self-Care

- You can speed relief from sudden cramps by massaging and gradually stretching your cramped muscle.

- If your doctor diagnoses superficial thrombophlebitis, you may get some relief from self-care. Lie down with your leg elevated. Apply a moist-heat pad, or warm, moist towel for 15 to 20 minutes, three to four times a day. If moist heat isn't available, take a warm bath or shower. Don't rub or massage the area.

164

Prevention

- Warm up and stretch before exercising. Drink plenty of water before, during and after exercise.
- To keep your circulatory system healthy, stop smoking, eat healthfully and maintain a healthy weight (see Page 17).

SEEK EMERGENCY HELP

▶ You have leg pain and a new onset of shortness of breath.

▶ You have sudden paralysis, weakness or loss of feeling in one leg.

▶ You have a painful, red or swollen calf especially after a prolonged period of inactivity.

▶ You have severe pain after an injury and can't bear weight on your leg.

▶ Your leg may show signs of impaired circulation—pale, blue or gray, and feels cold.

▶ You have a history of blood clots.

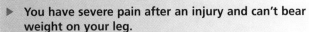

SEE YOUR DOCTOR

▶ You have leg pain and you're pregnant or taking birth control pills.

CALL YOUR NURSE INFORMATION SERVICE OR DOCTOR

▶ The pain occurs regularly during even mild exercise or continuous walking, and disappears when you rest.

▶ The pain started after taking a diuretic, or water pill.

TRY SELF-CARE

▶ The pain started gradually after unusually strenuous exercise.

YOUR CHILD'S SYMPTOMS

Seek emergency help if your toddler has injured herself and can't bear weight on her leg.

Leg pain or cramps and your child. Toddlers can break their bones even without a hard fall. An injury that simply twists the lower leg the wrong way can be enough to break the bone.

! *Don't give aspirin to anyone younger than age 19! It's linked to Reye's syndrome, a rare but sometimes fatal condition.*

LICE

Intense itching; some redness and flaking of the skin

About Lice

Lice are tiny bugs, or parasites, that pass from one person to another. They don't fly or jump, but crawl or fall off one person, or "host," and onto the next. Although annoying, they rarely pose a health risk. Try self-care.

Head lice are especially common for children. Lice leave red spots that may be extremely itchy. You're more likely to notice the nits—small, pale eggs on the hair shafts, close to the scalp.

Pubic lice, or "crabs," can be passed from one person to another by sexual contact or contact with infested bed linens or towels. Pubic lice look like little pieces of sand firmly attached to the base of pubic hair (see page 128).

Body lice live in and lay eggs on clothing and bedding. They only crawl onto the body to feed. If you have body lice, you'll notice tiny, itchy, red spots.

Self-Care

- There are many effective prescription and over-the-counter treatments. Ask your doctor for a recommendation. Follow the package directions exactly.

- If the medication doesn't remove all the lice and nits, try applying equal parts vinegar and water to your hair. Wrap your head in a towel for 15 minutes, and then comb.

- Comb your hair from your scalp outward with a fine-toothed comb until lice and nits are removed.

- Disinfect all combs, brushes and hair accessories. Soak them for one hour in anti-lice shampoo, rubbing alcohol or a disinfectant cleaning product. Keep these solutions out of the reach of children. Rinse thoroughly with water.

- Wash bedding and clothing in very hot water—at least 130° F. Dry on a high-heat cycle for at least 20 minutes.

- Dry-clean or seal exposed garments in an airtight plastic bag. Don't open the bag for at least two weeks. Then open it outdoors, and shake vigorously.

- Thoroughly vacuum all mattresses, pillows, stuffed animals, rugs and upholstered furniture. Dispose of the vacuum cleaner bag.

- Treat all affected family members. Call your nurse information service or doctor before treating anyone who is pregnant, nursing or younger than age 2 years.

- Check for nits in eyebrows and eyelashes. Apply petroleum jelly twice a day, for eight days, if affected.
- Repeat treatment for lice in seven to 10 days.
- If you have pubic lice, avoid sexual contact until you've completed treatment. All sexual partners in recent months should be informed.

Prevention

- Bathe daily and shampoo often.
- Avoid wearing the same clothing for more than one to two days.
- Change bed linens frequently.
- Don't share combs, brushes, hats or headgear.

CALL YOUR NURSE INFORMATION SERVICE OR DOCTOR

▶ **You have open wounds caused by scratching, or a fever, redness, swelling or oozing.**

▶ **You're pregnant or nursing a baby.**

▶ **You've tried self-care but your symptoms haven't improved after one week.**

TRY SELF-CARE

▶ **You see lice or nits on hair shafts, in your pubic area, or on bed linens or clothing.**

YOUR CHILD'S SYMPTOMS

Call your nurse information service or doctor if your child has lice and is age 2 years or younger, has allergies or other health concerns, or if you find lice or nits in his eyebrows or eyelashes.

Lice and your child. Check your child for head lice regularly, especially during peak season— August through November. Do so especially if you notice head scratching.

If your child has head lice, let his friends' parents and the school nurse know. You can treat your child with over-the-counter remedies.

MOLE

Small, somewhat circular spot on the skin that's much darker than the skin surrounding it; may be brown, black or blue, and may have coarse hair growing out of it

About Moles

It's not known why people develop moles. They usually aren't present at birth, but develop as people get older. They often fade away on their own after many years. Most moles are harmless. But, they should be watched carefully. Any change could be a warning sign of melanoma, a serious type of skin cancer.

Your risk of skin cancer is related to the amount of sun exposure you've had during your lifetime. Try using the "ABCDE" rule to determine if your mole is harmless or if it requires medical attention (see illustration). Call your doctor if you notice the following:

Asymmetrical   *Irregular Border*   *Diameter*

These are three examples of possible signs that a mole may require medical attention.

Asymmetry. One half of your mole looks different than the other.

Border. The edges of your mole are irregular, notched or scalloped.

Color. Your mole has blue, white or red patches, or a mixed brown or black color, or a change in color.

Diameter. Your mole is the size of a pencil eraser or larger. Or, your mole has grown noticeably.

Elevation. Your mole has become raised.

Be sure to tell your doctor if you experience any bleeding or itching, as well. These are also warning signs.

Self-Care

- Regularly examine your skin from head to toe. You're more likely to remember if you do it at a regular time, for instance on the first day of each season or month. Look for any changes in size, color, shape or appearance of your moles. Use a hand mirror for areas that you can't see easily.

- Have your skin examined by a doctor during health exams.

- Don't worry unnecessarily. If you do notice a change in a mole, call your doctor.

Prevention

You can't prevent moles from forming. However, you can protect your skin by avoiding unnecessary exposure to the sun:

- Wear sunscreen with a sun protection factor (SPF) of at least 15 that blocks both UVA and UVB rays.

- Wear a hat with a wide brim when outdoors.

CALL YOUR NURSE INFORMATION SERVICE OR DOCTOR

▶ You've developed a new mole that has grown rapidly.

▶ You have a mole that first appeared after age 35.

▶ You have a mole on the palm of your hand, on the sole of your foot, or under a nail.

▶ One of your moles has changed in size, shape or color.

▶ You have a mole on the inside of your mouth.

▶ You have a mole on the surface of your vagina.

▶ You have a lot of moles.

▶ You have a mole that burns, itches, hurts, stings or bleeds.

▶ You've had a mole reappear after it was removed.

▶ You have a mole that's irregularly shaped, or its color is mixed brown, black or blue.

MOUTH OR TONGUE SORENESS

Painful area on the lips, tongue or on the insides of the cheeks

Causes

Canker sore. You may have a small, shallow, but very painful sore on your lip, gum, inner cheek, tongue, palate or throat. Canker sores are extremely common. They usually heal on their own within a few days to two weeks. Try self-care.

Cold sore. You may have a painful sore on your lip, or perhaps inside your mouth. It probably started as a blister and now may have ruptured. Cold sores, or "fever blisters," are caused by the herpes simplex virus (see Page 64). They're common and very contagious. They generally clear up, but may recur. Try self-care.

Traumatic ulcer. You have a sore area inside your cheek or on your tongue. You may have poorly fitting dentures or a jagged broken tooth. Perhaps you've been burned by hot food or coffee. Mouth sores often are caused by a source of irritation. You'll need to correct the source of the problem in order to eliminate the sore. Call your doctor or dentist.

Oral thrush. You may have creamy, yellow, slightly raised patches on the insides of your cheeks and on your tongue. If you rub them off when brushing your teeth or eating, they leave a painful, raw area. Oral thrush is caused by the fungus Candida albicans, one of the many microscopic organisms normally present in your mouth. When you take antibiotics, use inhaled or oral steroids or if you're immuno-compromised, the fungus may get out of control. You may need a prescription medication. See your doctor.

Other causes may include allergies (see Page 303), cancer (see Page 264)—especially if you have a history of alcohol use and smoking—or dry mouth.

Self-Care

- Drink plenty of water each day. Keep your mouth moist. Dry mouth can cause mouth and tongue soreness and aggravate symptoms.

- To ease discomfort, gargle with 1/4 teaspoon of salt stirred into 8 ounces of water.

- Don't smoke or chew tobacco. Both irritate the lining of your mouth.

- Take a multivitamin supplement that contains B vitamins and vitamin C.

- Cold liquids and ice pops can be soothing. Choose soft foods that won't scrape against the inside of your mouth. Avoid salty or citrus foods, which may irritate sores.
- Be careful not to touch the cold sores and then touch your eyes. The virus could spread, causing a herpetic corneal ulcer.
- Avoid intimate contact.

Prevention

- See your dentist twice a year.
- Brush twice a day, or more often if directed by your dentist. Floss daily.
- If you wear dentures, make sure they fit properly. Fix broken or cracked teeth right away.

CALL YOUR NURSE INFORMATION SERVICE, DOCTOR OR DENTIST

- ▶ You have a mouth sore that hasn't healed after one week.
- ▶ You have creamy, yellow patches on the insides of your cheeks or the roof of your mouth that scrape off easily.
- ▶ You have poorly fitting dentures, or a tooth that's broken and jagged.
- ▶ You've started a new medication.
- ▶ You have a mouth ulcer on your gum, or a toothache.
- ▶ You have oral pain that limits your ability to eat or drink.
- ▶ You have red, swollen gum tissue.
- ▶ You've tried self-care but your symptoms haven't improved after one to two weeks.

TRY SELF-CARE

- ▶ You have mouth or tongue soreness but no other symptoms.

YOUR CHILD'S SYMPTOMS

Mouth or tongue soreness and your child. The coxsackievirus causes hand-foot-mouth syndrome and other diseases. It's a common, contagious virus that can cause mouth sores accompanied by spots on the hands and feet. Your child may have a fever, but may feel perfectly well. This infection should clear up on its own within a week.

Another common childhood infection is oral thrush, which can clear up on its own, but sometimes may require prescription treatment. Thrush may look similar to milk on your baby's tongue. But milk is easily removed from the tongue—thrush isn't.

NAIL PROBLEM

Discolored, split or thickened fingernail or toenail, which may be crumbling at the edges, or pitted; or pain, swelling or redness around a fingernail or toenail

Causes

Onychomycosis or fungal infection. Your nail may be thick and yellow. There may be a slight separation at the end of your nail. A crumbly material may be building up beneath it. If untreated, your entire nail may become separated, misshapen or destroyed. Fungus may affect fingernails after an injury. Or, it may be related to another skin disease. Toenails can be infected without an injury occurring. It may take six months for fingernails to clear up, and as long as one to two years for toenails. Self-care can help, but you may need a prescription medication.

Nail splitting. You may have cracks along your nails or flaking at the edges. This is generally painless. The condition may improve, but it may never completely disappear. It tends to run in families, and sometimes is caused by injury.

Paronychia. You may have red, swollen skin alongside your nail. This may be the result of a superficial yeast, herpes or staphylococcal infection. These infections may be caused by pulling off a hangnail or pushing back your cuticle.

Other causes may include nutritional deficiency, psoriasis (see Page 192), thyroid disease (see Page 308), trauma or vascular insufficiency.

Self-Care

- If you have an ingrown fingernail, push your skin back from the corner gently with a cotton swab twice a day. Keep the area clean.

- For fungal infections, keep your feet and hands clean and dry. Be sure to dry them thoroughly after bathing. Don't wear socks or shoes made of synthetics. Wear cotton-lined latex or rubber gloves during dishwashing, cleaning or activities that involve chemicals. Avoid heat and excessive sweating. Over-the-counter treatments usually are ineffective.

- If an ingrown toenail is the cause, see Page 224.

- Clear nail polish may help keep split nails under control. Don't remove it often. Nail polish removers can cause further damage. Rub hand cream on the skin around your nails.

- If paronychia is the cause, try hot soaks twice daily, for five to 10 minutes, to reduce inflammation. Then use an antibacterial medication or 1 percent gentian violet for fungal infections.

Prevention

- Keep your nails clean. Trim them weekly. Don't trim them too short. They should be even with the tips of your fingers or toes. Avoid biting, picking or tearing your nails or cuticles.
- Use nail polish remover sparingly. And, avoid nail strengtheners, artificial nails and cuticle removers. They can damage your nails.

CALL YOUR NURSE INFORMATION SERVICE OR DOCTOR

▶ You have pitted nails, or itchy and slightly raised patches of skin around the nails that have red borders and white-silver scales.

▶ Your nails have become easy to bend, opaque, white and thickened.

▶ You have red, swollen areas on the skin around your nail. You've tried self-care but now have pain, pus or red lines that appear along the skin.

▶ You have painless cracks running along the length of your nails that are severe.

▶ You've tried self-care but your symptoms haven't improved after six months.

TRY SELF-CARE

▶ You have painless cracks running along the length of your nails that aren't severe.

▶ You have flakes chipping off the ends of your nails.

▶ You have red, swollen areas on the skin around your nail but no signs of infection.

NAUSEA OR VOMITING

Feeling queasy; throwing up

Causes

Gastroenteritis. You may have several bouts of nausea and vomiting. You also may have diarrhea, headache or fever. Viral gastroenteritis is the most common cause of nausea and vomiting in children and young adults. As miserable as it is, this condition usually passes on its own very quickly, often within 24 hours. But, it may last as long as five days. Viral gastroenteritis can't be treated. It has to run its course. You can try self-care to feel better and prevent dehydration—the most serious risk of this condition.

Food poisoning. You may feel sick after eating food that might not have been thoroughly cooked or handled properly. Many different kinds of bacteria can cause food poisoning. Nausea and vomiting usually start within six to 48 hours. Symptoms generally go away on their own within one to two days. Until then, use self-care to prevent dehydration. Call your nurse information service or doctor.

Other causes may include bowel obstruction (see Page 80), brain tumor, gall bladder disease, gastritis (see Page 298) due to the use of non-steroidal anti-inflammatory drugs or alcohol, glaucoma (see Page 267), head trauma (see Page 9), hepatitis (see Page 156), kidney failure, migraine (see Page 290), motion sickness, peptic ulcer disease (see Page 298) or pregnancy (see Page 321).

Self-Care

- Dehydration is always a risk of vomiting. Be sure to drink plenty of fluids, but avoid alcohol or caffeinated drinks. Ginger ale and decaffeinated tea may help settle your stomach.

- You may want to wait an hour or two after vomiting before trying to keep food down. Try the BRAT diet—bananas, rice, applesauce or toast. Eat small amounts. Avoid spicy or fatty foods.

- If pregnancy is the cause, try eating crackers or plain toast. Eat small, frequent meals throughout the day.

Prevention

- To prevent motion sickness, try an over-the-counter medication. Take it at least an hour before you travel. But, don't take it if you'll be driving. These drugs can make you very drowsy.

■ Follow safe food-handling procedures. Keep hot foods hot and cold foods cold. Wash your hands often while cooking. Don't place any other food on a surface where raw meat has been. Cook all meats thoroughly, until the juices run clear.

SEEK EMERGENCY HELP

▶ You recently had a head injury and you have a severe headache.

▶ You have black or bloody vomit that looks like it has coffee grounds in it, or severe abdominal pain.

▶ You have severe pain around one eye, or your vision is blurred.

▶ You have a fever along with drowsiness or confusion, pain when you bend your head forward and pain in your eyes from bright light.

▶ You have a headache or stiff neck.

CALL YOUR NURSE INFORMATION SERVICE OR DOCTOR

▶ You've had a decrease in urine output, and your mouth and lips are very dry.

▶ You've been vomiting and can't keep liquids down.

▶ You're taking medication.

▶ You're pregnant.

▶ You've tried self-care but your symptoms haven't improved after three days.

TRY SELF-CARE

▶ You also have diarrhea but none of the symptoms or situations listed above.

Seek emergency help if your child is vomiting and has any of the following symptoms: continuous pain for more than two hours; dry tongue; abnormal drowsiness; or vomit that's yellowish-green.

NECK PAIN OR STIFFNESS

Pain or stiffness in the neck

Causes

Muscle strain and spasm. You may have pain and stiffness in your neck, but no other symptoms. Muscle strain and spasm are the most frequent causes. An old neck injury also may be a factor. Try self-care.

Arthritis (see Page 255). You may have pain and stiffness in your neck. You also may have a limited range of motion. Symptoms of arthritis vary depending on the type. See your doctor.

Pinched nerve. You may have pain in your neck that extends down your arm and is limited to one side. You also may have numbness or tingling in your arm or hand. See your doctor.

Herniated disk. You may have neck pain that's worse with movement. You may feel pain, numbness or tingling. A herniated, or slipped, disk is a protrusion of the central part of one of the flat, circular pads found between the bones of the spine. See your doctor.

Meningitis. You may have intense neck pain, accompanied by fever, severe headache, nausea or vomiting, drowsiness or confusion, and pain in your eyes when you look at bright light. Your neck may be so stiff that it's difficult to touch your chin to your chest. Meningitis is a rare but serious cause of neck pain. Seek emergency help.

Other causes may include central nervous system bleeding, mumps, strep throat or swollen glands.

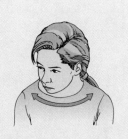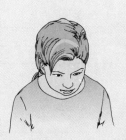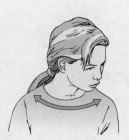

This exercise may help prevent neck stiffness. Gently rotate your head to one side. Slowly bring your head back to the center position. Then gently rotate to the other side. Repeat as needed. Check with your doctor about exercises that are right for you.

Self-Care

- For neck pain you've had a while or that has returned, warmth may help. Apply a moist-heat pad, or warm, moist towel for 15 to 20 minutes, three to four times a day. If moist heat isn't available, take a warm bath or shower.

- Try an over-the-counter pain reliever such as acetaminophen, ibuprofen, naproxen sodium or aspirin.

Prevention

- Sleep on a firm mattress. If you wake up with neck pain in the morning, sleep on a thin, feather pillow (not foam rubber), or try using none at all.

- When you feel your muscles tense up, take a break from what you're doing. Massage your neck, rotate your head and take deep breaths.

- Try gentle neck exercises (see illustration).

SEEK EMERGENCY HELP

▶ You have severe neck stiffness and any of the following: fever, nausea, drowsiness or confusion, or severe headache.

▶ You injured your neck recently, and you have a new weakness in your arms or legs.

CALL YOUR NURSE INFORMATION SERVICE OR DOCTOR

▶ You have pain, numbness or tingling that extends down your arm, and is limited to one side of your body.

▶ You have visible swelling of your neck.

▶ You've tried self-care but your symptoms haven't improved after one week.

TRY SELF-CARE

▶ You have neck pain or stiffness but no other symptoms.

Seek emergency help if your child has severe neck pain and fever, vomiting, irritability or lethargy. These may be signs of meningitis.

! *Don't give aspirin to anyone younger than age 19! It's linked to Reye's syndrome, a rare but sometimes fatal condition.*

NOSE, CONGESTED OR RUNNY

Stuffed up nose, or mucus or clear liquid running from the nose

Causes

Common cold. Your nose may be congested or running with clear to whitish mucus. You may be sneezing and coughing. You also may have mild body aches and a low-grade fever. Colds often are accompanied by minor sinus pain. Try self-care.

Vasomotor rhinitis. You may have a stuffy nose and some nasal discharge, though you may not be sneezing. Nasal stuffiness can be relieved by avoiding humidity and changes in temperature. Overuse of nasal decongestants may make symptoms worse.

Hay fever (see Page 303). You may have a stuffy or runny nose, itchy eyes and sneezing, but no other signs of illness. This probably is an allergy. Try self-care.

Other causes may include a foreign object in the nose.

Self-Care and Prevention

- If allergies are the cause, see Page 303.
- Use a cool-mist vaporizer or humidifier. Clean it daily or as instructed by the manufacturer.
- Drink plenty of fluids to stay hydrated.
- Hand washing can help prevent the spread of bacteria and viruses.

CALL YOUR NURSE INFORMATION SERVICE OR DOCTOR

▶ You have facial pain. You have a fever and yellowish-green mucus. Or, you're using an over-the-counter decongestant spray.

▶ You have thick, cloudy mucus from your nose, and your face feels tender above your eyes or across your cheeks.

▶ You're taking medication for another condition.

▶ You've tried self-care but your symptoms haven't improved after one week.

TRY SELF-CARE

▶ You're sneezing and coughing. You have a mild headache, muscle aches, fever, watery or itchy eyes, sore throat or postnasal drip.

YOUR CHILD'S SYMPTOMS

Call your nurse information service or doctor if your child's congestion is caused by a foreign object in his nose. Also call if your child has a fever of 102° F or higher, rapid or noisy breathing, or if he has a rash, earache or sore throat.

! *Don't give aspirin to anyone younger than age 19! It's linked to Reye's syndrome, a rare but sometimes fatal condition.*

NOSE, OBJECT IN

Foreign object lodged in the nose

Causes

Children do the most unexpected things—including putting or inhaling objects into their noses. Parents may not even be aware of a problem until their child complains of discomfort or sneezes a lot. If the object remains unnoticed for a long time, the inner walls of the nose will become swollen and the nose will become stuffed up. It may become infected with foul-smelling or bloody discharge. See your doctor.

Self-Care

Don't try to remove an object from your child's nose yourself. See your doctor.

Be extremely careful when trying to remove an object from an adult's nose. You may cause the object to be inhaled into the lungs. These tips and warnings may help:

- Don't try to remove the object by poking at it with a cotton swab or other implement.
- Don't try to remove an object that has been in the nose more than one or two hours.
- Don't try to remove a small round object, such as a bead, with tweezers.

- Breathe through your mouth while the object remains in your nose.
- Try to gently blow out through the affected nostril to dislodge the object, while holding the other nostril closed. Don't blow hard or more than a few times.
- If the object is visible and you're confident that it can be grasped with tweezers, try once to carefully remove it.

If these techniques don't work, call your doctor.

Prevention

- Keep small objects away from young children.
- Don't put small or sharp objects into your nose.

180

CALL YOUR DOCTOR

▶ You've tried self-care but couldn't remove the object in your nose after one attempt.

TRY SELF-CARE

▶ You have trouble breathing through one nostril, watering nose and eyes, or frequent sneezing.

Call your nurse information service or doctor if your child has an object in her nose. Don't try to remove it yourself.

NOSEBLEED

Bleeding from one or both nostrils

Causes

Nosebleeds can have several causes. Very often, self-care is effective. However, if the bleeding is severe and won't stop, see your doctor.

Injury or minor trauma. Your nose is bleeding after a blow to your nose or head. Or, it started bleeding after picking or scratching it.

Dry air. Your nose may start bleeding when the climate is hot and dry, or if you're inside a heated building in the wintertime. Dry air can cause delicate nasal tissue to crack and bleed.

Colds or allergies. You may have an infection or allergy, which can cause nasal inflammation and increase the likelihood of a nosebleed.

Certain medications. Some prescription and over-the-counter medications thin the blood and prevent clotting. In some cases, this may result in nosebleeds. Call your nurse information service or doctor.

Other causes may include a blood vessel problem in the nose, a deviated septum, exposure to certain chemicals or irritants, or lack of blood-clotting cells.

Self-Care

- Sit up straight and lean your head slightly forward. Don't tilt your head back—this can cause blood to flow down your throat. Firmly pinch your nose just above your nostrils. Hold it shut for 10 minutes and breathe through your mouth.

- If your nosebleed is caused by a minor trauma or injury, apply ice wrapped in a towel directly to your nose for 30 minutes. After the bleeding has stopped, avoid strenuous activity for six to eight hours.

Prevention

- Use a cool-mist vaporizer or humidifier to moisten the air. Clean it daily or as instructed by the manufacturer.

- Apply a small amount of petroleum jelly to the inside of your nose.

- Avoid using aspirin, ibuprofen and naproxen sodium, and overuse of steroidal nose sprays.

- Be gentle when you blow your nose.

- Don't pick or scratch your nose.

SEEK EMERGENCY HELP

► You have uncontrolled bleeding, severe weakness, lethargy, severe headache, confusion or any symptom of shock.

SEE YOUR DOCTOR

► The nosebleed started with blood draining down your throat rather than out through your nostrils.

► You're taking aspirin or an anticlotting medication, or you have nosebleeds often.

► You've tried self-care but your nose continues to bleed.

TRY SELF-CARE

► You have a nosebleed but no other symptoms.

NUMBNESS OR TINGLING

Lack of feeling in part of the body; feeling that a body part is "asleep" or has a "pins and needles" sensation

Causes

Nerve or blood vessel compression. You've been sitting or leaning in an awkward position, or sleeping on one part of your body for too long. Also, leaning on your elbow may compress the ulnar nerve—or "funny bone"— causing tingling and numbness in your fourth and fifth fingers. When you move, you may feel prickly tingling as the body part "wakes up," then the numbness goes away.

Carpal tunnel syndrome (see Page 248). You may have numbness and tingling that often worsens at night in your wrists and hands from the thumb to the ring finger.

Raynaud's disease. In cold weather, your fingers or toes may become numb and turn white, then blue. When they warm up, they become red and painful.

Cervical osteoarthritis. You may have numbness and tingling in part of your hands. You're probably age 50 or older, and your neck sometimes is stiff and painful. If the neck pain spreads to your shoulders, the numbness and tingling move into your arms, and you walk unsteadily, you may have cervical spondylosis.

Herniated disk. You may have lower back pain that's worse with movement. You may feel pain, numbness or tingling in your legs or buttocks. A herniated, or slipped, disk is a protrusion of the central part of one of the flat, circular pads in the joints between the bones of the spine. See your doctor.

Stroke or transient ischemic attack (TIA) (see Page 16). You may have numbness or tingling on one side of your body; weakness in your arms or legs; slurred speech; blurred or double vision; confusion or dizziness. Seek emergency help.

Other causes may include excessive use of alcohol, nutritional deficiency, or peripheral neuropathy from diabetes.

Self-Care

- Move the affected body part.
- Loosen your clothing.
- If you have Raynaud's disease, warm your hands or feet by soaking them in warm water.
- If you have a slipped disk, lie on a firm surface with a small pillow under your knees. Or, lie on your side with a pillow between your knees. Lying on a heating pad may help, too.

- Try an over-the-counter pain reliever such as acetaminophen, ibuprofen, naproxen sodium or aspirin for neck or back stiffness.

Prevention

- Avoid staying in one position for too long.

- Improve your posture.

- Quit smoking (see Page 25). It impairs your circulation.

- Break up repetitive tasks by resting, or alternating activities.

- Be sure your computer keyboard allows optimal hand, wrist and arm positioning.

SEEK EMERGENCY HELP

▶ **You have numbness or tingling on one side of your body, or weakness, dizziness, blurred vision, slurred speech or confusion.**

CALL YOUR NURSE INFORMATION SERVICE OR DOCTOR

▶ **You have numbness or tingling in your hands, legs or feet, plus a stiff or painful neck or lower back.**

▶ **You have redness and pain when the numbness goes away, and your fingers turn blue or white with cold.**

▶ **Your symptoms are worse at night, and you also have hand or wrist pain, or a weak grip.**

TRY SELF-CARE

▶ **You have numbness or tingling in your feet or hands after sitting or lying in one position for a long time.**

YOUR CHILD'S SYMPTOMS

! *Don't give aspirin to anyone younger than age 19! It's linked to Reye's syndrome, a rare but sometimes fatal condition.*

PENIS PAIN OR SWELLING

Painful or sore penis

Causes

Paraphimosis. If you haven't been circumcised, your foreskin may be pulled back and stuck behind the head of your penis. The swelling may be painful and severe. See your doctor.

Balanitis. The tip of your penis may be inflamed or irritated. This may be caused by a fungal or bacterial infection, or skin irritation from soaps or detergents. This condition often occurs in men who are uncircumcised or have diabetes. Treatments may include antibiotics, antifungal creams or ointments. Call your nurse information service or doctor.

Priapism. You may have an erection that lasts for no apparent reason and isn't related to sexual desire or activity. It usually is caused by a sudden, often unexplained obstruction that won't allow the blood in your penis to drain. See your doctor.

Cancer. You may have had a small, painless, pimple-like growth. It may have turned into a lump that now is bleeding or oozing. You also may have lumps in your groin, and urination may be painful. Cancer of the penis is rare. It often is curable if diagnosed early. See your doctor.

Other causes may include injury, certain medications, sexually transmitted diseases (see Page 311) or sickle cell disease.

Self-Care

Self-care isn't appropriate for most cases of penis pain. For instance, don't try to force the foreskin to its normal position if it's painful or swollen. Don't try to clean under the foreskin if it's irritated.

- If you have pain only during or after intercourse, it might be caused by your partner's vaginal dryness. Lubricants and longer foreplay may help. If you're using condoms, use water-based lubricants.

Prevention

- You can avoid minor irritations and inflammations with good hygiene, especially after sexual activity or if you're uncircumcised. Wash your genitals with soap and water.
- If you or your partner has a sexually transmitted disease, avoid sexual intercourse until treatment is complete.

SEEK EMERGENCY HELP

▶ You have an erection that lasts for no reason and is painful.

▶ Your uncircumcised foreskin is stuck behind the head of your penis so that it can't be brought forward, and there is severe swelling.

CALL YOUR NURSE INFORMATION SERVICE OR DOCTOR

▶ You have pain or bleeding, or discharge from a lump or sore on your penis, discomfort when urinating and lumps in your groin.

▶ The tip of your penis is inflamed and irritated.

▶ You have one or more blisters, ulcers or sores on your penis.

▶ You have pain with ejaculation, or blood in your semen.

▶ You've tried self-care but your penis pain and swelling have returned.

TRY SELF-CARE

▶ The pain only occurs during intercourse or on the tip of your penis after intercourse.

YOUR CHILD'S SYMPTOMS

Penis pain or swelling and your child. If your newborn son's penis was circumcised, talk with your doctor about how to care for it. Follow all instructions carefully.

RASH, DIAPER

Red, spotty, moist, sore skin in the diaper area

Causes

Skin sensitivity. Diaper rash is a common irritation that most often results from sensitive skin coming in contact with urine and feces. By changing diapers more frequently, this rash often goes away without treatment.

Infections. Fungal or bacterial infections also can cause diaper rash. The rash may be bright red and appear scalded. If there are large, fluid-filled pimples, the rash may be caused by bacteria and needs a doctor's attention. If the diaper rash doesn't respond to self-care, call your nurse information service or doctor.

Other causes may include allergies to food, detergents, diaper material or baby wipes.

Self-Care

- Your baby's doctor should diagnose diaper rash caused by a fungal infection. Over-the-counter creams can treat this condition.

- Keep the diaper area as dry as possible. Change diapers frequently.

- Use absorbent, disposable diapers until the rash clears.

- Expose your baby's bottom to the air. For instance, during a nap, leave your baby's diaper off. Have him or her lay on a waterproof sheet covered by soft towels.

- Avoid using baby wipes that contain alcohol. They may irritate the skin. Instead, use a clean, soft cloth moistened with lukewarm water.

- Don't use cornstarch-based powder. It promotes the growth of fungal organisms.

- Every day, bathe your baby with a mild soap. Tub soaks after bowel movements also can help. Dry gently after washing.

- If diaper rash occurs around the anus after several episodes of diarrhea, apply a thin layer of over-the-counter, petroleum- or zinc-based ointment or cream.

- When laundering cloth diapers, double rinse and avoid using softeners.

Prevention

- Keep your baby as clean and dry as possible.

- Change diapers frequently.

- Expose the diaper area to air.

- Avoid excessive scrubbing.

- Use absorbent, disposable diapers.

SEE YOUR DOCTOR

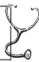

▶ The rash is very raw or bleeding.

CALL YOUR NURSE INFORMATION SERVICE OR DOCTOR

▶ Your child has a fever.

▶ There are fluid-filled blisters in the area of the rash.

▶ You've tried self-care but the symptoms have lasted more than three days.

TRY SELF-CARE

▶ The rash is bright, fiery red, with a sharp, distinct border. Or, there are small, red patches outside the diaper area.

▶ The rash is confined to the diaper area.

RASH, ITCHY

Itchy and red, spotty, blotchy, bumpy, scaly, rough or blistered skin

Causes

Contact dermatitis. You may have been in contact with an allergen or irritant—such as jewelry, detergent, perfume, cosmetics or poison ivy. Now you have an itchy rash. Scratching may leave narrow, raised red lines. Once the allergen or irritant is removed, the symptoms should fade.

Eczema. You may have itchy skin with redness or bumps, or skin thickening, scaling or color changes. You also may have asthma or allergies such as hay fever. Eczema refers to conditions that cause skin inflammation. For instance, hand eczema often is related to excessive hand washing. Nummular eczema refers to round patches of irritated skin. See your doctor or dermatologist if you have chronic eczema.

Pityriasis rosea. You may have one oval, itchy, scaly patch on your chest or back. You also may have similar, smaller patches on your upper arms, trunk or thighs. This may last up to three months and then disappear without treatment. Your doctor may prescribe medication to relieve the itch.

Other causes may include fifth disease, fungal infections or heat rash.

Self-Care

- Unless you have an infection, try hydrocortisone cream or calamine lotion. Follow directions carefully. Avoid calamine lotions that contain analgesics or antihistamines such as diphenhydramine hydrochloride.

- Oral antihistamines may help relieve itching. If you have a health condition, or if you're pregnant or breast-feeding, talk with your doctor before taking any medication.

- For heat rash, take cool baths without soap, and air dry. Try calamine lotion.

- Wash skin exposed to poison ivy with soap and water (not hot) as soon as possible. Wash any clothing that was exposed. Apply loose, cold compresses. Try calamine lotion.

- If you have dry skin, avoid overwashing and using harsh soaps.

- If you have eczema, bathe with a water-soluble cleanser instead of soap. Apply water-soluble moisturizing cream or lotion. Oatmeal products can be soothing, too.

- Staying cool will ease the itch. Heat will aggravate it.

Prevention

- Identify and eliminate irritants or allergens.
- Avoid exposure to extreme temperatures.

SEEK EMERGENCY HELP

► You have weakness, sweatiness, difficulty breathing or swallowing, a stiff neck and eye pain in bright light; you feel extremely sick.

► You have a fever of 104° F or higher.

SEE YOUR DOCTOR

► There's a painful, blistery rash on one side of your body or face.

► The rash is on the palms of your hands or soles of your feet.

► You've developed a red bull's-eye rash with a pale center, followed by a fever, chills, fatigue or headaches; you probably have a mild to moderate itch, but it's possible you have no itch.

► The rash burns or itches intensely. It's surrounded by swelling, blisters or pus. You have other symptoms besides the rash, such as a fever.

CALL YOUR NURSE INFORMATION SERVICE OR DOCTOR

► You're pregnant or immunocompromised.

► You started a new medication within the past four weeks.

► You have a sore throat and your rash is rough like sandpaper.

► You have a widespread rash.

► You've tried self-care but your symptoms haven't improved.

TRY SELF-CARE

► You have a rash but no other symptoms.

YOUR CHILD'S SYMPTOMS

See your doctor if your child's rash has red, black or purplish dots.

Call your nurse information service or doctor if your child has a facial rash that spreads to his body; or if he has a fever, sore throat, runny nose, cough or sore eyes.

Rash and your child. If your child gets chickenpox, give him plenty of fluids. Use calamine lotion for itching. Don't use topical medications containing diphenhydramine or lidocaine. Bathe him in cool water with baking soda or colloidal oatmeal—but no soap—every three to four hours for the first few days. Trim his fingernails. Wash his hands three times a day with antibacterial soap. Be aware that your child even may have sores in his mouth. Eating some foods may be uncomfortable, such as those that are salty, acidic or hot. If diagnosed in the first 24 hours, ask your doctor about prescription medication.

Avoid exposing your child with chickenpox to other people. Ask your doctor how long your child should be confined.

A chickenpox vaccine is recommended for all children ages 12 months or older.

! *Don't give aspirin to anyone younger than age 19! It's linked to Reye's syndrome, a rare but sometimes fatal condition.*

RASH, NON-ITCHY

Red, spotty, blotchy, bumpy, scaly, rough or blistered skin

Causes

Psoriasis. Your skin may be inflamed, scaly and thickened—especially on the knees, elbows, scalp and around the hairline. You also may have fingernail abnormalities, such as indentations or thickening. There are different types of psoriasis, based on the rash's location and appearance. See your doctor.

Rosacea. The skin on your face may be red, as though you're blushing or have a sunburn. You also may have small, red, and solid or pus-filled pimples. Rosacea is a skin condition that most often occurs in adults between ages 30 and 60. See your doctor and try self-care.

Tinea versicolor. This is a type of fungal infection. It causes tan-colored, oval patches with defined borders. It has an irregular shape and fine scaliness. You may notice it on your trunk and upper arms. This condition is caused by an overgrowth of Pityrosporum, a yeast normally found on skin. Although tinea versicolor isn't a serious condition, you should see your doctor.

Lyme disease. You've been bitten by a tick, and now you have a bull's-eye rash. You also may have aching muscles, fever, fatigue, or swelling of your knees or other joints. See your doctor.

Rocky Mountain spotted fever. You've been bitten by a tick, and now you have a rash, severe headache, a fever of 103° F or higher, severe muscle aches and weakness. Seek emergency help.

Other causes may include infections such as fifth disease or scarlet fever.

Self-Care

Rashes have many possible causes. Talk with your doctor about self-care that's right for you.

- If you have tinea versicolor, wash your skin daily with an antidandruff shampoo. The salycylic acid may clear the rash and prevent recurrence.
- Bathe with mild soap or a soap substitute. Use cool or lukewarm water.

Prevention

- Identify and eliminate irritants or allergens.
- Keep your skin dry and cool.
- While you're being treated for tinea versicolor, you may want to wash towels and bedding. This may help you avoid even a remote chance of reinfecting yourself.

- If you have rosacea, avoid touching or rubbing your face. Use face products that are noncomedogenic—they're less likely to clog your pores.

- If you've spent time outdoors or in wooded areas, check yourself and your pets for ticks.

SEEK EMERGENCY HELP

▶ You feel very sick and have sweatiness; difficulty breathing or swallowing; diarrhea; a stiff neck, and eye pain in bright light; or muscle and joint pain.

▶ You have a fever of 104° F or higher.

▶ You have severe pain even though the rash doesn't look severe.

▶ You have a sunburn-like rash, sudden fever, vomiting, diarrhea or muscle pain, and recent use of tampons.

SEE YOUR DOCTOR

▶ There's a painful, blistery rash on one side of your body or face.

▶ The rash is on the palms of your hands or soles of your feet.

▶ You've developed a red bull's-eye rash with a pale center, followed by fever, chills, fatigue or headaches.

CALL YOUR NURSE INFORMATION SERVICE OR DOCTOR

▶ You're pregnant or immunocompromised.

▶ You started a new medication within the past four weeks.

▶ You have a sore throat and your rash is rough like sandpaper.

▶ You've tried self-care but your symptoms haven't improved.

TRY SELF-CARE

▶ You have a rash but no other symptoms.

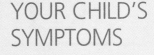

YOUR CHILD'S SYMPTOMS

See your doctor if your child's rash has red, black or purplish dots.

Call your nurse information service or doctor if your child has a red rash; or a facial rash that spreads to her body; or if she has a fever, sore throat, runny nose, cough or sore eyes.

▮ *Don't give aspirin to anyone younger than age 19! It's linked to Reye's syndrome, a rare but sometimes fatal condition.*

RECTAL BLEEDING

Blood in the toilet, on the toilet paper, or in the stool after a bowel movement; blood may be bright red, burgundy or black

Causes

Bismuth-containing medications. Some antidiarrheals or iron supplements can cause black stools. Some red foods such as beets also can cause red stools. This is not the same as blood in the stool.

Hemorrhoids. After you have a bowel movement, you may notice bright-red blood on the toilet paper, in the toilet bowl or on the stool itself. You also may have pain during bowel movements. Hemorrhoids are the most common cause of rectal bleeding. They occur when the veins around the anus become engorged and enlarged. Pregnant women and people who strain to have bowel movements commonly get them. They may protrude through the anal opening, or be inside and invisible. Symptoms usually disappear on their own. Surgical treatment rarely is necessary. Call your nurse information service or doctor if the pain or bleeding is severe.

Fissure. You may have bleeding, itching or pain during and right after bowel movements. Anal fissures are crack-like sores around the opening of the anus. They often are associated with constipation or hemorrhoids. Fissures usually can be treated with self-care but occasionally require surgery.

Infectious diarrhea. You have sudden diarrhea, nausea and vomiting, headache, abdominal cramps, low-grade fever, and fatigue. Diarrhea may be caused by bacteria in spoiled food.

Colorectal cancer. You have dark, black, burgundy- or rust-colored stools. See your doctor. Or, you may have bright-red rectal bleeding, along with one or more of these symptoms: changes in bowel habits; diarrhea; constipation; bleeding between bowel movements; narrow stools; lower abdominal pain; bloating; cramps; excessive gas; loss of weight and appetite; or chronic fatigue.

Colorectal cancer isn't a frequent cause of rectal bleeding. However, it's a consideration, especially if you're age 50 or older, or have a family history. If you have any of these symptoms that don't go away, call your doctor.

Other causes may include diverticulitis (see Page 262), certain medications, polyps or ulcers (see Page 261).

Self-Care

■ If hemorrhoids are the cause:

• Call your nurse information service or doctor before using any over-the-

194

counter creams or ointments, especially if you're pregnant.

- Take a sitz bath twice daily—sit in a bathtub with enough warm (not hot) water to cover your anal area. Sitz baths help speed healing, keep the area clean and provide comfort.
- Clean your anal area after a bowel movement. Use soft toilet paper moistened with water, or over-the-counter, disposable cleansing pads.

■ If anal fissures are the cause, stool softeners may help. Also, take a sitz bath every day.

Prevention

■ Straining during bowel movements is often the cause of hemorrhoids and anal fissures. Avoid constipation by drinking plenty of water each day; eating high-fiber foods such as fruits, vegetables, beans and whole-grain cereals; and exercising regularly.

■ Gently clean your anal area every day.

■ Talk with your doctor about colorectal cancer screenings (see Page 31).

SEEK EMERGENCY HELP

▶ **You have severe abdominal pain or tenderness, and a fever.**

▶ **There is a large amount of blood which may look dark-red, bright-red or tarry. The blood is mixed with your stool.**

SEE YOUR DOCTOR

▶ **Your stool is dark-red, burgundy, black, tarry or rust-colored.**

CALL YOUR NURSE INFORMATION SERVICE OR DOCTOR

▶ **You have a small amount of rectal bleeding, or you see bright-red blood on the toilet paper.**

YOUR CHILD'S SYMPTOMS

See your doctor if you notice rectal bleeding in your baby or child who also feels sick or has little or no appetite.

Rectal bleeding and your child. The normal, frequent, yellow stools of infants can irritate the skin in and around the anus, causing small amounts of bleeding. Constipation frequently is the cause of rectal bleeding in young children.

Pinworms (see Page 196), which cause anal itching, very rarely may cause a little bleeding.

RECTAL PAIN OR ANAL ITCH

Pain or itching in the rectal or anal area

Causes

Hemorrhoids (see Page 194). You may have veins around your anus that have become engorged and enlarged. Pregnant women and people who strain to have bowel movements commonly get hemorrhoids.

Fissure (see page 194). You may have bleeding, itching or pain during and immediately after bowel movements. Anal fissures are crack-like sores that develop around the opening of the anus.

Perirectal abscess. You may have a collection of pus under the skin that surrounds the anus. Glands in this area sometimes become blocked, causing pus to form. If left untreated, it can lead to pain, fever and painful bowel movements. Call your nurse information service or doctor. For severe pain that persists, seek emergency help.

Pinworms. You may have anal itching that worsens at night, along with restless sleep or irritability. Pinworms generally infect young children, but can spread to other family members, too. To determine if the cause of the itching is pinworms, get a specimen by wrapping a piece of transparent tape (sticky side out) around a flat, small object such as a Popsicle stick.

Spread the buttocks, and press the tape firmly and flatly over the anal opening for two minutes. Seal the sample in a plastic bag, and see your doctor.

Muscle spasm. You may have a sharp, stabbing pain in your rectum. It may occur at any time. This condition, proctalgia fugax, is common among women ages 45 and younger. It's believed to be caused by an intense spasm of the muscles near the rectum. This condition isn't serious, and often disappears on its own.

Fungal infection. Anal itching can be caused by a fungal infection—usually Candida, or yeast. This condition also can be associated with a vaginal yeast infection (see Page 236), diabetes (see Page 281), obesity or compromised immune system.

Other causes may include bowel disorders (see Page 261) or poor hygiene.

Self-Care

■ Cleanse your anal area after each bowel movement. Use soft toilet paper moistened with water. Or, use over-the-counter, disposable cleansing pads. Gently pat dry.

196

- Don't use feminine hygiene deodorant sprays or powders.
- Wear cotton underpants.
- Don't drink more than two cups of coffee a day. Coffee beans contain oils that can't be digested. They may irritate the skin around your anal area when excreted.
- Use perfume- and dye-free toilet paper.

Prevention

- Keep the anal area clean and dry.
- Don't strain during bowel movements.
- Avoid using medicated or perfumed powders and sprays.
- Wear cotton underpants.

SEE YOUR DOCTOR

▶ You have a tender lump in your anal area, or a fever.

CALL YOUR NURSE INFORMATION SERVICE OR DOCTOR

▶ You have diabetes or any of the following: frequent urination, increased thirst or appetite, weight loss or fatigue.

▶ You've tried self-care but your symptoms haven't improved after one week. Or, the intense itching has gotten worse.

TRY SELF-CARE

▶ You have rectal pain or anal itching but no other symptoms.

Call your nurse information service or doctor if your child has anal itching that's worse at night. He also may have irritability or restless sleep.

SCRAPE OR ABRASION

A shallow injury in which the top layers of the skin have been scraped off

About Scrapes or Abrasions

Scrapes or abrasions result when one or several layers of skin get rubbed off by contact with something sharp or rough. Since they aren't deep wounds, scrapes and abrasions tend to heal rather quickly. They can be treated effectively with self-care.

Self-Care

- Wash the wound thoroughly with soap and warm water. If washing doesn't remove all the dirt, soak the wound in clean, warm water.

- Once clean, if the wound hasn't stopped bleeding, apply pressure with a clean gauze pad or cloth.

- If the scrape has created a flap of skin, trim it away to minimize the risk of infection.

- If the abrasion is small or isn't likely to bleed, leave it uncovered. If the wound is bleeding, cover it with a bandage. Remove the bandage once a scab has formed.

- Applying antibiotic creams or ointments may help. Follow package directions. Don't use these products for more than five consecutive days.

- To reduce swelling and ease discomfort, wrap crushed ice in a thin towel and place on the wound. Use for 20 minutes on and 20 minutes off until the pain subsides. Do this within 24 hours of the injury.

- Try an over-the-counter pain reliever such as acetaminophen, ibuprofen or naproxen sodium for pain relief, if needed. Don't use aspirin—it can cause bleeding.

- If your last tetanus shot was more than five years ago, or you're unsure of your tetanus status, you may need a booster. Call your doctor.

- Watch for signs of infection such as redness, swelling, pus or fever.

Prevention

- Many scrapes and abrasions occur while playing sports. Wear appropriate protective gear, such as knee and elbow pads, helmets and shinguards.

SEE YOUR DOCTOR

▶ You were injured more than 24 hours ago and now have signs of infection such as redness, swelling, pus or fever.

▶ You can't remove dirt and debris from the wound after washing and soaking it for 15 minutes.

CALL YOUR NURSE INFORMATION SERVICE OR DOCTOR

▶ The scrape or abrasion covers an extremely large area.

▶ Your last tetanus shot was more than five years ago or you're unsure of your tetanus status.

▶ You've tried self-care but the wound hasn't steadily improved or healed after one week.

TRY SELF-CARE

▶ You have a scrape or abrasion but no other symptoms.

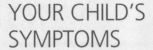

YOUR CHILD'S SYMPTOMS

Scrapes or abrasions and your child. Make sure children wear helmets and other protective gear as appropriate.

SHOULDER PAIN

Pain or tenderness in the shoulder

Causes

Arthritis (see Page 255). You may have pain, along with swelling or stiffness in your shoulder or other joints. Symptoms of arthritis vary depending on the type. See your doctor.

Bursitis. Your shoulder may be tender and painful, or swollen. The twinges of pain can become severe in a few hours, making it difficult to lift your arm. Bursitis is an inflammation of the bursae—fluid-filled sacs around joints. These sacs limit friction and make movement easier. See your doctor.

Tendinitis. You may have muscle spasms and pain. Tendinitis is inflammation of a tendon, which connects muscle to bone. Try self-care.

Frozen shoulder. Your shoulder may be painful or inflamed for no apparent reason or from overuse. If you keep your arm still, your shoulder's range of motion becomes restricted. You may need physical therapy. See your doctor.

Other causes may include diaphragmatic irritation, injury or trauma, nerve compression, or neurological disorders due to neck or spine pain.

Self-Care

- If you have bursitis, avoid using your affected shoulder and arm for one to four days. To ease the pain, wrap crushed ice in a thin towel, apply to your shoulder for 15 to 20 minutes, three to four times a day for the first 48 to 72 hours. Perform normal range-of-motion movements several times a day to restore mobility.

- If you have tendinitis, rest the affected area for a day or so. Wrap crushed ice in a thin towel. Apply for 15 to 20 minutes, three to four times a day.

- If you have a frozen shoulder, try an over-the-counter pain reliever such as acetaminophen, ibuprofen, naproxen sodium or aspirin.

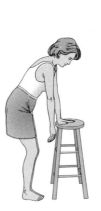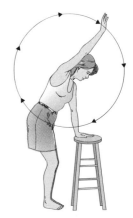

Keep your shoulders limber with exercise. With knees slightly bent, extend your arm and gently rotate it in a full circle. Alternate arms. Check with your doctor about exercises that are right for you.

- Avoid extreme movements.
- After three to four days, if the pain has lessened, apply a moist-heat pad, or a warm, moist towel, for 15 to 20 minutes, three to four times a day. If moist heat isn't available, take a warm bath or shower.
- Massage your shoulder with lotion or balm. This can increase blood flow and relax your muscles.
- Rest—but avoid complete inactivity.

Prevention

- Avoid repetitive shoulder movement. Vary your activities.
- Try gentle exercise to keep your shoulders limber (see illustration).

SEEK EMERGENCY HELP

▶ You're in your first trimester of pregnancy, and you have vaginal bleeding and abdominal pain.

▶ The pain resulted from an injury and you can't move your shoulder.

▶ The pain began suddenly. You have a fever and you feel sick.

▶ You can't move your arm at the shoulder joint.

SEE YOUR DOCTOR

▶ Your shoulder is red and swollen, and you have a fever.

▶ You have pain only when you move, and your shoulder has become increasingly sore and difficult to move.

▶ You have serious pain and swelling that started after athletic activity or chores.

▶ You have severe or nagging pain, swelling, stiffness, stabbing or radiating pain, numbness or tingling.

TRY SELF-CARE

▶ You have shoulder pain but no other symptoms.

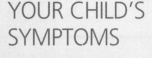

! *Don't give aspirin to anyone younger than age 19! It's linked to Reye's syndrome, a rare but sometimes fatal condition.*

201

SINUS PAIN

Severe nasal congestion with thick mucus; pressure around the eye and in the head; a headache that's worse in the morning or when bending forward; or pain over the cheeks—possibly accompanied by low-grade fever and upper tooth pain

Causes

Common cold. Your nose may be congested or running with clear to whitish mucus. You may be sneezing and coughing. You also may have mild body aches and a low-grade fever. Colds often are accompanied by minor sinus pain. Try self-care.

Sinusitis (see Page 303). If you have a cold with moderate to severe sinus pain, you may have sinusitis, an inflammation of the sinus passages. This condition usually is caused by a bacterial infection which may require prescription medication. See your doctor.

Other causes may include allergic rhinitis, or hay fever (see Page 303), or certain medications such as beta blockers.

Self-Care

If your sinus pain is caused by a bacterial infection, use self-care in addition to taking prescription medication.

- Use a cool-mist vaporizer or humidifier. Clean it daily or as instructed by the manufacturer.

- To help your sinuses drain during the night, place a pillow or foam wedge under the mattress to elevate the head of the bed.

- Over-the-counter oral or spray decongestants can help. Don't use nasal sprays for longer than three days. Overuse can cause a "rebound" effect that will make your congestion worse.

- If your sinus pain is caused by a cold, try an over-the-counter pain reliever such as acetaminophen, ibuprofen, naproxen sodium or aspirin to reduce fever and muscle aches. Drink plenty of fluids and get lots of rest.

Prevention

- Allergies often set the stage for sinus infections. Avoid exposure to allergens. Treat your allergies with prescription or over-the-counter medications recommended by your doctor.

- Avoid cigarette smoke—it's a severe sinus irritant.

- Drink plenty of water to stay hydrated and keep mucous membranes moist.

202

SEEK EMERGENCY HELP

▶ You have vision problems, or red, painful or bulging eyes.

SEE YOUR DOCTOR

▶ You have a fever, severe headache or swelling.

CALL YOUR NURSE INFORMATION SERVICE OR DOCTOR

▶ You have a thick, yellowish-green nasal mucus, headache, pressure in your head, pain in your cheeks and forehead, and a fever.

▶ You have seasonal allergies, itchy eyes, clear nasal mucus and frequent sneezing.

▶ You've tried self-care but your symptoms haven't improved after three to four days.

TRY SELF-CARE

▶ You have thick nasal mucus, and pain in your cheeks and forehead.

▶ You have seasonal allergies, itchy eyes, clear nasal mucus and frequent sneezing.

YOUR CHILD'S SYMPTOMS

Call your nurse information service or doctor if your child has a persistent nighttime cough that lasts longer than two weeks and a thick, yellowish-green nasal discharge. She may have a sinus infection.

Sinus pain and your child. Children can develop sinusitis, especially if they have allergies. When your child has a cold, help nasal secretions drain by using a cool-mist vaporizer or humidifier. Clean it daily or as instructed by the manufacturer.

Over-the-counter oral decongestants may help. Only use those made specifically for children.

! *Don't give aspirin to anyone younger than age 19! It's linked to Reye's syndrome, a rare but sometimes fatal condition.*

SKIN, ITCHY OR DRY

Dry, itchy, cracked or irritated skin

Causes

Pruritis, or "winter itch." Your skin may itch—especially your lower legs, upper arms or thighs. You may have cracked or irritated patches of skin, or no visible irritation. There may not be enough humidity in your environment. Try self-care.

Aging. As people age, the number of oil glands in their skin tends to decrease. The result may be dry skin. Lack of humidity in the air during the winter months can further aggravate dry skin. Try self-care.

Irritants. You may have tried a new detergent, soap or cosmetic product. Now your skin is dry or itchy. You might have an allergic reaction. Call your nurse information service or doctor, and try self-care.

Medications. You may be using topical acne treatments, beta blockers, lithium or a medication for high cholesterol. Dry, itchy skin can be a side effect of certain medications. Call your nurse information service or doctor.

Self-Care

■ Avoid skin irritants such as perfumes or antiperspirants. They can dry out your skin.

■ Bathe only once a day using warm—not hot—water. Use glycerine soap. Gently pat—don't rub—your skin dry.

■ Use a moisturizing lotion as necessary.

■ Use a cool-mist vaporizer or humidifier. Clean it daily or as instructed by the manufacturer.

Prevention

■ Avoid excessively dry air, if possible.

■ Identify and avoid allergens and irritants.

■ Use a moisturizing lotion as needed.

■ Drink plenty of water each day to stay hydrated.

CALL YOUR NURSE INFORMATION SERVICE OR DOCTOR

▶ You have skin that's very itchy, with tiny gray lines or red spots between your fingers or on your wrist.

▶ You're taking medication.

▶ You have itchy, raised, light red patches with clearly defined edges.

▶ You've tried self-care but your symptoms haven't improved after seven days.

TRY SELF-CARE

▶ Your skin is itchy, but not red or flaking.

▶ You have itchy, red, flaky skin.

YOUR CHILD'S SYMPTOMS

Call your nurse information service or doctor if your child has itchy, raised red spots that turn into blisters (see Page 191).

SPLINTER

A sliver of wood or other material stuck under the skin

About Splinters

Unless they're very large, or embedded deeply under a nail, nearly all splinters can be removed and treated with self-care. The primary concern is infection, which you can avoid by keeping the area clean.

Self-Care

Call your nurse information service or doctor if you have diabetes, have a large or deeply embedded splinter, or if the splinter is made of treated wood. You may need a tetanus shot if your last one was more than five years ago, or you're unsure of your tetanus status.

- Don't get a wood splinter wet. Water will cause the splinter to swell and make it more difficult to remove.

- Small splinters can be removed with a sterile pair of tweezers and a sharp needle. Wash your hands. Sterilize the tweezers and needle by boiling them in water, soaking them in rubbing alcohol or holding them over an open flame. Cool before using. Try to grab the splinter with the tweezers. If you can't, try to lift the splinter with the tip of the needle. Don't persistently poke with the needle, especially if the area becomes red and painful, or begins to bleed.

- After removing the splinter, wash the area with soap and warm water. Use an antibiotic cream or ointment that contains bacitracin. Cover the area with a bandage and change it daily. During the next few days, watch for signs of infection such as redness, swelling, pus or fever. Soak the area three to four times a day in warm, soapy water. Apply antibiotic cream or ointment, and a bandage for the next four to five days. Don't use bacitracin for more than five consecutive days.

- If the splinter is very small, you may wait for it to come out on its own. Keep the area clean to avoid infection.

Prevention

- Wear shoes when walking on wood floors or decks.

- Don't rub wood surfaces against the grain.

206

SEE YOUR DOCTOR

▶ You have signs of infection such as redness, swelling, warmth, increased pain or discomfort, pus and red streaks at the splinter site, and a fever.

▶ The splinter is very large or deeply embedded.

CALL YOUR NURSE INFORMATION SERVICE OR DOCTOR

▶ You have diabetes.

▶ Your last tetanus shot was more than five years ago or you're unsure of your tetanus status.

▶ You've tried self-care but can't remove the splinter completely.

TRY SELF-CARE

▶ You have a splinter but no other symptoms.

SPRAIN OR STRAIN

Injury to a joint by sharply twisting or overusing it; pain or tenderness, and possibly swelling, redness or bruising; difficulty moving the injured area

About Sprains and Strains

Sprains and strains are injuries to the tissues that connect the bones of a joint. These tissues provide stability when the joint moves.

A sprain is a stretched and torn ligament. A strain is a stretched muscle. Sprains and strains occur when a trauma, such as a sudden twist or stretch, causes a joint to move outside its normal range of movement. They occur most often in the ankles, knees and fingers, although any joint is susceptible.

Many sprains and strains are minor and can be treated with self-care. When serious, they may require surgery.

Self-Care

- Stop what you're doing as soon as you feel pain. Try the PRICE remedy—protect, rest, ice, compression and elevation. Protect the affected body part from further injury. Rest it for a day or so. Wrap crushed ice in a thin towel, and apply for 15 to 20 minutes, three to four times a day. Use an elastic wrap or bandage around the injury.

Whenever possible, keep the body part elevated above the level of your heart to help reduce swelling.

- If you sprained a finger joint, remove rings from your finger immediately, before the joint swells.
- Try an over-the-counter pain reliever such as acetaminophen, ibuprofen, naproxen sodium or aspirin.

Prevention

- Check your house for conditions that could lead to accidents:
  - Put handrails on stairways.
  - Use rubber mats in bathtubs and showers.
  - Don't leave objects where people can trip over them.
- Before exercising or participating in sports:
  - Warm up with slow, gentle stretches before starting any strenuous physical activity.
  - Cool down for at least five minutes after exercising.
  - Don't overexert or overuse your muscles.

208

SEEK EMERGENCY HELP

▶ Your injured joint is deformed, crooked, or shows signs of impaired circulation—pale, blue or gray, and feels cold.

CALL YOUR NURSE INFORMATION SERVICE OR DOCTOR

▶ You can't move your joint; you feel severe pain with movement, or can't put weight on your injured limb.

▶ You have tingling, numbness, loss of sensation, severe swelling or pain when you press along the bone.

▶ You've tried self-care but your symptoms haven't improved after 48 hours.

TRY SELF-CARE

▶ You have mild pain but none of the symptoms or situations listed above.

Sprain or strain and your child. Children can't always express pain, so watch them for signs of sprains or strains. If your child suddenly stops his activity, begins to limp or favors one side of his body over another, he may have an injury that requires medical attention.

! *Don't give aspirin to anyone younger than age 19! It's linked to Reye's syndrome, a rare but sometimes fatal condition.*

STING OR BITE

Red lump or area on the skin that may be itchy, swollen or painful

About Stings and Bites

For most people, insect stings are rarely serious—except for tick, black widow spider and brown recluse spider bites. Typically, redness, itchiness and swelling develop one day after the sting or bite. However, if you have an allergic reaction to the sting or bite, you may have more serious symptoms.

Bee sting. A bee has stung you—or injected venom into your skin. The discomfort should disappear after several days. Symptoms of an allergic reaction include nausea or vomiting, difficulty breathing, swelling around the eyes, lips, tongue or throat, or unconsciousness. This can be deadly. Seek emergency help.

Black widow spider bite. Within hours of this bite, you may experience cramping in your abdomen, convulsions, difficulty breathing, chills, nausea or vomiting. Seek emergency help.

Brown recluse spider bite. You have a blue or purple spot with a white ring around it, surrounded by a larger red ring. It may blister and leave a deep ulcer. You also may have rash, nausea or listlessness. Seek emergency help.

Chigger bite. You have severe itching or red sores around your ankles, under your belt line or under openings in your clothes. You recently may have ventured into grassy or wooded areas. Call your nurse information service or doctor.

Other causes may include fire ants, horseflies, mosquitoes, scorpions or ticks (see Page 192).

Self-Care

- For all kinds of insect bites, use ice or cold compresses immediately, even if you've called for emergency help.

- Over-the-counter antihistamines, or pain relievers such as acetaminophen, ibuprofen, naproxen sodium or aspirin may help.

- Clean the affected area with soap and water.

- For stings, remove the stinger by gently scraping it out with a firm edge, such as a credit card.

- If you have a history of severe reactions to bee stings, talk with your doctor about carrying an injectable form of epinephrine for emergency treatment of allergic reactions.

210

- To remove a tick, use tweezers to grasp it by its body.
- Don't use kerosene, gasoline or alcohol on ticks.

Prevention

- Avoid high grass, woods, bushes and other places where you may come in contact with insects. Wear protective clothing. Use insect repellents containing DEET (diethyltoluamide). Don't use DEET on children ages 2 years and younger.
- Avoid wearing brightly colored clothing and using scented products such as perfume and hairspray.
- Regularly inspect yourself, children and pets for ticks after being outdoors.

SEEK EMERGENCY HELP

▶ You have faintness, confusion, paleness, clamminess, lethargy or difficulty breathing.

▶ You have a headache, nausea or vomiting, excessive sweating, or a tingling sensation at the site of the bite or sting.

▶ You were bitten by a spider. You have eye, lip or genital swelling, abdominal pain, muscle twitch or jerking limbs.

▶ You were bitten by a spider. You have blue or purple splotches near the bite, or a widespread rash or hives.

▶ You were stung in the mouth or on the tongue.

CALL YOUR NURSE INFORMATION SERVICE OR DOCTOR

▶ You've tried self-care but the bite or sting is oozing, or developing a deep sore. Or, it's still painful after 24 hours.

▶ The site of the bite or sting is red, swollen, painful and streaky, or you have a fever.

TRY SELF-CARE

▶ You've been bitten or stung by an insect but have none of the symptoms or situations listed above.

YOUR CHILD'S SYMPTOMS

Seek emergency help if your child has been bitten by a poisonous spider. Spider bites are far more dangerous for children than adults. Put ice or a cold compress on the bite.

❗ *Don't give aspirin to anyone younger than age 19! It's linked to Reye's syndrome, a rare but sometimes fatal condition.*

STOMACH PAIN

Pain in the stomach

Causes

Irritable bowel syndrome (IBS) (see Page 262). You may have abdominal cramping and stomach pain, diarrhea, constipation or bloating. The cause of IBS is unknown, but stress, and high-fat or gas-producing foods may make it worse. Your doctor may prescribe medication to help control symptoms.

Small-bowel obstruction. You may have pain that comes in waves, and centers around your navel, along with nausea, vomiting and abdominal tenderness. This may indicate a small-bowel obstruction that requires hospitalization or surgery. See your doctor immediately.

Pancreatitis. You may have mid- to upper-abdominal pain, which can range from mild to severe. The pain may radiate to your back, chest or lower abdomen. See your doctor.

Gall bladder disease. You may have steady pain in your abdomen just under the rib cage on your right side. You also may have nausea or vomiting. You may need surgery to remove gallstones. See your doctor.

Other causes may include gastritis or peptic ulcer disease (see Page 298), gastroesophageal reflux disease (GERD) (see Page 144), or referred stomach pain due to kidney stones (see Page 232) or infection.

Self-Care

If you have severe or lasting stomach pain, don't use self-care. See your doctor immediately.

For mild stomach pain caused by something you ate:

- Sip on water or suck on crushed ice for a few hours. Stay hydrated and avoid solid foods. When you feel better, try the BRAT diet—bananas, rice, applesauce or toast.
- Passing gas or having a bowel movement often brings relief. However, don't use laxatives. They may aggravate your condition.

Prevention

- Avoid long-term use of aspirin, ibuprofen or naproxen sodium, unless otherwise directed by your doctor.
- Limit alcohol consumption.
- Avoid high-fat foods.

SEEK EMERGENCY HELP

▶ The pain is severe and you're pregnant or you think you might be.

▶ The pain is constant, localized or rapidly getting more intense.

▶ The pain has lasted more than two hours, repeated vomiting hasn't relieved the pain, or your abdomen is swollen and tender.

▶ You have excessive thirst, fast breathing or rapid heartbeat.

CALL YOUR NURSE INFORMATION SERVICE OR DOCTOR

▶ You have bloody or painful urination.

▶ You've tried self-care but the mild stomach pain hasn't improved. You may have no other symptoms, or diarrhea that's lasted more than 24 hours.

TRY SELF-CARE

▶ You have relatively mild pain but no other symptoms except possibly diarrhea for less than 24 hours.

YOUR CHILD'S SYMPTOMS

Seek emergency help if your child screams in pain at the slightest movement or touch, or has blood in his stool.

Call your nurse information service or doctor if your baby stops eating and seems to have stomach pain.

! *Don't give aspirin to anyone younger than age 19! It's linked to Reye's syndrome, a rare but sometimes fatal condition.*

SUNBURN

Red, swollen, painful and possibly blistered skin, due to sun exposure; if severe, may include chills, fever, nausea or vomiting

About Sunburn

Sunburn is caused by too much exposure to ultraviolet (UV) light. This exposure may be from the sun or artificial sources such as tanning beds.

UVA and UVB are two main types of UV rays. UVB rays are the primary cause of sunburn. Everyone who spends a lot of time in the sun is at risk of sunburn. But, those with fair skin, blond or red hair, and light eyes are at highest risk. Certain medications also can increase sensitivity to the sun.

Limiting your exposure to the sun's harmful rays is extremely important. Sunburn and general overexposure to UV light, especially during childhood, can greatly increase your risk of developing skin cancer.

Self-Care

- To reduce heat and pain, make cool compresses. Dip towels or strips of gauze in cool water and lay them on the burned areas.

- Soak in a cool bath with over-the-counter oatmeal preparations, or 1/2 cup of baking soda.

- Avoid using products containing benzocaine unless directed by your doctor. They may temporarily numb the skin, but can be irritating. They may delay healing by triggering an allergic reaction.

- Try an over-the-counter pain reliever such as acetaminophen, ibuprofen, naproxen sodium or aspirin.

- If blisters develop, avoid touching or breaking them.

- Drink plenty of water to replace lost fluids.

- Stay out of the sun until your sunburn has healed.

Prevention

- Avoid the sun between 10 a.m. and 4 p.m. This is when the sun's rays are strongest.

- Use sunscreen with a sun protection factor (SPF) of 15 or higher, even when it's cloudy or overcast. Make sure it protects against both UVA and UVB rays. Reapply sunscreen at least every two hours, especially if you're swimming or sweating.

- Wear a wide-brimmed hat and sunglasses to protect your eyes from bright light and ultraviolet (UV) rays. Tightly woven clothes can help prevent penetration of the sun's rays.
- Avoid tanning beds and lamps.

SEEK EMERGENCY HELP

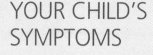

- ▶ **You have severe sunburn and fever, vomiting, diarrhea, confusion or visual disturbance.**
- ▶ **You have blistering on your eyelids.**

SEE YOUR DOCTOR

- ▶ **You have blisters larger than 2 inches.**
- ▶ **You have large blisters on your face, hands, feet or ears.**
- ▶ **You have multiple blisters.**
- ▶ **You've tried self-care but your symptoms haven't improved after 48 hours.**

TRY SELF-CARE

- ▶ **You have sunburn and possibly some minor blistering but no other symptoms.**

Sunburn and your child. Children need extra protection from the sun. Just a few serious sunburns can significantly increase your child's risk of skin cancer later in life. Make sure she wears sunscreen with an SPF of at least 15 that blocks both UVA and UVB rays. She also should wear a hat and protective clothing.

Ask your doctor if sunscreen is appropriate for your infant.

! *Don't give aspirin to anyone younger than age 19! It's linked to Reye's syndrome, a rare but sometimes fatal condition.*

SWALLOWING DIFFICULTY

Discomfort or pain when swallowing; difficulty getting food to go down at all

Causes

Infection. You may have difficulty swallowing. You also may have a sore throat, fever, headache, fatigue or loss of appetite. This could indicate a viral or bacterial infection in your upper respiratory tract. See your doctor.

Gastroesophageal reflux disease (GERD). You may have difficulty swallowing, heartburn, pain in your chest or upper abdomen, or a sour or bitter taste in your mouth. GERD is a digestive disorder in which the stomach's juices flow back up into the esophagus. Self-care can help. But, see your doctor if your symptoms persist.

Esophageal motility disorder. You may have difficulty swallowing food. This could be a symptom of esophageal spasms—when the muscles that move food down the esophagus become uncoordinated. You also may have achalasia, a condition in which the valve in the lower esophagus doesn't open properly. See your doctor in either case.

Other causes may include dry throat or a foreign object lodged in the throat.

Self-Care

- If you have a dry throat, drink plenty of water each day. Try a cool-mist vaporizer or humidifier. Clean it daily or as instructed by the manufacturer.

- If GERD is the cause, try an over-the-counter antacid.

- If you have a cold or upper respiratory tract infection, suck on lozenges. Don't give small children lozenges—they can cause choking.

Prevention

- Lifestyle changes can help prevent GERD. Avoid coffee, chocolate, and fatty or spicy foods to help prevent acid reflux. Eat smaller, more frequent meals. Don't drink alcohol or smoke. Lose excess weight. Also, place a pillow or foam wedge under the mattress to elevate the head of the bed. This may prevent stomach acid from backing up into your throat.

SEEK EMERGENCY HELP

▶ You're having difficulty swallowing, associated with difficulty breathing.

▶ You're drooling uncontrollably.

▶ You've had a recent onset of severe sore throat and you're having trouble swallowing your saliva.

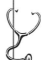

SEE YOUR DOCTOR

▶ You may have swallowed something small and sharp that got lodged in your throat.

▶ Your swallowing has been getting worse. You've lost more than 10 pounds in the past month without trying.

CALL YOUR NURSE INFORMATION SERVICE OR DOCTOR

▶ You've tried self-care for any of the following symptoms but they haven't improved: sore throat and a fever; headache; muscle aches; fatigue; nasal mucus or congestion; a burning feeling in your chest; a feeling like your stomach contents are backing up into your mouth; or feeling like there's a lump in your throat.

TRY SELF-CARE

▶ You have a sore throat and fever, headache, muscle aches, fatigue, nasal mucus or congestion for less than three to four days.

▶ You have a new onset of a burning feeling in your stomach. It feels like your stomach contents are backing up into your mouth.

▶ You swallow normally but have been feeling like there's a lump in your throat, for less than one week.

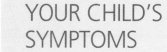
Seek emergency help if your child shows any of these signs of dehydration: small amounts of urine for more than 12 hours; unusual lethargy or irritability; lack of skin elasticity; dry mouth; sunken eyes; and very little saliva or tears.

Call your doctor if your child complains of swallowing difficulty, or has throat pain and fever that doesn't subside after two days.

Swallowing difficulty and your child. Children can dehydrate much more quickly than adults. Make sure that any difficulty swallowing isn't interfering with your child's ability to drink.

! *Don't give aspirin to anyone younger than age 19! It's linked to Reye's syndrome, a rare but sometimes fatal condition.*

SWEATINESS

Excessive perspiration

Causes

Obesity. Your weight falls in the obese range (see Page 24). Extra weight puts stress on your body and can cause excessive sweating. Talk with your doctor about healthy ways to lose weight.

Menopause (see Page 317). You're age 38 or older, and your menstrual periods may be irregular. You may become warm suddenly and begin to sweat profusely. This is known as a hot flash. You also may have night sweats. Though uncomfortable, these are normal symptoms of menopause. Call your nurse information service or doctor.

Hyperthyroidism (see Page 308). In addition to excessive sweating, you may have unexplained weight loss; an increase in appetite; weakness or trembling; bulging eyes or rapid heartbeat. Call your nurse information service or doctor.

Other causes may include anxiety (see Page 330), hyperhidrosis or certain medications.

Self-Care

Sweating is natural—it helps regulate your body temperature. Try these tips to help minimize sweating:

- Dress in natural, light, loose-fitting fabrics, such as cotton. They absorb perspiration and allow air to circulate. Avoid man-made fibers such as rayon, nylon and polyester.

- Use a deodorant that contains antiperspirant. Choose roll-on or stick. They tend to provide more protection than sprays. Dry yourself thoroughly before applying antiperspirant. Moisture can dilute its effectiveness.

- Avoid hot, spicy food.

- Don't smoke. If you drink alcohol, do so in moderation. These both can increase sweating.

- If you think you have symptoms of menopause, ask your doctor if hormone replacement therapy or other treatments may be right for you (see Page 318).

Prevention

- Shower at least once a day. Though it won't stop perspiration, it will help eliminate odor and cool you off.

CALL YOUR NURSE INFORMATION SERVICE OR DOCTOR

▶ You have three or more of the following: bulging eyes, rapid heartbeat, unexplained weight loss, weakness or trembling, increased appetite, more frequent bowel movements, or heat intolerance.

▶ You sweat mostly at night and have a cough, or you've lost weight.

▶ You're taking a new medication.

▶ You've tried self-care but your sweatiness hasn't improved after three to four days.

▶ You're a woman age 38 or older and your periods are irregular.

TRY SELF-CARE

▶ You have a fever and you feel achy and sick.

YOUR CHILD'S SYMPTOMS

Sweatiness and your child. If your teen complains of sweatiness, let him or her know that it's perfectly normal. This can be embarrassing for teens. Try to be supportive. Regular showers and an antiperspirant can help prevent unpleasant body odor.

THIRST, EXCESSIVE

Very dry mouth; possibly dry lips and skin

Causes

Dehydration. You may be sweating excessively or vomiting, or you may have diarrhea. As a result, you now have severe thirst, along with dry lips and tongue, lack of energy, or muscle cramping. These are signs of dehydration. Mild dehydration can be treated by increasing your intake of water.

Seek emergency help if you notice symptoms of severe dehydration—decreased urine output, rapid and shallow breathing, skin that lacks its normal elasticity, low blood pressure, rapid heartbeat or loss of consciousness.

Diabetes (see Page 281). You may have excessive thirst, hunger and urination, and weight loss. These symptoms may signal diabetes. See your doctor, especially if you have a family history of diabetes. People with diabetes have an increased risk of dehydration, so drink plenty of fluids as recommended by your doctor.

Heatstroke or heat exhaustion (see Page 11). After spending time in strong sunlight or high heat, your temperature is 103° F or higher. You aren't sweating and your skin is dry. You may be confused or cranky; feel faint; have muscle cramps; lose consciousness; or have a seizure (see Page 14). Seek emergency help.

Other causes may include aging, certain medications or mouth breathing.

Self-Care

- If you think you're dehydrated—you have severe thirst, or dark yellow urine—suck on ice chips. Also, sip clear fluids such as water or sports drinks. As you begin to feel better, work your way up to juices, soups, gelatin and applesauce.

Prevention

- Drink plenty of water each day to stay hydrated.
- Avoid caffeine and alcohol.
- Drink water before, during and after exercise. Don't overexert yourself.

SEEK EMERGENCY HELP

▶ You have low urine output, dry mouth and lethargy.

CALL YOUR NURSE INFORMATION SERVICE OR DOCTOR

▶ You're experiencing increased appetite and excessive urination.

▶ You're taking a prescription or over-the-counter medication.

▶ You have a chronic illness, such as diabetes.

▶ You feel weak and fatigued.

TRY SELF-CARE

▶ You have excessive thirst but none of the symptoms or situations listed above.

YOUR CHILD'S SYMPTOMS

Seek emergency help if your child is vomiting or has diarrhea and shows any of these signs of dehydration: small amounts of urine for more than 12 hours; unusual lethargy or irritability; lack of skin elasticity; dry mouth; sunken eyes; and very little saliva or tears.

Excessive thirst and your child. Infants and young children can dehydrate much more quickly than adults. Also, children often ignore thirst because they're easily distracted. Make sure your child drinks plenty of fluids, especially when he's playing outside in hot weather.

When your child is vomiting or has diarrhea, it's very important to keep him hydrated.

THROAT PAIN

Red, painful throat; swallowing may be painful

Causes

Pharyngitis. Your throat may be inflamed and sore. You may have a fever, swollen glands and difficulty swallowing. This common condition is caused by a virus or bacteria.

Strep throat. You may have a fever, painful swallowing, swollen glands under your jaw and white spots on the back of your throat. Strep throat is caused by streptococcus bacteria. This condition is treated with antibiotics—if left untreated, complications can be serious. See your doctor.

Laryngitis. Your vocal cords may be inflamed and swollen. You also may be hoarse or have lost your voice. The cause usually is a virus, allergy or overuse of your voice. Laryngitis can be treated with self-care.

Other causes may include gastroesophageal reflux disease (GERD) (see Page 144), mononucleosis (see Page 126), postnasal drip from allergies (see Page 303), or thyroiditis (see Page 309).

Self-Care

- Try an over-the-counter pain reliever such as acetaminophen, ibuprofen, naproxen sodium or aspirin.

- To soothe your throat:
  - Suck on hard candy or lozenges. Don't give small children lozenges—they can cause choking.
  - Drink fluids. Try soup, or tea with honey or lemon.
  - Gargle with a mixture of 1/4 teaspoon salt in 8 ounces of warm water.
  - Rest your voice.
  - If dry air is the cause, try a cool-mist vaporizer or humidifier to moisten the air and provide relief. Clean it daily or as instructed by the manufacturer.
  - Quit smoking (see Page 25).

Prevention

- Don't smoke.
- Use a cool-mist vaporizer or humidifier. Clean it daily or as instructed by the manufacturer.
- Hand washing can help prevent the spread of infection.
- Don't overuse your voice.

SEEK EMERGENCY HELP

▶ You can't swallow or you have difficulty breathing.

CALL YOUR NURSE INFORMATION SERVICE OR DOCTOR

▶ You have a fever, and white spots or pus in the back of your throat, or a red skin rash.

▶ You have a fever and you've had close contact with someone recently diagnosed with strep throat.

▶ You have severe pain when swallowing.

▶ You've tried self-care but your symptoms haven't improved after 48 hours.

TRY SELF-CARE

▶ You have a sore throat but no other symptoms.

YOUR CHILD'S SYMPTOMS

Seek emergency help if your child has trouble swallowing or is drooling more than usual.

Throat pain and your child. Almost all respiratory illnesses are spread through saliva. Therefore, it's important to avoid sharing eating utensils. Wash hands frequently.

Most respiratory illnesses last seven to 10 days. But some, such as infectious mononucleosis (see Page 126), may cause throat pain for weeks.

! *Don't give aspirin to anyone younger than age 19! It's linked to Reye's syndrome, a rare but sometimes fatal condition.*

TOE PAIN

Soreness in one or more toes

Causes

Hammertoe. One of your toes may be painful and bent, with an arched, claw-like appearance. This condition can occur with age, or from poorly fitting shoes. It also affects people who've had diabetes for a long time and now have nerve damage. Call your nurse information service or doctor.

Mallet toe. Your toe may be painful and curled under at the tip. Mallet toe usually is caused by shoes with high heels and pointy toes that squeeze the front of your foot. Call your nurse information service or doctor.

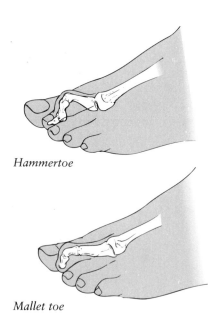

Hammertoe

Mallet toe

Ingrown toenail. The skin around your toenail may be red, swollen or painful, and possibly has green or yellow discharge. An ingrown toenail occurs when the sharp end of a toenail grows into the skin of the toe. It can result from poorly fitting shoes or from improperly cutting your toenails. Try self-care.

Gout. Your big toe becomes red, feels hot and hurts, usually at night. Gout is a type of arthritis that is caused by too much uric acid in the joints. See your doctor—he or she may prescribe medication to reduce the pain and swelling.

Bunion. You have a painful, enlarged, bony bump at the base of your big toe. Your toe may be pushed inward and may overlap your second toe.

Other causes may include dislocation, fracture or trauma to the toe.

Self-Care

If you have diabetes or a circulatory condition, or if your toe is infected, call your doctor before trying self-care.

- Reduce pressure on your toes by wearing sandals or other comfortable shoes. Or, try using a toe pad insert to push your toe back in its proper position. Surgery may be an option for hammertoe, mallet toe or bunions, if you're in pain.

■ If you have an ingrown toenail, soak your foot for 15 to 20 minutes in warm salt water. Gently massage the skin away from the trapped nail. Place a small piece of cotton between your nail and skin for a few days, until the nail grows out, and the skin heals.

■ If you have gout, keep your weight off your affected joint. Put a hot pad or ice pack on it.

Prevention

■ Wear comfortable shoes that fit well. Have your feet measured each time you buy shoes.

■ Cut your toenails straight across using toenail clippers—after you bathe, when your nails are soft.

SEEK EMERGENCY HELP

▶ Your toe is painful and blue, and your foot is cold.

CALL YOUR NURSE INFORMATION SERVICE OR DOCTOR

▶ You have diabetes, or circulatory problems in your legs.

▶ Your toe pain followed an injury.

▶ You have pain and tenderness in your toe—usually the big toe—and the joint is red, warm and swollen.

▶ You have an ingrown toenail with a yellowish-green discharge.

▶ You've tried self-care but your symptoms haven't improved after five days.

TRY SELF-CARE

▶ You have toe pain but none of the symptoms or situations listed above.

TOOTH PAIN

Dull, throbbing or sharp pain in one or more teeth

Causes

Tooth decay. You may have throbbing pain in your tooth. The pain can be triggered by hot or cold food or liquid, or by inhaling cold air through your mouth. You may have a deep cavity, loose filling, or injured tooth. Sugary foods and poor dental hygiene are common causes of tooth decay. See your dentist for treatment.

Gum disease. Your gums may bleed easily and they may be receding, a red-purple color, swollen or shiny. Your teeth may be sensitive to hot or cold, and you may have bad breath. These symptoms indicate gingivitis (see Page 130), a disease that causes the gums to shrink away from the base of the teeth, leaving sensitive areas exposed to temperature shock. See your dentist for treatment. Untreated gum disease can result in tooth loss.

Abscess. You have continuous pain, an uncomfortable bite, a loose tooth or a fever. You could have an abscess, which is the result of pus building up around a tooth with a cavity. An abscess also can be caused by an injury or gum disease. See your dentist.

Other causes may include injury or sinus pain (see Page 303).

Self-Care

- To relieve pain, use ice packs.
- Try an over-the-counter pain reliever such as acetaminophen, ibuprofen, naproxen sodium or aspirin.
- Try toothpaste specifically intended for sensitive teeth. Use it as directed. See your dentist if the pain persists.

Prevention

- See your dentist twice a year for cleanings and preventive checkups.
- Brush twice a day, or more often if directed by your dentist. Floss daily.
- Limit your intake of sugary foods. If you eat something sweet, rinse your mouth with water afterward. Or, snack on nuts or cheese, which neutralize the acid formation triggered by sugar. But keep in mind, these foods can be high in fat and sodium.

SEEK EMERGENCY HELP

▶ You have pain in your lower teeth or neck. You also have chest discomfort and pain in your shoulder, and you're sweating.

CALL YOUR NURSE INFORMATION SERVICE, DOCTOR OR DENTIST

▶ You have pain when you open your mouth wide, an earache and a fever.

▶ You have tenderness over your cheekbones, a fever and nasal congestion.

▶ You have bleeding gums, a fever, swelling, bad breath—even after brushing—or pain all night.

▶ Your tooth hurts only when eating or drinking hot or cold liquids.

TRY SELF-CARE

▶ You have tooth pain but no other symptoms.

YOUR CHILD'S SYMPTOMS

Teething and your child. Children "teethe" until mid-adolescence. The first tooth erupts, on average, at age 6 months. Earlier or later is quite normal, too.

Whether or not babies experience pain when teeth erupt is debatable. Children who can't talk yet, naturally can't explain why they are fussing. Caregivers may then attribute this to teething. Verbal children generally don't complain when teeth erupt.

It's a normal part of oral development for a 4-month-old child to drool, gum, chew on her hands or put objects in her mouth. This occurs months before the first tooth appears.

Check with your doctor before using topical or oral teething medications.

! *Don't give aspirin to anyone younger than age 19! It's linked to Reye's syndrome, a rare but sometimes fatal condition.*

URINARY INCONTINENCE

Inability to hold back urine; dribbling or leaking urine

Causes

Urinary incontinence is a very common problem that has many possible causes. It's important to get a diagnosis from your doctor before trying self-care.

Stress incontinence. You may have urine "leaks" during exercise, coughing, sneezing, laughing, lifting heavy objects or other body movements that put pressure on your bladder. This is common, especially in women. It usually can be treated effectively. Call your nurse information service or doctor.

Uninhibited bladder contractions. You may feel an urgency to urinate that's so strong you may not be able to wait long enough to reach the bathroom. This sometimes is called urge incontinence. It's the most common type of incontinence among older people. It often is managed well with bladder training or medication. Call your nurse information service or doctor.

Bladder infection. You may have urgent, painful, frequent, but not very productive, urination. You also may have blood in your urine, fever, or lower back or pelvic pain. Bladder infections and cystitis are among the most common causes of incontinence. They usually can be treated with antibiotics. Call your nurse information service or doctor.

Prostate condition (see Page 300). You're male and may have difficulty urinating. You often may get up at night to urinate. You may be going more frequently, but with less volume. These could be signs of a prostate condition. Call your nurse information service or doctor.

Estrogen deficiency. You're female and approaching or going through menopause (see Page 317). You may be having embarrassing episodes of leakage. Incontinence has been linked to a decline in estrogen production by the ovaries, which can lead to thinning of the tissues lining the urethra. Hormone replacement therapy may help (see Page 318). Call your nurse information service or doctor.

Other causes may include certain medications, neurological disorders, pregnancy (see Page 321) or recent childbirth, surgery or trauma.

Self-Care

- Use adult diapers or pads only if recommended by your doctor. They may offer security—but they also can irritate your skin. Moreover, you may be tempted to use them instead of seeking professional care. You may need other treatment.

- Try to regain some control over your bladder by going to the bathroom often and regularly.

- Women can learn Kegel exercises to strengthen their pelvic floor muscles. Contract the muscles around your vagina and anus. Hold for a couple of seconds, then relax. Do this throughout the day. You may have heard that one way to practice this exercise is by stopping your urine flow midstream—don't do this. Doing Kegels during urination can increase your risk of urinary tract infections.

- Try "double voiding." Empty your bladder as completely as possible. Then, a couple of minutes later, try to empty it again.

- Practice good hygiene.

Prevention

- Don't drink anything between your dinner and bed-time—especially alcohol or caffeinated drinks.

- Talk with your doctor about any medications you may be taking. They may be contributing to your incontinence.

CALL YOUR NURSE INFORMATION SERVICE OR DOCTOR

▶ You have a fever or pain during urination, or a general feeling of illness.

▶ You have burning during urination, frequent and urgent urination, decreased urine volume, or blood in your urine.

▶ You have lower abdominal pain and a fever. If you're male you also may have pain during ejaculation.

▶ You're a female who has a small leakage of urine when you cough, sneeze, laugh or run.

▶ You're a male who dribbles a small amount of urine after you finish urinating.

URINATION CONCERNS

Pain, burning or discomfort during urination; discolored, cloudy or foul-smelling urine; abnormally large or small amounts of urine; inability to urinate at all, or urinating too frequently

Causes

Diabetes (see Page 281). You may have excessive urination, thirst and hunger. You also may have weight loss. These symptoms may signal diabetes, especially if you have a family history of the disease. See your doctor.

Infection of the kidney, bladder, urinary tract or urethra. You may have a burning sensation during urination. You also may have frequent and urgent urination with only small amounts of urine passed; blood in the urine; lower abdominal pain; pain during intercourse or ejaculation; or a low-grade fever. In addition, you may have sudden fever; shaking chills; severe fatigue; cloudy, bloody, or foul-smelling urine; nausea; or vomiting. You may have one of several kinds of infections. Women are especially likely to develop cystitis, or urinary tract infections. See your doctor. Self-care along with treatment can be helpful.

Blocked urethra. You have sudden urges to urinate but can't pass any urine. This condition most often affects men. See your doctor immediately.

Sexually transmitted disease (see Page 311). You have pain or burning during urination, along with pain during intercourse, discharge from your penis or vagina, or itching around your genital area. These symptoms may indicate a sexually transmitted disease. See your doctor.

Other causes may include bladder disorders or prostate conditions (see Page 300).

Self-Care

- If you have symptoms of an infection, drink plenty of fluids, especially cranberry juice.

Prevention

- Women always should wipe from front to back after a having a bowel movement or urinating. Urinate before and after sexual intercourse. Avoid bubble baths, perfumed soaps or douches. Drink plenty of water each day, and avoid caffeine.

- If you need to urinate frequently at night, limit the amount of liquid you drink late in the day.

- Drink cranberry juice. It may help prevent urinary tract infections.

- Use latex condoms or practice abstinence to help prevent sexually transmitted diseases.

Call your nurse information service or doctor if your child is urinating more often than usual or whimpering when urinating. Or, he has a fever.

SEE YOUR DOCTOR

▶ You're having difficulty urinating, and you have a fever, vomiting, back pain or shaking chills.

▶ You're having difficulty urinating and you're pregnant.

▶ You're having difficulty urinating. You also have had a trauma in the past week, blood in the urine, foul-smelling urine or a history of kidney disease.

▶ You're male and you have a dull, heavy ache in your groin, and a fever.

▶ You have discomfort when urinating, and pain in one side of the small of your back, just above the waist.

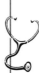

CALL YOUR NURSE INFORMATION SERVICE OR DOCTOR

▶ You have to wait a few moments for urine to flow every time you urinate.

▶ You're passing abnormal amounts of urine. You also are experiencing unexplained fatigue, weight loss and increased thirst.

▶ You have urgent, frequent, burning urination.

URINE, BLOOD IN

Red, pink or brown urine, or red streaks or clots in urine

About Blood in Urine

Color pigments in food, such as beets, and certain bismuth-containing medications, can cause urine to turn red. This isn't the same as blood in your urine—and it's nothing to worry about.

Causes

Bladder infection. You may have urgent, painful, frequent or unproductive urination; blood in the urine; fever; and lower back and pelvic pain. Bladder infections are treated with antibiotics. See your doctor.

Bladder stone. Along with blood in your urine, you urinate often but pass very little, and only when you're in a certain position. You also may have abdominal or lower back pain, and a low-grade fever. See your doctor.

Kidney stone. You may have spasms of pain in your lower back, spreading to your lower abdomen and groin. You also may have an urge to urinate, but only pass a small amount of blood-tinged urine. See your doctor.

Glomerulonephritis. You may have blood in your urine, along with swelling of your ankles or around your eyes, shortness of breath, and fatigue. You may have a sudden or chronic inflammation of the structures in your kidneys that filter blood. See your doctor.

Hemolytic anemia. There may be blood in your urine, and you're tired, weak or short of breath. Your skin may be jaundiced, or yellow. Hemolytic anemia sometimes is caused by a genetic abnormality in the red blood cells. It also can be caused by certain medications and infectious diseases that destroy red blood cells. When these cells are destroyed, bone marrow can't produce replacement cells quickly enough. For people who have a genetic deficiency of a certain enzyme, some medications may trigger hemolytic anemia. See your doctor.

Benign hematuria. You may have blood in your urine but no other symptoms. This is a nonprogressive condition that can appear and then disappear. Call your nurse information service or doctor.

Other causes may include sexually transmitted diseases (see Page 311) or a urinary tract tumor.

Taking Care: Self-Care for You and Your Family

Self-Care

Self-care isn't appropriate if you have blood in your urine.

Prevention

- Drink plenty of water each day.
- Use latex condoms or practice abstinence to help prevent sexually transmitted diseases.
- Urinate before and after sexual intercourse.
- Take showers instead of baths, and use mild soaps.

SEE YOUR DOCTOR

▶ You have blood in your urine and you have any of the following: swelling of the ankles or around the eyes; shortness of breath; vomiting; fever; impaired vision; back pain; or chills.

CALL YOUR NURSE INFORMATION SERVICE OR DOCTOR

▶ You have passed pink, red, or smoky- or clear-brown urine.

▶ You have fatigue, nausea or loss of appetite.

▶ You have itching, headaches, or a frequent or urgent need to urinate.

VAGINAL BLEEDING

Bleeding between menstrual periods, during pregnancy or after menopause

Causes

Menopause (see Page 317). You're age 38 or older. Your menstrual periods may be coming more frequently than usual. Or, you may be bleeding after a few months of no periods at all. Irregular bleeding is normal prior to menopause. Ask your doctor if hormone replacement therapy is right for you. Any postmenopausal bleeding should be reported to your doctor.

Birth control (see Page 319). You recently may have had an intrauterine device (IUD) inserted. Perhaps you're taking birth control pills. These contraceptive methods may cause spotting between periods. Call your nurse information service or doctor if you're concerned.

Miscarriage. Bleeding during pregnancy may be a sign of miscarriage. However, some women bleed throughout the first trimester of pregnancy. See your doctor if you're pregnant and spotting.

Ectopic pregnancy. You may have bleeding along with abdominal pain, and you're pregnant. This may be a sign of an ectopic pregnancy—a pregnancy developing outside the uterus (see illustration). Seek emergency help.

Other causes may include cervical polyps, cervicitis or dysfunctional uterine bleeding.

Self-Care

- Use pads or tampons as you would during a normal period.
- Avoid regular use of aspirin and extended ibuprofen use. They can affect blood clotting and may cause prolonged bleeding.

Prevention

- If your birth control device causes spotting between periods, consider switching to another method.
- Get preventive health exams.

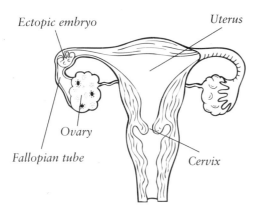

Ectopic embryo

Uterus

Ovary

Fallopian tube

Cervix

SEEK EMERGENCY HELP

▶ You could be pregnant, and you have bleeding and abdominal pain.

▶ You have shaking chills—not just shivering.

▶ You have severe abdominal pain.

▶ You feel faint since bleeding began.

▶ You have been soaking a sanitary pad every hour, or a tampon every 15 minutes, for four hours or more.

SEE YOUR DOCTOR

▶ You've had unexplained vaginal bleeding of any kind.

▶ You're pregnant, and you have bleeding but no pain.

▶ You had your last period one year ago or more.

CALL YOUR NURSE INFORMATION SERVICE OR DOCTOR

▶ Your last period was more than six months ago, and you're age 38 or older.

▶ You're experiencing a heavy, watery vaginal discharge.

▶ You have vaginal bleeding after intercourse or douching.

▶ You have an intrauterine device (IUD) in place or you're taking birth control pills; or you're on hormone replacement therapy.

YOUR CHILD'S SYMPTOMS

Vaginal bleeding and your child. A female infant may have bloody discharge from her vagina in the first weeks of life. This is due to the normal decrease in hormones.

On average, menstruation begins between ages 12 to 14 years. However, many girls start earlier or later. During the first three years, irregular periods are normal (see Page 316).

In children, vaginal bleeding sometimes can be a sign of sexual abuse or the presence of a foreign object, whether or not menstruation has begun. Call your nurse information service or doctor.

VAGINAL DISCHARGE OR ITCH

Vaginal itching; or excessive, discolored, foul-smelling discharge

Causes

Yeast infection. You may have a thick, white, foul-smelling discharge. You also may have irritation or itching around the vagina. A yeast infection is a fungal infection. It often develops in women with diabetes; during pregnancy; or after taking antibiotics or birth control pills. If this is the first time you're experiencing these symptoms, see your doctor for a diagnosis, then try self-care.

Trichomoniasis. You may have greenish or foul-smelling discharge. Trichomoniasis is caused by a microscopic organism. It can result in vaginal infections and inflammation of the urethra. See your doctor.

Pelvic inflammatory disease or salpingitis. You may have a discolored, foul-smelling vaginal discharge and pelvic pain. You also may have a low-grade fever and chills; fatigue; low back pain; irregular menstrual bleeding; and loss of appetite. You may have pelvic inflammatory disease (PID). Or, you may have salpingitis—an infection of your fallopian tubes. See your doctor immediately.

Other causes may include atrophic vaginitis, a forgotten tampon or diaphragm, or sexually transmitted diseases (see Page 311).

Self-Care

- If you have vaginal itching, try a sitz bath—sit in a bathtub of enough warm (not hot) water to completely cover your genitals. These baths help speed healing, keep the area clean and provide comfort.

- Avoid scratching.

- If you have a yeast infection, try an over-the-counter treatment.

- Wear cotton underpants. Avoid wearing pantyhose and tight pants.

Prevention

- Use latex condoms or practice abstinence to help prevent sexually transmitted diseases.

- If you're prone to yeast infections and you're using an antibiotic, eat yogurt with live, active cultures.

SEEK EMERGENCY HELP

▶ You have heavy, foul-smelling discharge two or more days after childbirth.

▶ You have shaking chills, not just shivering.

SEE YOUR DOCTOR

▶ You're pregnant and notice a change in the color or consistency of your vaginal discharge.

CALL YOUR NURSE INFORMATION SERVICE OR DOCTOR

▶ You have vaginal discharge with abnormal color or odor. You also have lower pelvic or back pain, irregular menstrual bleeding or other signs of being sick.

▶ Your discharge is thick, and white or yellowish-green. You're taking birth control pills or using an intrauterine device (IUD).

▶ It's possible you've forgotten to remove a tampon or diaphragm.

▶ You have vaginal itching plus any of the following: unexplained weight loss, increased thirst or hunger, or frequent urination.

▶ You're age 38 or older. You have irregular periods, and feel sore, itchy or a burning sensation around your vagina, or are experiencing painful intercourse.

▶ You've tried self-care but the discharge or itching hasn't improved after five days.

TRY SELF-CARE

▶ Your vagina feels irritated, sore or itchy for no apparent reason.

YOUR CHILD'S SYMPTOMS

Call your nurse information service or doctor if your child hasn't reached puberty and she has unusual discharge, itching or soreness. Vaginal discharge is unusual in girls before puberty. In such a case, possible sexual abuse should be considered. Other causes include streptococcus, other bacteria or yeast.

Vaginal discharge and your child. In infants, a mucousy, white vaginal discharge during the first weeks of life is normal.

If your child has vaginal discharge, these tips may make her more comfortable:

■ Gently wash the area twice a day with plain water.

■ Have her wear cotton underpants. Be sure to wash them with perfume-free, additive-free detergent.

■ Teach her to wipe from front to back after using the toilet.

■ Be sure that she avoids long periods in a wet bathing suit.

VISION PROBLEM

Ability to see has worsened; symptoms may include blurring, seeing double images, flashing lights or floating spots

Causes

Aging. You're age 50 or older, and your vision has worsened. Some visual changes are normal with age.

Retinal detachment. You may have a sudden appearance of "floaters," and you see brief, bright flashes of light. You may have lost some central or peripheral vision. See your doctor or ophthalmologist immediately. Prompt treatment can help prevent permanent damage. If you have floaters but no other symptoms, you probably don't have retinal detachment.

Dry macular degeneration. You may have started having slightly blurred vision. It then progressed to a blurred spot in the center of your vision. Dry macular degeneration is a disease that develops slowly in older adults. Though there isn't a proven treatment yet, research is ongoing. People with this condition still can lead active lives for many years. See your doctor.

Cataracts (see Page 267). You may have cloudy, blurry or double vision, or frequent (yearly) changes in your eyeglass prescription. You also may have sensitivity to light and glare. Cataracts are extremely common in older adults. They can be treated successfully with surgery. See your doctor.

Glaucoma (see Page 267). You notice your side vision worsening or completely disappearing. You may have open-angle glaucoma. See your doctor for diagnosis and treatment.

Other causes may include diabetes (see Page 281), eye strain, migraines (see Page 290), optic neuritis, temporal arteritis or wet macular degeneration.

Self-Care

- Rest your eyes if you spend a lot of time using a computer or reading small print. Focus your eyes on something else every 10 to 15 minutes.

- If you're seeing floaters, try rapidly moving your eyes up and down. This action stirs up the eyeballs' fluid, causing the floaters to settle outside your line of vision.

Prevention

- Get regular preventive eye exams once a year, especially if you're age 50 or older.

- Wear sunglasses to protect your eyes from bright light and ultraviolet rays.

- Don't smoke.

- Eat a balanced diet that includes dark, leafy green vegetables such as spinach, broccoli and brussels sprouts.

SEEK EMERGENCY HELP

▶ **You have blurred or double vision with a severe, sudden headache and loss of consciousness.**

▶ **You have paralysis on one side of your face or body.**

SEE YOUR DOCTOR

▶ **You have blurred vision and pain in one eye.**

▶ **Your vision is suddenly blurred, or you've started seeing halos or rainbows around lights.**

▶ **You've been seeing flashing lights or the sudden appearance of numerous floating spots.**

CALL YOUR NURSE INFORMATION SERVICE OR DOCTOR

▶ **Your vision has gradually blurred, and you're age 50 or older.**

YOUR CHILD'S SYMPTOMS

Call your nurse information service or doctor if your child's vision suddenly seems to change. For example, he may blink or squint often; complain of not being able to see the blackboard in school; or doesn't seem to recognize familiar people from several feet away. Also, call for information about "lazy eye"— an eye that wanders, especially when your child is tired.

Vision problems and your child. Children may not be able to tell you when they're having problems with their vision. A child who always watches television with his head turned to one side may have a vision problem in one eye.

WART

Small, raised, painless, rough bump on the skin; same color as the surrounding skin or slightly darker

About Warts

Warts are an extremely common skin condition. Many warts are harmless, and most disappear within two years. Warts are caused by the human papillomavirus (HPV), of which there are more than 60 types. The virus is contagious and enters the skin through tiny breaks in the skin's surface.

- Common warts most often appear on the hands and fingers.
- Plantar warts appear on the soles of the feet.
- Periungual warts are found around the fingernails and toenails.
- Digitate warts are small, finger-like projections that are located on the scalp.
- Flat warts cluster in groups of as many as several hundred.
- Genital and anal warts result from sexual transmission of HPV (see Page 311). See your doctor.

Self-Care

- Over-the-counter wart removers usually are effective. Follow the package directions exactly. Don't use wart removers on your face or genitals, or on any area that's infected or red. See your doctor if you have diabetes or poor blood circulation. He or she can remove your warts safely.

Prevention

- Don't bite or pick at warts. This causes them to spread to other areas of your skin.
- Wear sandals in public showers.
- Don't touch someone else's wart.
- Use latex condoms or practice abstinence to help prevent sexually transmitted diseases.

SEE YOUR DOCTOR

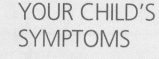

▶ You or your sexual partner has genital or anal warts.

▶ You have many warts on your body.

▶ You have warts on your face.

▶ You're immunocompromised.

▶ You've tried self-care but your symptoms haven't improved after three months.

TRY SELF-CARE

▶ You've just developed a new wart and you have none of the symptoms or situations listed above.

YOUR CHILD'S SYMPTOMS

Warts and your child. Warts are more common in children and teens than in adults. Reassure your child that warts are nothing serious. Unless they hurt or are on the bottom of her feet, consider waiting for the warts to go away on their own.

WEIGHT GAIN

Steady or sudden weight gain without having changed eating or exercise patterns

Causes

Medication. You may have gained weight after taking steroids—which you may know as cortisone drugs—oral contraceptives, antidepressants or nonsteroidal anti-inflammatory drugs (NSAIDs) including ibuprofen or naproxen sodium. Call your nurse information service or doctor.

Edema. You've gained weight and your ankles, legs or abdomen may appear swollen. You also may be urinating less, or more often, during the night. You may be suffering from fluid accumulation in your tissues due to congestive heart failure (see Page 275) or kidney disease. If left untreated, these are life-threatening conditions. See your doctor immediately.

Hypothyroidism (see Page 308). Along with weight gain, you may have increased sensitivity to cold; dry skin; drowsiness or exhaustion; or thinning hair. Hypothyroidism, or underactive thyroid, is a condition in which the thyroid doesn't produce enough thyroid hormone. Synthetic hormones can treat this condition successfully. See your doctor.

Other causes may include depression (see Page 332).

Self-Care

■ If you've recently quit smoking, healthy lifestyle choices can help you control your weight. Exercise regularly. Eat a balanced diet. Drink plenty of water each day. And, try to eat healthy snacks as you cope with your cravings (see Page 17).

Prevention

■ Work closely with your doctor to develop a safe weight control plan.

CALL YOUR NURSE INFORMATION SERVICE OR DOCTOR

► You have swelling of your ankles, legs or abdomen.

► You have insomnia, fatigue, heart problems, shortness of breath, dry skin, or you've started a new medication.

► You urinate more at night, feel colder than usual, or your hair is thinning.

TRY SELF-CARE

► You've recently quit smoking.

YOUR CHILD'S SYMPTOMS

See your doctor to determine if your child's weight is appropriate for her age.

WEIGHT LOSS

Sudden or unexplained loss of weight

Causes

Eating disorder (see Page 333). Anorexia nervosa is intentional starving. Bulimia is binge eating followed by purging—forced vomiting or the intentional misuse of laxatives. These are two very common eating disorders. They are most common in teen girls and women, but they can affect boys and men, too. You may be underweight according to height and weight charts. Yet, you still limit food intake because you feel you need to lose more. Or, your weight may be normal but you're afraid of gaining weight. You may exercise excessively or to extreme in order to lose weight. Eating disorders can be life-threatening. See your doctor immediately.

Depression (see Page 332). You've recently lost weight. You also may have feelings of sadness, guilt, worthlessness or anxiety. Your sleep patterns may have changed. You may feel easily irritated. These are symptoms of depression. See your doctor or a counselor. If you or someone you know has thoughts of suicide, seek emergency help.

Chronic infection. You may have weight loss plus drenching night sweats, recurring fever, persistent or bloody cough, and a general feeling of being sick.

These symptoms may be caused by a number of chronic infections. See your doctor for a diagnosis.

Other causes may include inflammatory disorders, malignancies, metabolic disorders, nutrient malabsorption or thyroid conditions (see Page 308).

Self-Care

Self-care isn't appropriate if you have any unexplained weight loss. See your doctor.

Prevention

- Eat a balanced diet (see Page 17).
- Get preventive health exams (see Page 31).

CALL YOUR NURSE INFORMATION SERVICE OR DOCTOR

► Your bowel movements have become irregular. You've had diarrhea or constipation, or have seen blood in your stool.

► You have any of these symptoms: fatigue; night sweats; a fever or cough with or without blood; unusual thirst or frequent urination.

► You have persistent diarrhea or unusually pale, floating stools.

► You have any of the eating disorder symptoms listed on the previous page.

WOUND, PUNCTURE

Injury caused by a sharp, pointed object

About Puncture Wounds

The primary concern with puncture wounds is infection. See your doctor if you have a puncture wound. Because it can take about 24 hours for signs of infection to show, your doctor may prescribe antibiotics right away to avoid any complications. You also may need a tetanus shot, especially if your last tetanus shot was more than five years ago or you're unsure of your tetanus status.

If you have a puncture wound and there's a great deal of blood loss, or blood is spurting from the wound, seek emergency help.

Self-Care

- If the object that caused the puncture is small and still in the wound, remove it. Soak tweezers for 20 minutes in rubbing alcohol. Remove the object with the tweezers, being careful not to cause more injury. Clean the wound with warm water and soap. Leave it uncovered unless there's a chance it will get dirty.
- Clean the wound in warm, soapy water two to three times a day for five days.

- If the object that caused the puncture is large and still in the wound, seek emergency help.

Prevention

- Safely store sharp tools and kitchen utensils.
- Wear heavy gloves when doing construction or repair work.
- Wear shoes when walking outside.
- Make sure to get your tetanus booster shots on schedule.

SEEK EMERGENCY HELP

▶ The puncture wound is to your head, neck, abdomen or chest.

▶ The puncture wound is from a needle used by another person.

▶ The puncture wound has penetrated a joint.

▶ You have difficulty moving your arms, legs, fingers or toes. The wound spurts blood, or has rapid swelling or foreign material that won't wash out.

SEE YOUR DOCTOR

▶ You have symptoms of infection—a fever, pus, extensive redness and swelling, or red streaks leading away from the injury.

▶ You feel numbness or tingling below the site of the wound.

▶ The wound is deep, contaminated or dirty.

▶ The puncture wound is on your hand.

▶ You have diabetes or circulatory impairment.

CALL YOUR NURSE INFORMATION SERVICE OR DOCTOR

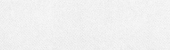

▶ The wound isn't deep.

▶ Your last tetanus shot was more than five years ago or you're unsure of your tetanus status.

▶ The wound is on the sole of your foot.

WRIST PAIN

Pain, or numbness and tingling in one or both wrists

Causes

Arthritis (see Page 255). You may have pain and swelling or stiffness in your wrist or in other joints. You also may have limited movement in your wrist. Symptoms of arthritis vary depending on the type. See your doctor.

Carpal tunnel syndrome and repetitive motion injuries. You may have pain, numbness and tingling that often gets worse at night, in your wrists and hands from the thumb to the ring finger. Parts of your hands may be weak. Carpal tunnel syndrome is common among people who do repetitive work or activity with their hands, such as keyboarding, assembly-line work, knitting, golfing or sewing. It occurs when the tendons between the arm and hand become inflamed and swollen. They then begin to close in on the major nerve of the wrist. See your doctor.

Injury. You may have pain and throbbing in your wrist, possibly after falling. You also may notice a clicking or grinding sound coming from the joint. Sprains and strains are the most common wrist injuries. Dislocations and fractures also can cause wrist pain. See your doctor if the pain is severe.

Infection. You may have pain in your wrist, along with swelling that developed rapidly, and a fever. You may need antibiotics if you have a bacterial infection. See your doctor.

Other causes may include ganglion cyst (see Page 134) or tendinitis (see Page 134).

Self-Care

- If carpal tunnel syndrome is the cause, break up repetitive tasks by resting or alternating activity. Be sure your computer keyboard allows optimal hand, wrist and arm positioning.

- Splint your wrists so they remain stable. Wear the splint constantly for three to four days, then just at night for a few more weeks, as needed.

- If the wrist pain is caused by an injury, elevate the wrist, and apply a cold pack for 10 to 15 minutes to decrease pain and swelling. Do this three to four times a day for the first 24 to 48 hours. Once the swelling has gone down, apply warm, moist heat for 15 to 20 minutes, three times a day. Securely, but not too tightly, wrap an elastic bandage around your wrist to reduce swelling and to help protect it.

- Try an over-the-counter pain reliever such as acetaminophen, ibuprofen, naproxen sodium or aspirin.

Prevention

- Take frequent breaks from any strenuous work or activity that requires repetitive hand motions. Vary your movements so that your wrists aren't constantly bent.

- Use a wrist-support pad while typing or keyboarding.

- Wear protective gear such as wrist guards when playing sports.

SEEK EMERGENCY HELP

▶ You've had an injury and your wrist looks deformed.

▶ Your wrist shows signs of impaired circulation—pale, blue or gray, and feels cold.

▶ You feel a sudden weakness, paralysis or loss of feeling in your wrist.

SEE YOUR DOCTOR

▶ After an injury, your wrist is discolored or sore to the touch.

CALL YOUR NURSE INFORMATION SERVICE OR DOCTOR

▶ You have severe pain in your wrist even when you rest it. You also have swelling and a fever.

▶ You have a persistent lump in your wrist.

▶ You can't move your wrist through the normal range of motion.

▶ You can't make a fist or button a shirt, and you're frequently dropping things.

TRY SELF-CARE

▶ You have numbness or tingling, pain in your forearm or hand, or the pain gets worse at night.

YOUR CHILD'S SYMPTOMS

! *Don't give aspirin to anyone younger than age 19! It's linked to Reye's syndrome, a rare but sometimes fatal condition.*

Long-Term Conditions

Our lives can be profoundly affected by long-term health conditions. Perhaps you've recently been diagnosed with an illness. Maybe you've been coping with a health issue for a long time. Or, you may be a caregiver whose loved one has chronic health concerns. The physical and emotional aspects of a long-term condition can be challenging.

The following pages provide valuable information about 22 long-term conditions. You and your loved ones can learn helpful tips and strategies for day-to-day living.

This chapter can help you:

- Recognize signs and symptoms
- Learn about prevention techniques and treatments
- Stay active as you learn more about managing your condition
- Develop an open discussion with your doctor
- Cope with your condition or cope as a caregiver

Use this information as a starting point for a conversation with your doctor. Also, be sure to refer to the Resources section of this book for the additional information and support you may need.

ALZHEIMER'S DISEASE

What is Alzheimer's disease?

Alzheimer's is a progressive, degenerative disease that affects the brain. It causes impaired memory and mental abilities. Alzheimer's is the most common form of dementia—the loss of mental abilities so severe that daily functioning becomes difficult. Researchers haven't found a way to cure or prevent it. However, great progress is being made in understanding and treating this complex condition.

What are the causes?

Scientists still are unclear as to the exact cause of Alzheimer's disease. However, some theories include genetic predisposition and environmental toxins.

What are the symptoms?

Being forgetful from time to time—no matter what your age—is normal. But Alzheimer's causes more than forgetfulness. People with this disease experience dramatic changes in thinking, reasoning and behavior. Symptoms include:

Increasing forgetfulness—trouble remembering recent events, the names of close friends and relatives, and common, everyday objects

Disorientation—losing a sense of time or day; or getting lost in familiar surroundings, such as your street or home

Poor judgment—increased difficulty planning or making decisions; or making inappropriate decisions such as wearing a bathrobe to the store

Problems with language—forgetting simple words; or using improper words or phrases to complete sentences

Difficulty doing routine things—once-simple tasks such as cooking or brushing teeth become challenging

Changes in behavior, personality or mood—experiencing rapid mood swings for no reason, or dramatic personality changes

Misplacing objects—putting things in inappropriate places, such as storing an iron in the refrigerator

Occasionally misplacing your keys or forgetting someone's name doesn't mean you have Alzheimer's disease. Alzheimer's symptoms are much more severe and debilitating.

See your doctor if you have symptoms that concern you. He or she may conduct physical, psychiatric or neurological evaluations, and blood or urine tests.

252

But don't assume that Alzheimer's disease will be the diagnosis. Some people may have symptoms of dementia due to depression, drug interactions, thyroid problems, stroke or Parkinson's disease. That's why it's important to see your doctor whenever you have any symptoms.

How is Alzheimer's treated?

When someone has Alzheimer's disease, lifestyle changes often need to be made. In the early stages, it may be beneficial to modify the home environment, including lighting, color and noise. Use easy-to-read clocks and calendars. Maintaining a dependable daily routine also may help. This may provide solace and reduce confusion or frustration.

Your doctor may prescribe medications such as cholinesterase inhibitors to enhance memory. Other medications can decrease symptoms such as sleeplessness, agitation, anxiety and depression. Your doctor may recommend antioxidant vitamins. Talk with him or her about which treatments are right for you or your loved one. An open, honest relationship with your health care provider can help ease your fears.

How can I cope?

In the early stages of Alzheimer's disease, you still can lead a normal life. Staying active and enjoying yourself can be therapeutic and comforting. This is also a good time to start thinking about the future.

Preparing for the transitions that will take place can give you peace of mind. Discuss these changes with your spouse, family and friends. There are things you can do to maximize your quality of life, and help your loved ones, too.

- Continue doing the things you enjoy. However, you may need to modify these activities to match your abilities. Use calendars and reminder notes to help you remember things.
- Discuss caregiver services with your spouse or family members. Talk openly about preferences or concerns. Review financial and legal issues with loved ones, as well.
- Maintain your health. Get regular checkups and follow your doctor's advice. Eat healthfully and rest when you're tired. Avoid any unnecessary prescription and over-the-counter medications. Don't smoke, and limit how much alcohol you drink.
- Take care of your mental health. Don't keep your emotions to yourself. Attend support groups and counseling sessions—alone, and with your loved ones. Let friends and family members help you.

How can caregivers cope?

Being a caregiver to someone with Alzheimer's disease requires time, dedication and patience. It's important to keep the bond with your loved one strong. But don't forget that your own health and well-being are important, too. These tips may help:

- Be aware of your nonverbal language. Regardless of how you feel, convey calmness by smiling, hugging or holding hands with your loved one.

- Provide a safe, structured environment. Unfamiliar situations can cause anxiety and distress to a person with Alzheimer's.

- Speak slowly and clearly. To avoid confusion, use simple sentences that present only one idea.

- Accept help from family, friends and home health aides. Let someone take some of the weight off your shoulders—this can help you feel more relaxed and refreshed. Check out local community resources that provide respite care.

- Don't keep your emotions bottled up—share them. Join a caregiver support group, or simply talk with those close to you about your feelings.

- Acknowledge that you can't do it all. There may be a time when you'll need to rely on outside help. Prepare for this possibility by researching adult day care programs and housing options such as assisted living or nursing homes.

Undeniably, Alzheimer's disease can be a physically and emotionally draining condition. Whether it's you or a loved one living with Alzheimer's, remember you're not alone. Working with your doctor, family and friends can help you face the challenges ahead.

WHEN TO SEEK HELP

Call your nurse information service or doctor if:

▶ **You notice increasingly frequent or severe memory lapses.**

▶ **You notice persistent and unexplained personality or behavioral changes.**

For related information, see: Anxiety, Page 330; Caregiver's Concerns, Page 331; Confusion and Forgetfulness, Page 78; Depression, Page 332; Insomnia, Page 154; Parkinson's Disease, Page 296; Stroke, Page 305; Thyroid Conditions, Page 308

ARTHRITIS

Arthritis is characterized by joint pain, swelling and stiffness. There are more than 100 types. Osteoarthritis and rheumatoid arthritis are the two most common adult forms. The most common type affecting children is juvenile rheumatoid arthritis.

What is osteoarthritis?

Osteoarthritis (OA) occurs when the cartilage that cushions joints becomes irregular. This is known as degenerative—or wear-and-tear—arthritis. With this breakdown of cartilage, bones rub together. This can cause pain and difficulty moving. OA most often occurs in middle-aged and older adults. It affects joints in the fingers, knees, hips, feet and spine. OA may occur with repeated episodes of gout.

Causes. Age is a major risk factor for OA. But, OA isn't an inevitable part of aging. Other risk factors include:

- Heredity
- Obesity
- Previous joint infections
- A history of joint injuries or overuse
- Repeated episodes of gout
- Certain metabolic disorders such as hemochromatosis

Symptoms. OA may develop in one or more joints on one or both sides of your body. Signs and symptoms include:

- Stiffness or pain after inactivity that improves after 30 to 60 minutes
- Joint pain and sometimes swelling as a result of too much activity
- Grinding sensation or cracking noise during movement
- Bony bumps at the end or on the middle joint of fingers

Prevention. Maintaining muscle strength and optimal weight may help prevent OA. If possible, avoid activities with repetitive movements, or those that overuse your joints.

Treatment. See your doctor regularly if you have arthritis. He or she may prescribe medication or suggest an over-the-counter pain reliever such as acetaminophen. In certain cases, your doctor may inject a corticosteroid drug to decrease inflammation around your joint.

To help relieve pain and stiffness:

- Try exercises such as swimming, water aerobics, yoga or tai chi. They can help keep joints flexible, and supporting muscles strong. Before exercising, check with your doctor.

- Soak in a warm bath.
- Apply heat to stiff or painful joints.

What is rheumatoid arthritis?

Rheumatoid arthritis (RA) causes pain, stiffness, warmth, redness and swelling around the joints. RA is an autoimmune disease. This means that the body's immune system attacks healthy tissue—in this case, joint tissue. This results in inflammation and joint damage. RA generally affects more than one joint at a time. Typically, it may affect elbows, shoulders, knees, neck, hands, wrists, feet and ankles. Often, joints are affected symmetrically—on both sides of the body. More women than men have RA. It usually develops in middle-age.

Causes. The cause of RA is unknown. But some theories include genetics and viruses.

Symptoms. If you have RA, you may experience:

- Pain, swelling, limited motion, and warmth around affected joints
- General fatigue and soreness
- Stiffness after inactivity—known as gelling—lasting more than one hour
- Painless lumps below the skin—especially around the elbows
- Weight loss
- Loss of mobility

Prevention. Unfortunately, because RA is an autoimmune disease, it can't be prevented.

Treatment. Treatment of RA aims to reduce swelling, pain, inflammation and stiffness. Your doctor may prescribe medications including nonsteroidal anti-inflammatory drugs (NSAIDs) such as ibuprofen, naproxen sodium or aspirin. Some prescription drugs can slow or stop the disease. For some people, combining medications with exercise, rest, and physical and occupational therapy can control RA. Your doctor will know what's best for your situation. He or she also may refer you to a rheumatologist.

What is juvenile rheumatoid arthritis?

Juvenile rheumatoid arthritis (JRA) is an autoimmune disease. It generally occurs in children ages 16 years and younger. JRA often affects joints in the knees, hands and feet. It can hinder bone growth and development. Symptoms include persistent joint swelling, pain and redness. If your child limps in the morning, especially along with having a fever, see your doctor.

Unlike adult rheumatoid arthritis, JRA is a condition children can outgrow. Your child's doctor may recommend treatments to reduce swelling, relieve pain and prevent complications.

How can I cope?

Work with your doctor to develop a plan for living life to the fullest. Read up on the latest arthritis developments. Research is ongoing and may result in new treatments that offer relief. Talk with your doctor about exercises that may help ease your discomfort. Connect with a support group or arthritis-related organization. By talking with others, you may learn how to perform daily activities more easily.

If your child has arthritis, he may feel angry, discouraged or frustrated. Allow your child to express his or her emotions. Interacting with peers who also have arthritis may help, too.

WHEN TO SEEK HELP

Call your nurse information service or doctor if:

▶ Joint pain interferes with your normal activities, is severe or won't go away.

For related information, see: Caregiver's Concerns, Page 331; Chronic Pain, Page 273; Complementary Medicine, Page 335; Dry Eye, Page 104; Fatigue, Page 114; Joint Pain, Page 160; Maintain a Healthy Weight, Page 21; Medications, Page 37

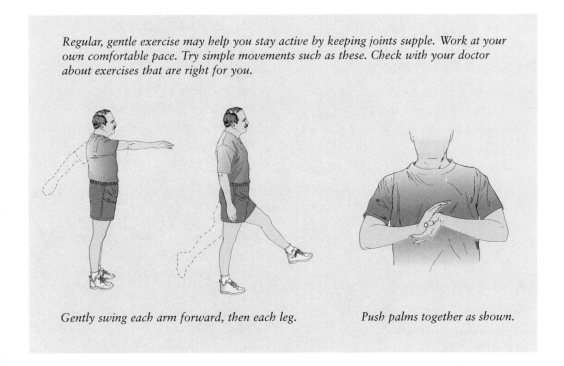

Regular, gentle exercise may help you stay active by keeping joints supple. Work at your own comfortable pace. Try simple movements such as these. Check with your doctor about exercises that are right for you.

Gently swing each arm forward, then each leg.

Push palms together as shown.

ASTHMA

What is asthma?

Asthma is a chronic inflammatory condition in which airflow into and out of the lungs becomes blocked. This is due to changes that occur in the bronchial tubes, such as inflammation, overproduction of mucus, swelling of the air passages and tightening of the muscles in the air passages. When this happens, airways narrow, and breathing becomes difficult.

What causes asthma attacks?

Asthma attacks may start suddenly or take days to develop. Either way, they often are triggered by factors that set off a reaction in your lungs. Asthma triggers and irritants include:

- Allergens such as dust and dust mites, pollen, mold and pet dander—tiny flakes of hair, feathers or skin
- Irritants such as tobacco and wood smoke, chemical fumes, poor air quality, strong odors or scents, and certain weather conditions such as cold air or extreme winds
- Viral or sinus infections, including colds, flu or pneumonia
- Exercise or physical activity
- Certain medications and foods
- Gastroesophageal reflux disease (GERD)

What are the symptoms?

Most asthma attacks are mild to moderate. Taking your medication should relieve symptoms. You may experience:

- Tightness in your chest
- Wheezing or making whistling sounds when you breathe out
- Coughing or spitting up sputum
- Shortness of breath
- Restlessness or trouble sleeping

If you experience any severe symptoms, seek emergency help.

Can asthma attacks be prevented?

If you have asthma, work with your doctor to identify what's triggering your attacks. That way, you can prevent attacks from happening in the first place. Of course, certain triggers may be more difficult to control than others.

The following tips may help:

- Don't own a pet. If you do, have someone bathe it weekly to minimize dander. If possible, keep your pet outdoors or restrict it to certain areas of the house.
- Change air conditioner and furnace filters often.

258

- To help get rid of dust mites, use air-tight mattresses and pillow covers. Wash bedding weekly in hot (at least 130° F) water. Remove carpeting from your bedroom. Dust and mop as often as possible. Use a High Efficiency Particulate Arresting (HEPA) filtered vacuum cleaner. Replace window blinds with shades, which don't collect as much dust. Store off-season clothes in plastic garment bags.

- To prevent mold and mildew, use dehumidifiers in basements and rooms where humidity is high. Don't place rugs or carpeting in the basement or bathroom.

- Don't use perfume, cleaning supplies, deodorizers or other substances that have strong fumes or odors.

- Don't smoke, and avoid secondhand smoke.

- Avoid wood stoves and fireplaces.

- To keep from getting sick, wash your hands often. Don't spend too much time around others who are ill.

- If you're outdoors in cold weather, cover your face with a scarf to avoid breathing in cold air.

- If you have asthma attacks while exercising, tell your doctor. He or she may prescribe medication you can take before exercising to help prevent attacks.

- If your doctor prescribes controller medication, follow instructions carefully and don't skip any doses.

- After your doctor teaches you how to use a peak flow meter, use it regularly to monitor your progress.

Practicing these and other habits can help keep asthma attacks at bay. Your doctor can provide additional information and tips.

How can asthma be monitored?

Along with seeing your doctor regularly, asthma can be monitored with a hand-held device called a peak flow meter, which measures your ability to push air out of your lungs.

This measurement helps your doctor determine which medications to prescribe. It can indicate whether you need to change your dosage or the way you're using your medicines. A peak flow meter can show whether your asthma is under control. It also can warn if an attack is coming.

Discuss with your doctor how to use your meter, how to chart your peak flow rates and how you can determine what your normal peak flow rate is.

How is asthma treated?

The goal of asthma medications is to reduce inflammation, reverse symptoms and prevent attacks. Controller medications are designed for overall asthma management. It's important to note that controller medications aren't effective in acute situations. Rescue medications are used for those sudden, acute attacks that call for quick action.

Asthma medications come in many forms—including sprays, pills and liquids. With careful monitoring, you and your doctor can choose the best form for you. Medications include:

Anti-inflammatories—prevent attacks from starting. They keep air passages open, reduce swelling and decrease the amount of mucus.

Bronchodilators—help stop asthma attacks that already have started. They relax the muscles in your air passages and make breathing easier.

Leukotriene modifiers—fight the chemicals that are responsible for causing inflammation in air passages.

How can I cope?

With lifestyle changes and careful management, you can keep your asthma under control. See your doctor regularly—your triggers and symptoms may change.

Remember to take your medications as directed by your doctor. Don't skip doses just because you feel well. Also, make sure your family and friends know how to help you in case you have an asthma attack. Wear a medical identification bracelet.

If you have asthma, learn as much as possible about this condition. Remember, the more educated and empowered you are, the better you'll feel—physically and mentally.

If you're a parent whose child has asthma, encourage her to learn about it. This will help increase her confidence level. Create an action plan for your child's school nurse. Include information about triggers and how to help your child if she has an attack.

WHEN TO SEEK HELP

If you have a severe asthma attack, take your asthma medication and *seek emergency help immediately.* During a severe attack, you may experience:

▶ **Gasping for air and extreme breathlessness**

▶ **Rapid pulse**

▶ **Sweating and anxiety**

▶ **Tightness in neck or chest muscles**

▶ **Gray or blue lips or fingernails**

For related information, see: Breathing Difficulty, Page 70; Gastroesophageal Reflux Disease (GERD), Page 144; Insomnia, Page 154; Staying Healthy, Page 17

BOWEL CONDITIONS

What are bowel conditions?

Normal bowel function varies from one person to another. Bowel movements range from as many as three stools a day to three a week. A normal bowel movement is formed, but not hard or bloody. It's passed without pain or cramping.

A chronic bowel condition is a long-lasting disease or disorder in the digestive tract that results in abnormal bowel function. Common conditions include inflammatory bowel disease, irritable bowel syndrome and diverticular disease.

Bowel conditions often are uncomfortable. You may feel embarrassed to talk about them. But, getting a diagnosis is the first step toward finding—and possibly preventing—more serious illness.

What is inflammatory bowel disease?

Inflammatory bowel disease (IBD) refers to a group of chronic disorders that cause inflammation or ulceration in the small or large intestines. Crohn's disease and ulcerative colitis are the most common. Crohn's disease usually causes inflammation in the small intestine and colon. But, it can affect any part of the digestive tract from the mouth to the anus. Ulcerative colitis is limited to the colon and rectum.

Causes. The exact cause of IBD is unknown. It may have a genetic component. About 25 percent of people with IBD have a relative with the disease. Viruses or bacteria also may play a role. While some people feel stress aggravates their symptoms, there's no clinical evidence that it causes IBD.

Symptoms. IBD symptoms include abdominal pain, diarrhea, constipation, rectal bleeding, weight loss, fever, and nausea or vomiting. Because these same symptoms are seen in a number of health conditions, you should see your doctor for a diagnosis.

Prevention. There's no known way to prevent IBD. However, eating a well-balanced, nutritious diet can help you stay healthy. By storing up vitamins and nutrients, you can decrease complications from malnutrition such as weight loss or low blood count.

Treatment. Treatment aims to control the inflammation; correct nutritional deficiencies; and relieve symptoms of abdominal pain and diarrhea. Medication, nutritional supplements, surgery or a combination of these options may provide relief. Work closely with your doctor to develop a treatment plan that's right for you.

Ulcerative colitis may increase your risk of colon cancer. Have your colon checked regularly for signs of cancer.

What is irritable bowel syndrome?

Irritable bowel syndrome (IBS) is a common disorder in which the nerves and muscles in the bowel are extra-sensitive. IBS can cause a great deal of discomfort. However, it doesn't cause permanent harm to the intestines, intestinal bleeding or serious disease, such as cancer.

Causes. The cause of IBS is unknown. For some people, certain foods may spur painful spasms. Some common triggers include beans and other gas-producing foods, fatty foods, alcohol and caffeine. While stress doesn't cause IBS, it may trigger symptoms.

Symptoms. People with IBS usually have crampy, abdominal pain with constipation or diarrhea. Often, having a bowel movement relieves the pain. Sometimes, mucus is passed as part of the bowel movement.

Prevention. Because the cause is unknown, it's difficult to prevent IBS. Symptoms may be prevented with careful attention to diet and other factors such as stress.

Treatment. The goal of IBS treatment focuses on reducing symptoms. This may include diet changes, medicine or stress relief. Keep track of and avoid foods that trigger your symptoms. Add fiber to your diet—unless you have acute diarrhea. Relaxation techniques such as breathing exercises or meditation also may help.

IBS can be disabling for many sufferers. For people with severe symptoms, going to social events, traveling or getting through a day of work can be distressing. Talk with your doctor if your symptoms are disrupting your life or causing you to withdraw from normal activities.

What are diverticulosis and diverticulitis?

Diverticula are weak spots or pouches in your colon that bulge out. Having these pouches is called diverticulosis. Diverticulitis occurs when the pouches become inflamed or infected.

Causes. No one really knows the cause of diverticular disease. A low-fiber diet might be a factor. Some scientists believe there may be a genetic link.

Symptoms. Diverticulosis—or simply having the pouches—often causes no symptoms or discomfort. However, you may have bloating, constipation and mild cramps.

Steady, abdominal pain—usually in the lower left abdomen—is the most common symptom of diverticulitis. You also may experience fever, nausea, vomiting, chills, cramping and constipation.

262

Prevention. A high-fiber diet may reduce the risk of diverticular disease. Fiber also helps prevent constipation, which may contribute to the formation of diverticula.

Try to get 20 to 35 grams of fiber a day, preferably from fruits, vegetables and whole grains. Your doctor also may recommend a fiber supplement. Talk with him or her before taking one. Stay physically active to help prevent constipation.

Treatment. Increasing the amount of fiber in your diet may reduce symptoms of diverticulosis and prevent diverticulitis. Treatment for diverticulitis focuses on clearing up the infection and inflammation, resting the colon and preventing complications. Antibiotics can treat the infection. Bed rest and a liquid diet, along with a pain reliever to control muscle spasms, may help the colon rest. In severe cases, hospitalization and surgery may be necessary.

How can I cope?

If you have a chronic bowel condition, there may be times when you experience few or no symptoms. Other times, your symptoms may flare up. Most people with bowel conditions have a good quality of life. If you have a chronic bowel condition, it can be helpful to:

- Know your body and how your condition affects you.
- Learn to care for yourself—take control of things you can change.
- Develop a strong support system of family and friends.
- Work closely with your doctor.

WHEN TO SEEK HELP

Seek emergency help if you have:

▶ **Severe abdominal pain; may be accompanied by vomiting, dizziness or fainting**

▶ **A large amount of rectal bleeding, or uncontrollable bleeding**

See your doctor if you have:

▶ **Fever**

▶ **Bleeding from the rectum**

▶ **Blood in your stool**

▶ **Persistent abdominal pain**

▶ **Abdominal pain accompanied by vomiting, dizziness or fainting**

▶ **Unexplained weight loss**

For related information, see: Abdominal Cramping, Page 48; Constipation, Page 80; Diarrhea, Page 90; Eat Well, Page 17; Fever, Page 116; Gas or Flatulence, Page 122; Nausea or Vomiting, Page 174; Rectal Bleeding, Page 194; Reduce Stress, Page 28; Weight Loss, Page 244

CANCER

What is cancer?

A diagnosis of cancer can be frightening. If you or a loved one has cancer, you may feel anxious, uncertain and overwhelmed. These emotions are normal—but remember, there is hope. Learning more about cancer and understanding treatment options can help ease your initial fear and lead you on a healthy path toward recovery.

Cancer isn't a virus or bacterium. It's a group of many related diseases characterized by the uncontrolled growth and spread of abnormal cells. These cells multiply and form tumors that may attack and destroy normal cells.

If cancerous cells break away from the tumor, they can travel through the bloodstream or lymph system to other areas of the body. They may settle there and form new tumors. This is called metastasis. However, even when cancer spreads, it's named after the part of the body where it started. For instance, if breast cancer spreads to the lungs, it still is called breast cancer.

What are the causes?

The exact cause of cancer remains a mystery. However, some lifestyle and genetic factors may increase your risk of developing the disease. Risk factors vary among different forms of cancer. Some people may have several risk factors and never get cancer, while others may have none but still develop the disease.

Some habits are known to be dangerous and unhealthy. For instance, smoking has been linked to a variety of diseases, including lung and many other cancers. Other risk factors include:

- Family history of cancer
- Heavy use of alcohol
- Overexposure to the sun
- Using any form of tobacco
- Overexposure to cancer-causing chemicals or radiation
- Genetic predisposition

Whether or not you have risk factors, leading a healthy lifestyle can help boost your immune system, reduce stress and ward off disease.

What are the symptoms?

Symptoms vary with each type of cancer. But some common symptoms include unexplained weight loss, fatigue or lumps. However, these symptoms can signal a variety of other illnesses, too. Don't be afraid to talk with your doctor about anything unusual you may be experiencing. He or she can help determine the cause of your symptoms.

Remember, early detection is key to beating cancer, so see your doctor right away.

To remember the seven signs of cancer, think CAUTION:

C Change in bowel or bladder habits

A A sore that doesn't heal

U Unusual bleeding or discharge

T Thickening or lump in your breast or other body part

I Indigestion or swallowing difficulty

O Obvious change in a wart or mole

N Nagging cough or hoarseness

Source: American Cancer Society

Can cancer be prevented?

Practicing a healthy lifestyle is one of the best ways you can help prevent cancer—and many other health conditions.

Don't start smoking. If you do smoke, quit now. Avoid the sun's harmful rays. If you go out in the sun, wear sunscreen with a sun protection factor (SPF) of 15 or higher that protects against both UVA and UVB rays. Wear sunglasses that protect against the sun's harmful ultraviolet rays, too. Eat a well-balanced diet high in fiber, fruits and vegetables. Exercise also is important—try to be active at least five days a week.

Talk with your doctor about scheduling preventive screenings. These tests can help find cancers of the breast, colon, rectum, cervix, prostate, testicles and skin in their early stages.

How is it treated?

Treatment depends on the type of cancer you have and what stage it's in. Some common treatments:

Surgery is performed on approximately 60 percent of people with cancer. Often, the tumor is removed as a first step in treatment.

Radiation uses beams of high energy waves or particles to destroy cancer cells. Radiation can be used to treat many kinds of cancer and often is combined with other treatments. Some people may experience side effects, but it depends on the dose and the part of the body that's being treated. Some general side effects include fatigue and skin irritation. If you have any worrisome side effects, tell your doctor about them. He or she can help ease your discomfort.

Chemotherapy destroys cancer cells by stopping them from growing and multiplying. These anticancer drugs most commonly are given intravenously, by mouth or through an injection. In the process of killing cancer cells, chemotherapy also may harm healthy cells. The damage to healthy cells is what causes possible side effects, such as fatigue, nausea, vomiting, hair loss and infection. Whether or not you have side effects has nothing to do with the success of the treatment. Your doctors can determine if the chemotherapy is successful through exams and tests.

Hormone therapy also is used to kill cancer cells or slow their growth. Often, doctors prescribe drugs that interfere with hormone production to accomplish this. Some people may have hormone-producing glands removed, too.

Biological therapy, or immunotherapy, uses the body's own defense system to either fight cancer or prevent it from spreading. This therapy sometimes is used in combination with other cancer treatments to help reduce side effects. When specific antibodies and immune system substances are produced in a laboratory for these purposes, they're called biological response modifiers. These include interferons, interleukins and monoclonal antibodies. Talk with your doctor to learn more about this promising therapy.

How can I cope?

There may be times when you find it difficult to cope with cancer. Illness can sometimes put a strain on relationships. At times it can be hard to stay optimistic. Talk with your doctor about anything that's worrying you—he or she is there to help every step of the way. You also may find assistance from family, friends, counselors and support groups. Sharing your thoughts with others who have had similar experiences can be therapeutic. Ask your doctor for recommendations.

Plan activities to lift your spirits. Do things that interest you—get involved in old or new hobbies. If your doctor says it's OK, exercise. Some good choices include walking, yoga and tai chi. But be careful not to push yourself. Exercise can help relieve pain, boost your immune system, restore energy and help you keep a positive outlook during this challenging time.

WHEN TO SEEK HELP

Call your doctor if:

▶ **Your symptoms worsen.**

▶ **You experience any new symptoms.**

For related information, see: Caregiver's Concerns, Page 331; Chronic Pain, Page 273; Complementary Medicine, Page 335; Cough, Page 84; Fatigue, Page 114; Hoarseness or Loss of Voice, Page 152; Mole, Page 168; Prevention and Early Detection, Page 31; Rectal Bleeding, Page 194; Staying Healthy, Page 17; Sunburn, Page 214; Weight Loss, Page 244

CATARACTS OR GLAUCOMA

What is a cataract?

A cataract is the clouding of the normally clear lens of your eye. Cataracts reduce the amount of light that passes through the lens, resulting in impaired vision. They can occur in one or both eyes.

Causes. Cataracts develop as a result of aging, trauma, or endocrine or metabolic disease. They also may result as a side effect of certain medications. Most people who have cataracts develop them between ages 40 and 50. But, they usually don't affect vision until after age 60. Other risk factors include exposure to ultraviolet (UV) radiation and smoking.

Symptoms. If the cataract is small, you may not notice vision changes right away. But, as it grows, you may notice:

- Cloudy, blurry or double vision
- Frequent (yearly) changes in your eyeglass prescription
- Sensitivity to light and glare
- Halos around lights
- Colors seem faded

Prevention. At this time, it's not certain how to prevent cataracts. But, taking care of your eyes throughout your life can help keep them healthy. Limit your exposure to UV radiation. Wear sunglasses that block UV rays. Wear them even on cloudy days. Eat a healthy diet rich in fruits and vegetables. Leafy, green vegetables, in particular, contain vitamins that benefit your eyes. And, don't smoke.

Treatment. Cataracts generally can be treated with surgery. This is one of the most frequently performed procedures in the United States. And, it's effective—resulting in dramatically improved vision in more than 90 percent of cases. The surgery is a short, outpatient procedure that can be done under local anesthetic. Talk with your doctor or eye specialist about whether cataract surgery is right for you.

In some cases, your doctor may recommend ways you can cope with cataracts on your own. For instance, he or she may suggest that you avoid bright sunlight and wear special sunglasses when you go outdoors.

What is glaucoma?

Glaucoma is a disease wherein pressure builds and can possibly damage the optic nerve. Pressure builds up when the clear liquid—aqueous humor—that flows in and out of your eye doesn't drain properly. Glaucoma can lead to severe vision loss or blindness.

There are two primary types of glaucoma—open-angle and closed-angle. Open-angle glaucoma results from an imbalance between production and drainage of aqueous humor. Closed-angle, or acute, glaucoma is not as common. It causes a sudden and rapid increase in eye pressure. If left untreated, it can lead to vision loss in as little as one to two days.

Causes. Glaucoma develops when a drainage network inside your eye becomes clogged. However, the cause of this blockage is unknown. While anyone can develop glaucoma, those at higher risk have a family history, are ages 60 or older, or are African-American.

Symptoms. At first, open-angle glaucoma has no symptoms. There's no change in vision, and there's no pain. But over time, you may notice your side vision worsening or completely disappearing. It may seem as though you're looking through a tunnel. Without treatment, central vision also may become affected.

The symptoms of closed-angle glaucoma are more dramatic and require emergency care. They include:

- Severe pain over the affected eye
- Blurred vision
- Headache
- Reddening in the eye
- Nausea or vomiting

Prevention. There's no way to prevent glaucoma. Unfortunately, glaucoma often is diagnosed after significant, irreversible damage has occurred. For this reason, it's important to get regular preventive eye exams to help detect it in its early stages. Talk with your doctor or eye specialist about getting screened for glaucoma.

Treatment. Open-angle glaucoma usually is treated with eye drops or pills that help lower the pressure inside your eye. Use these medications as directed by your doctor.

If medication doesn't work, your doctor may recommend laser or conventional surgery. These procedures help drain the fluid out of your eye.

Closed-angled glaucoma must be treated immediately to help prevent vision loss. Laser surgery often cures this condition. However, some people may need to use medicated eye drops to prevent future problems.

How can I cope?

If you have cataracts or glaucoma, you still can lead an active life. It's important, however, to see your doctor or eye specialist regularly. Carefully follow his or her instructions on caring for your eyes. Your doctor can suggest lifestyle changes that can help protect the health of your eyes. Also, ask your doctor about resources that offer information and support. Talking with others who have similar experiences can be comforting.

WHEN TO SEEK HELP

Seek emergency help if:

▶ **You experience severe eye pain or sudden vision loss in one or both eyes.**

Call your nurse information service or doctor if:

▶ **You notice blurry or double vision, halos around lights, or sensitivity to light.**

▶ **You experience side effects from your glaucoma medication.**

For related information, see: Eye Pain, Page 110; Headache, Page 138; Nausea or Vomiting, Page 174; Vision Problem, Page 238

CHRONIC OBSTRUCTIVE PULMONARY DISEASE (COPD)

What is COPD?

Chronic obstructive pulmonary disease, or COPD, refers to a group of disorders that block breathing passages. The two most common types are chronic bronchitis and emphysema.

Chronic bronchitis is inflammation and thickening of the walls of the bronchial tubes—the passageways that carry air to the lungs. This condition can induce coughing spells. It also can cause increased production of mucus.

Emphysema is a condition in which the tiny air sacs in the lungs—alveoli—are damaged. These sacs normally are elastic, but with emphysema, they lose their elasticity. Eventually, the sacs begin to rupture, making breathing difficult. Exhaling, in particular, may be a problem. If you have emphysema, you may feel breathless constantly.

What are the causes?

The main cause of COPD is smoking. If you smoke cigarettes, cigars or pipes, you may have up to a 25 percent chance of developing COPD. Other contributing factors include:

- Exposure to air pollution and second-hand smoke
- Occupational exposure such as chemical fumes, dust from cotton, mining hazards or other sources
- Genetic factors

What are the symptoms?

People with COPD usually have symptoms of both chronic bronchitis and emphysema. The main symptom of chronic bronchitis is a continuous cough that may produce mucus. Along with the cough, you may have breathlessness and rapid breathing.

Symptoms of emphysema include:

- Shortness of breath
- Wheezing
- Coughing
- Tightness in the chest
- Fatigue

In severe COPD, you may develop hypoxemia—a lack of oxygen in your blood. Symptoms of hypoxemia include:

- Fatigue
- Memory impairment

- Difficulty concentrating
- Acute shortness of breath on exertion

Report any of these symptoms to your doctor.

Can COPD be prevented?

You can drastically cut your chances of developing COPD by avoiding cigarettes, cigars, pipes and secondhand smoke. Look for tobacco cessation programs and support groups that can help.

You also can reduce your risk of COPD by staying indoors when air pollution levels are high.

How is COPD treated?

Treatment for COPD aims to prevent infections and relieve symptoms. The first step is to quit smoking. Cutting back on the number of cigarettes you smoke won't benefit you enough—you should quit entirely.

Your doctor also may suggest medication to ease your symptoms:

Bronchodilators—relax airway muscles, allowing freer breathing

Corticosteroids—reduce inflammation of the airways, and reduce mucus production

Oxygen therapy—corrects low blood-oxygen levels, and improves your body's overall functioning

Antibiotics—treat respiratory infections such as bacterial pneumonia

How can I cope?

While COPD can't be cured, practicing healthy lifestyle habits can help you feel better physically and emotionally.

- **Exercise.** Regular physical activity can help improve your lung function, as well as increase your energy levels and keep your spirits up. Talk with your doctor about what types of exercises are best for you.

- **Practice good nutrition.** Eating a healthy, balanced diet can strengthen your immune system and keep you strong. Be sure to drink plenty of water each day to help mucus drain.

- **Talk with your loved ones.** Explain COPD to your friends and family. Let them know how they can help you manage your condition—specifically by not smoking around you. Loved ones also can be a good source of comfort and support as you cope.

- **Join a support group.** Ask your doctor about support groups in your area. Talking with others in similar situations can be reassuring. Consider speaking with a counselor, who can help you cope with feelings of frustration or depression.

WHEN TO SEEK HELP

Seek emergency help if:

▶ **Your complexion turns blue or purple.**

▶ **You have chest pain.**

Call your nurse information service or doctor if:

▶ **You develop fever or swelling in your legs or ankles.**

▶ **You're short of breath when resting or doing light exercise.**

▶ **Your mucus is thick or discolored.**

For related information, see: Breathing Difficulty, Page 70; Cough, Page 84; Depression, Page 332; Fatigue, Page 114; Quit Your Tobacco Habit, Page 25; Staying Healthy, Page 17

CHRONIC PAIN

What is chronic pain?

When pain lasts for three months or longer, it's considered chronic pain. In the case of injury or acute disease, it's pain that lasts longer than expected.

Chronic pain may come and go, or it may be constant, continuing for several months or even years. Often, the pain is so intense that sleep patterns, appetite, mood, work and relationships are affected. You may feel depressed or exhausted. There may be an ongoing cause or a past injury that you can pinpoint as the source of your pain.

Chronic pain can be stressful. But, it also can be managed effectively and treated. Treatment can make a difference in your quality of life. You don't have to "get used to" the continuous pain.

How does chronic pain differ from acute pain?

Regardless how unpleasant it is, pain, for the most part, serves a purpose. It alerts you to injury or illness. Pain keeps you in check when your body needs to heal itself. Muscle aches may prevent you from overdoing it when you have the flu. Or, a sprained ankle may hurt to walk on. These are examples of acute pain, and it's necessary for survival.

When it stops being useful, however, and lingers long after you've been alerted to the distress, the pain itself can become debilitating. This is chronic pain. For millions of Americans, it's persistent, unrelenting and a source of great frustration.

What causes chronic pain?

You may have sustained a serious injury that has lingering effects long after the incident. Maybe you were in a car accident or you have an old football injury from college. Perhaps the work you do leaves you with an aching back each day. Or, your pain may be caused by a health condition such as cancer, arthritis or fibromyalgia. Pain even may be a side effect of your treatment.

Chronic pain conditions are common in older adults, but pain certainly doesn't discriminate. Men and women of all ages suffer from chronic pain. As life expectancy continues to increase, more people are likely to experience chronic pain at some point. With this in mind, research into how to best manage pain is making great strides.

How is it treated?

Pain management is an ongoing process that focuses on easing your suffering and helping you regain control of your life. Chronic pain isn't one-dimensional, and so, neither is the treatment. Pain management involves the whole person—physically, emotionally, intellectually and socially.

Taking charge of your treatment may be challenging at first. Your body might hurt, and you may be exhausted. Once a diagnosis is made, it may be tempting to just put your fate entirely in your doctor's hands. But, being actively involved can make a big difference. Work with your doctor—he or she will be better able to help if you're open about your concerns and honest about how you feel. It may help to keep a pain journal that you and your doctor can review together during your visits.

There are effective drugs that may help ease the physical pain. But, don't limit yourself to medication alone. There are things you can do that may improve your well-being. Exercise—loosen up your muscles through low-impact, gentle workouts. Your doctor can help you develop a program that will work best for you. Learn to relax. Try deep breathing, yoga, meditation or other relaxation techniques. Be sure to eat healthfully to help boost your energy.

How can I cope?

Think of pain management as a journey. Set realistic goals and try to keep things in perspective. What's most important to you? Is your pain standing in the way of enjoying time with your family? Are you worried about the effects it might have on your career or finances? All of your concerns are valid, and many of your goals may be reachable, but you may have to take small steps. Try not to get discouraged too quickly. Enjoy each victory—even small ones can be sweet.

Reach out to family, friends, counselors or support groups. You may want to ask your doctor about pain management programs. These sometimes are available through hospitals and rehabilitation centers. Specially trained professionals provide treatment that can help you manage your chronic pain.

WHEN TO SEEK HELP

Call your doctor if:

▶ **You're suffering with pain but aren't sure of the cause.**

▶ **You have pain that persists despite treatment.**

For related information, see: Arthritis, Page 255; Cancer, Page 264; Complementary Medicine, Page 335; Fatigue, Page 114; Medication, Page 37; Working With Your Doctor, Page 43

CONGESTIVE HEART FAILURE (CHF)

What is CHF?

Congestive heart failure, or CHF, occurs when the heart becomes so weakened that it no longer can pump enough blood to meet your body's needs. "Heart failure" doesn't mean that the heart has stopped, as it may in cardiac arrest. Rather, it's failing to pump effectively. The term "congestive" refers to the fluid buildup that occurs with the disease. How serious the condition is depends on how much pumping capacity the heart has lost.

Congestive heart failure can be classified as left- or right-side heart failure. Though, to some degree, both often exist at the same time. In left-side heart failure, the left ventricle isn't pumping effectively. This leads to fluid buildup in the lungs and shortness of breath. Right-side heart failure is characterized by fluid buildup in the liver, lungs and legs.

What are the causes?

CHF develops slowly. It usually is the result of an underlying disease or physical problem, such as:

- Coronary heart disease, which narrows the arteries that supply blood to the heart muscle
- Prior heart attack that has damaged the heart muscle
- High blood pressure, which makes your heart work harder
- Heart valve problems—valves regulate the flow of blood within the heart chambers
- Damage to the heart muscle—caused by disease or infection (cardiomyopathy or myocarditis)
- Congenital heart disease—heart problems that are present at birth
- Abnormal heart rhythms, or arrhythmias, making your heart beat too fast or too slow

Other potential risk factors include emphysema; chronic, untreated hyperthyroidism; anemia; or severe nutritional deficiencies.

What are the symptoms?

If your heart is damaged or weak, it'll pump less blood with each heartbeat. Blood returning to the heart may back up, causing congestion in the tissues. This results in swelling, or edema— often in the legs or feet. Fluid also may collect in the lungs. CHF also reduces the kidneys' ability to get rid of sodium and water.

Talk with your doctor if you experience any of these symptoms:

- Fatigue and weakness
- Shortness of breath when you exert yourself, or when lying down
- Wheezing or coughing up pinkish sputum
- Swollen legs, ankles or feet, particularly when you first wake up
- Swollen neck veins
- Rapid weight gain
- Dizziness

Can CHF be prevented?

The best defense against CHF is prevention. Make healthy lifestyle choices. Quit smoking. Maintain a healthy weight. Exercise regularly and eat nutritious foods. If you have diabetes or hypertension, take an active role in managing your condition to prevent complications.

How is CHF treated?

Treatment is based on the type of heart failure you have. Your doctor likely will recommend lifestyle changes to help relieve your CHF symptoms and prevent the disease from getting worse:

- **Reduce sodium and saturated fats.** Salt can contribute to water retention. So, limit your sodium intake. Excess saturated fat and cholesterol are major risk factors for developing other types

of heart disease. Carefully read nutrition labels. You may want to talk with a dietitian for menu ideas.

- **Limit alcohol.** Avoid alcohol or limit yourself to one drink, two or three times a week. Alcohol can reduce your heart's ability to pump, and it can interact with some medications.

- **Exercise.** While you may need to limit your physical activity, especially if your CHF is severe, moderate exercise can help your heart pump more efficiently. Ask your doctor about exercise that's right for you.

- **Stop smoking.** Quitting now can help your heart and lungs. Smoking damages your blood vessels, reduces the amount of oxygen your cells receive and makes your heart beat faster. Your doctor can help you quit.

- **Consider immunizations.** Ask your doctor if the pneumococcal vaccine and annual flu shots are right for you.

Your doctor also may prescribe medications—many patients take more than one. These may include:

Angiotensin-converting enzyme (ACE) inhibitors—expand blood vessels, increase blood flow and reduce blood pressure

Diuretics—help reduce the amount of fluid in the body

Digoxin—also called digitalis, increases the force of the heart's contractions

Beta blockers—slow your heart rate and reduce blood pressure

276

Some people with severe CHF may need oxygen therapy to help them breathe. In some cases, surgery, including a heart transplant, may be necessary.

How can I cope?

Pay close attention to your body and let your doctor know when you're feeling better or worse. Working closely with your doctor can result in developing a treatment plan that works best for you.

If you're having trouble sleeping, place a pillow or foam wedge under your mattress to elevate the head of the bed. You generally can get a better night's sleep if you avoid taking naps or eating meals right before bedtime.

Diuretics may make you urinate more often. Talk with your doctor about adjusting the timing of these medications. Taking them earlier in the day may minimize the need to get up in the middle of the night.

Living with CHF may be challenging at times. Family and friends can be wonderful sources of emotional support. They also can help with medical care issues and day-to-day activities. Find out about other resources that may be available to you. These may include meal delivery programs, errand services, visiting health aides and support groups.

WHEN TO SEEK HELP

Seek emergency help if:

▶ You experience severe breathlessness.

▶ You have any chest pain.

Call your doctor if:

▶ You're being treated for CHF and your symptoms, including breathlessness, and rapid or irregular heartbeat, get worse.

▶ You develop any of the following symptoms: dizziness, dry cough that won't go away, increased fatigue, decreased urine output, or weight increase of 3 to 5 pounds in one week.

For related information, see: Breathing Difficulty, Page 70; Caregiver's Concerns, Page 331; Dizziness, Page 92; Fatigue, Page 114; Hyperthyroidism, Page 308; If You Drink, Do So in Moderation, Page 25; Quit Your Tobacco Habit, Page 25; Weight Gain, Page 242

CORONARY HEART DISEASE (CHD)

What is CHD?

Coronary heart disease, or CHD, occurs when the arteries that carry blood to the heart muscle—coronary arteries—become stiff and narrow. This usually is due to atherosclerosis, a process in which deposits—called plaques—of fat, cholesterol, calcium and other matter build up inside the arteries, reducing the flow of blood.

Ischemia, or reduced blood supply, deprives the heart muscle of the oxygen and nutrients it needs to function. When this happens, you may feel pain in your chest. But, some people feel no symptoms and are unaware they have CHD.

What are the symptoms?

CHD develops slowly and its symptoms vary widely:

Chest pain. If your heart doesn't get enough oxygen and nutrients, you may have pain in the center of your chest. You also may have a feeling of pressure, tightness or burning. This is called angina, which can be brought on by physical or emotional stress. You also may feel pain or pressure in your arms, neck or jaw; shortness of breath; or palpitations. Angina symptoms usually are temporary and go away within a few minutes of stopping the stressful activity. Your doctor may prescribe medication, such as nitroglycerin, to relieve your symptoms.

Shortness of breath. Some people may experience shortness of breath, fatigue and swelling of the legs or ankles. Women more commonly have these types of symptoms rather than what might be considered classic symptoms of CHD, such as chest pain.

Heart attack. If a coronary artery becomes completely blocked—usually by plaque or a blood clot—part of the heart muscle dies. Pain from a heart attack can be excruciating and "crushing." Heart attacks generally last longer than the pain of angina—sometimes 30 minutes or more. The pain isn't relieved by rest or medication.

Know the warning signs of a heart attack:

- Uncomfortable pressure, fullness, squeezing or pain in the chest lasting longer than two minutes
- Pain spreading to the shoulders, arms, neck, jaw or back
- Dizziness, fainting, sweating, nausea or shortness of breath

Women often have fewer chest symptoms and more unusual symptoms, such as stomach or abdominal pain, nausea, dizziness or cold, sweaty skin.

Seek emergency help any time you think you may be having a heart attack.

No symptoms. You may notice no CHD symptoms. This is called silent ischemia.

Can CHD be prevented?

Some risk factors for CHD are beyond your control. These include advanced age, being male, or having a family history of heart disease. Changing your lifestyle, however, can help control angina and prevent heart attacks or recurrences.

Talk with your doctor about the following strategies:

Get regular health exams. Many risk factors for CHD—high cholesterol, hypertension and diabetes—have no symptoms in the early stages. You also may have CHD but no symptoms. Regular visits to your doctor can help identify and manage any conditions early to help prevent complications.

Stop smoking. Smoking and secondhand smoke are major risk factors for CHD. Check out a tobacco cessation program in your area. Many hospitals offer these resources.

Eat a heart-healthy diet. Too much saturated fat and cholesterol in your diet can clog your arteries. Sodium can raise

your blood pressure. Read food labels carefully when shopping.

Maintain a healthy weight. Obesity is a risk factor for CHD. Losing excess weight can help you lower cholesterol and keep your blood pressure in check—do so under your doctor's supervision.

Exercise. Regular physical activity can make your heart stronger, lessen arterial stiffness and reduce your danger of CHD. Check with your doctor before starting any exercise program.

How is CHD treated?

Lifestyle changes. Adopting healthy habits is the key to prevention and one of the best ways to keep CHD from progressing. If you smoke, quit now. Quitting smoking dramatically reduces your risk of a first or second heart attack. Eat a diet low in saturated fat and cholesterol, and high in fruits and vegetables. With your doctor's approval, exercise 30 minutes a day, five times a week. With severe CHD, you may need to restrict your physical activity. Talk with your doctor about lifestyle changes that are right for you.

Medication. Your doctor may prescribe medications to help ease your symptoms and prevent progression of the disease. These may vary depending on the nature and severity of your CHD, and whether you have other health conditions.

Prescription medications such as nitroglycerin, beta blockers and calcium channel blockers may improve your heart function and control irregular heartbeats. Your doctor also may prescribe medications that lower your cholesterol or blood pressure. He or she may advise you to regularly take aspirin to prevent blood clots. Ask your doctor about what each medication does and what possible side effects to expect.

If you have a heart attack, thrombolytic drugs can dissolve blood clots quickly. To be effective, these need to be given within six hours after heart attack symptoms begin.

Surgery. If your symptoms are frequent or severe, your doctor may recommend surgery. In angioplasty, a balloon is inflated inside the artery to flatten the layer of plaque. This widens the artery to help improve blood flow. Often, a small wire tube called a stent is inserted to hold the artery open. Another approach is coronary artery bypass, in which a blood vessel, usually taken from your leg or chest, is sewn into the coronary artery to bypass the blocked area.

How can I cope?

Once CHD is diagnosed, it requires lifelong management. Your lifestyle can significantly affect the health of your heart and the arteries that feed it. Adopting healthy habits and working closely with your doctor can help you feel better and prevent complications.

There may be times when you feel discouraged. This can be a natural reaction to chronic illness. Talking with family and friends is important, especially when you feel down. Your doctor can be a good source of support, too. He or she can help you connect with helpful resources if you begin to feel depressed.

WHEN TO SEEK HELP

Seek emergency help if:

▶ **You think you're having a heart attack. Don't assume the pain will go away. Medications can be given to dissolve blood clots and help prevent a heart attack from progressing. Get help immediately to reduce your risk of permanent damage, or death (see Page 10).**

▶ **You have any chest pain that lasts more than a few minutes.**

See your doctor if:

▶ **You have chest pain that begins due to activity and resolves promptly with rest.**

Call your doctor if:

▶ **Your symptoms worsen or become more frequent and you have previously been diagnosed with CHD.**

For related information, see: Breathing Difficulty, Page 70; Chest Pain, Page 76; Staying Healthy, Page 17

280

DIABETES

What is diabetes?

When you eat, your body transforms some of the food into glucose, a sugar that supplies cells with energy. Normally, glucose travels in the blood and enters cells with the help of insulin, a hormone produced by the pancreas. Diabetes is a condition in which glucose can't enter cells—either due to a lack of insulin, or a problem with the way the insulin functions. This can result in dangerously high blood glucose levels. Over time, this can cause damage to your eyes, kidneys, nerves or heart.

Type 1 diabetes is a disease in which the pancreas produces little or no insulin. It most often occurs in children and young adults—but can develop at any age. The cause of Type 1 diabetes is unknown—genetic and environmental factors may be involved. It accounts for 5 to 10 percent of diabetes cases in the United States. People with Type 1 diabetes need to take insulin every day.

Type 2 diabetes is much more common. About 90 to 95 percent of diabetes cases in the United States are Type 2. This form of diabetes is a metabolic disorder. It impairs the body's ability to make enough, or properly use, insulin. You have a higher risk of Type 2 diabetes if you're overweight, age 45 or older, physically inactive, or if you have a family history of the condition. Type 2 diabetes often can be managed with healthy eating, physical activity and blood glucose testing. Your doctor also may prescribe medication or insulin to help control your blood glucose levels.

What are the symptoms?

Often, there are no symptoms. Type 2 diabetes, in particular, develops slowly. See your doctor if you have any of these warning signs:

- Increased thirst
- Frequent urination
- Weight gain or loss
- Blurred vision
- Slow-healing sores or frequent infections
- Numbness or tingling in your toes or feet

What are the risks?

High blood sugar (hyperglycemia). Your blood sugar levels may become extremely high if you don't closely monitor them. High doses of steroids, large amounts of alcohol, stress, infection or illness also can cause glucose levels to rise. Symptoms of hyperglycemia include excessive thirst, increased urination, weakness, leg tingling, confusion and, rarely, convulsions and coma. If untreated, hyperglycemia can be fatal.

Low blood sugar (hypoglycemia). If you're taking insulin or medication to lower your blood sugar, and you skip a meal or exercise more strenuously than usual, your blood glucose level may drop too low. Symptoms of hypoglycemia are sweating, shakiness, weakness, hunger, dizziness, nausea, slurred speech, drowsiness or confusion. If you experience any of these symptoms, eat or drink something that will raise your blood sugar. Doctors sometimes prescribe a glucagon injection device to help counteract low blood sugar. Use of this device requires training.

Very low blood glucose levels can cause convulsions or coma. This is a life-threatening condition.

Increased blood acids (ketoacidosis). Your cells may become so starved for energy that they break down fat. This produces toxic acids known as ketones. Ketoacidosis most often occurs in people with Type 1 diabetes. If left untreated, it can lead to coma and possibly death. Seek emergency help if you have high blood sugar levels, and stomach pain or a sweet, fruity smell on your breath. Call your doctor if you experience loss of appetite, nausea, vomiting or fever. Talk with your doctor about self-tests that can help you measure the ketone level in your urine.

Other risks. Over time, diabetes can result in poor circulation that can lead to foot problems, severe nerve damage, kidney disease, heart disease, stroke, eye disease, blindness or death. Keeping your blood sugar levels close to normal can help you reduce your risk of complications.

How is diabetes managed?

There's no cure for diabetes, but you can live a healthy, active life if you take care of yourself.

Create a treatment plan. Work closely with your doctor to develop a diabetes care plan that's right for you. Discuss a plan of action for routine illnesses and emergencies. Ask about the value of medical-alert ID bracelets. Make sure you understand your doctor's instructions. Keep all medical appointments so that your doctor can monitor your long-term glucose control.

Monitoring your glucose levels. Checking your blood glucose levels is crucial to staying healthy and feeling your best. Your doctor will teach you how and when to take these measurements. Record your levels in a diary and bring it with you to medical appointments. Ask your doctor when to report results outside your normal range.

A healthy diet. Your doctor will help you plan the size and frequency of meals, as well as appropriate food choices. Follow this plan carefully to reduce your risk of excessively high or low glucose levels.

Maintaining a healthy weight also is important. Eat nutritionally balanced meals. Limit alcohol.

Exercise regularly. Exercise strengthens your heart and improves circulation. It also helps your body properly use food, including glucose. And, it can help you maintain a healthy weight. Ask your doctor to recommend an exercise program. Eat a snack 30 minutes before exercise, and have carbohydrates available during exercise. To reduce the risk of low glucose levels, avoid exercising when insulin injections have their peak effect or if you haven't eaten for several hours.

Take your prescribed medication. Whether you're taking insulin or oral medication, work with your doctor to control your glucose levels. Ask questions about your medications including how, when and why to take them.

Care for yourself. Keep snacks with you in case of low blood sugar—ask your doctor for ideas. It's extremely important to have annual eye exams with pupil dilation so your retina can be examined closely. Diabetic retinopathy is a leading cause of blindness. You also should take good care of your feet. And, be sure to see your dentist twice a year.

Talk with your doctor. Ask how often you should have health exams—follow his or her recommendations. Ask your doctor if annual flu shots and a pneumococcal vaccine are right for you.

How can I cope?

Diabetes is a complicated condition. At times, managing it may seem overwhelming. If you feel stressed, try relaxation techniques such as yoga or meditation. You occasionally may experience denial, anger or depression. Talk with your family and friends—they can be great sources of support. If your emotions get in the way of good self-care, talk with your doctor. Support groups also can provide comfort and assistance.

WHEN TO SEEK HELP

Seek emergency help if:

▶ **You have a diabetic emergency, such as severe hyperglycemia, hypoglycemia or ketoacidosis.**

Call your nurse information service or doctor if:

▶ **You have trouble controlling your glucose levels.**

▶ **You experience complications such as poor healing of wounds; weight concerns; numbness in your toes or feet; or any vision problem.**

For related information, see: Faintness, Page 112; Numbness or Tingling, Page 184; Staying Healthy, Page 17; Urination Concerns, Page 230; Vision Problem, Page 238

HIV INFECTION

What is HIV infection?

The human immunodeficiency virus, or HIV, lives and multiplies primarily in white blood cells called T lymph cells. These cells normally protect the body from disease. HIV weakens the immune system by destroying T cells. As the infection progresses, the immune system breaks down. The body then becomes vulnerable to infections and illnesses, ranging from pneumonia to cancer. Over time, untreated HIV infection progresses to acquired immune deficiency syndrome, or AIDS.

How is HIV transmitted?

A person infected with HIV carries the virus in body fluids. These include blood, semen, vaginal secretions and breast milk. The virus can be transmitted only if HIV-infected fluids enter the bloodstream through body openings, mucous membranes or skin breaks. Usually, HIV is transmitted through unprotected sexual contact. It also is spread through the use of infected hypodermic needles or syringes—this includes needles for steroids and illegal drugs such as heroin. Body piercings and tattoos possibly can spread this or other diseases through unsterilized needles. An infected mother can pass HIV to her baby during pregnancy, childbirth or breast-feeding. Transmission through blood transfusions is very rare because donated blood has been tested for HIV since 1985. However, HIV-infected body tissue can transmit the disease in corneal, cartilage or other transplants.

HIV isn't transmitted by sharing food utensils. Nor is it transmitted in the air through coughing or sneezing. There also is no evidence that HIV can be spread through casual contact with infected persons, towels, bedding, toilet seats, doorknobs or telephones. Mosquitoes, fleas and other insects don't transmit HIV.

What are the symptoms?

In its early stages, HIV infection often has no symptoms. Some people may experience a flu-like illness—with headache, fatigue or swollen lymph nodes. The only way to know your HIV status is to be tested for HIV antibodies—proteins the body produces to fight infection. If you think you may have been exposed, see your doctor immediately. Your doctor's office, local hospital, health department or clinic may offer tests, treatment or follow up. Many states offer anonymous HIV-related services. Home test kits, in which you mail a small blood sample to the manufacturer, also are available. Talk with your nurse information service or doctor.

284

Some people with HIV may not have symptoms for five, 10 or more years. The length of this symptom-free phase—called asymptomatic seropositivity—varies. Though no symptoms of HIV are noticeable, the person is still very contagious.

As the immune system deteriorates, a variety of complications may develop. Symptoms may include persistent swollen lymph glands; fungal or parasitic infections; a "hairy" growth on the tongue called hairy leukoplakia; skin problems such as acute psoriasis or severe seborrheic dermatitis; herpes infections; night sweats; weight loss and diarrhea.

HIV infection may cause the T-cell count to drop to 200 or below. The immune system may be so weakened that serious infections or illnesses develop. It's at this point that the HIV infection has progressed to AIDS. This phase includes severe infections; cancers; and illnesses of the lungs, heart, digestive system and central nervous system. Unfortunately, there currently is no known cure for AIDS, and the disease appears to be fatal. But, new research and treatments are helping people with HIV live longer, healthier lives.

Can HIV be prevented?

There is no vaccine to prevent HIV. Healthy lifestyle choices, therefore, are crucial. Avoid unprotected vaginal, oral and anal sex. Use a latex condom every time to help prevent transmission of the virus. Use only water-based lubricants. Oil- and petroleum-based lubricants reduce a condom's effectiveness. While sex with multiple partners increases risk, you also can get HIV through a single encounter.

If you use intravenous drugs, don't share needles. Talk with your doctor about seeking help for drug abuse.

If you're pregnant or planning a pregnancy, and you think you may have been exposed to HIV, seek testing and counseling. Special prenatal care and medications may help decrease the risk of passing HIV to your baby.

How is HIV treated?

Treatment for HIV has three goals: prevent infections and diseases from developing; relieve symptoms of medical problems that occur; and slow the progression to AIDS. Work with your doctor to develop a treatment plan.

People with HIV are susceptible to a range of illnesses. Vaccines offer protection against hepatitis A and B, tetanus, measles, flu and pneumonia. However, anyone with HIV should avoid all live-virus vaccines such as oral polio, typhoid and yellow fever. In people with weakened immune systems, these vaccines may cause the very diseases they're meant to prevent.

Your doctor may prescribe medications to treat or prevent specific infections or illnesses, such as herpes, fungal infections, or Kaposi's sarcoma—a form of cancer usually on the skin. This infection can spread to internal organs.

There are antiviral medications designed to make it harder for HIV to reproduce and destroy the body's immune system. Reverse transcriptase inhibitors attack an HIV enzyme called reverse transcriptase. Protease inhibitors attack protease, another HIV enzyme. Treatment for HIV is developing rapidly. Talk with your doctor about the most current and effective medications.

Your doctor may prescribe more than one medication. This combination regimen is called highly active antiretroviral therapy (HAART). Such "cocktails" may significantly reduce the level of HIV in the bloodstream. This can help people infected with HIV enjoy longer, healthier lives.

Unfortunately, many of these medications have severe side effects. But it's important to take them exactly as prescribed. If you have any concerns, talk with your doctor right away.

How can I cope?

The most important ways to stay healthy longer are to work closely with your doctor; take your medications; and make positive lifestyle choices. Eat healthfully, exercise

regularly and get enough sleep. Many people find that spirituality or meditation helps them cope with the stresses of being ill.

Living with HIV can be physically and emotionally draining. Friends and family can be wonderful sources of support. You also may want to talk with other people who have HIV. Ask your doctor about local support groups. There may be times when you feel it's difficult to cope. Don't hesitate to speak with a professional such as a counselor.

WHEN TO SEEK HELP

Call your doctor if:

▶ **You think you may have been exposed to HIV.**

▶ **You're pregnant, or planning a pregnancy, and think you may have been exposed to HIV.**

For related information, see: Caregiver's Concerns, Page 331; Complementary Medicine, Page 335; Fatigue, Page 114; Sexual Health, Page 311; Staying Healthy, Page 17; Swollen Glands, Page 126

HYPERTENSION (HIGH BLOOD PRESSURE)

What is hypertension?

As your heart pumps, your blood exerts pressure on the walls of your arteries. Hypertension, or high blood pressure, occurs when the pressure reaches high, unhealthy levels. If left untreated, hypertension can damage blood vessels throughout your body. This can lead to arteriosclerosis, kidney damage, heart attack, congestive heart failure and stroke.

Your blood pressure measurement has two numbers—systolic and diastolic. Systolic pressure is the force with which your heart pumps blood into your arteries when it squeezes, or contracts. Diastolic pressure is the pressure in your arteries when your heart relaxes. Your systolic pressure—the first number in the reading—is always higher than your diastolic pressure.

An average healthy blood pressure for most adults is about 120/80 mm Hg (millimeters of mercury). But, your doctor may adjust your target range depending on your age, gender and general health. Your blood pressure may vary throughout the day. But, if you have several readings of 140/90 or above during the course of a few weeks, you may have hypertension.

What causes hypertension?

Most cases of hypertension have no known cause. Doctors refer to this as primary, or essential, hypertension. In some cases, it may result from pregnancy or a medical condition, such as a kidney disorder or hormonal imbalance. Hypertension due to an identified underlying cause is called secondary hypertension.

What are the symptoms?

Most people with hypertension don't notice any symptoms. That's why it's so important to visit your doctor and have your blood pressure checked regularly. In severe cases of hypertension, you may experience dizziness, headaches or mental confusion. Some people have nosebleeds but the connection to hypertension is uncertain.

Can hypertension be prevented or controlled?

Some risk factors for hypertension are beyond your control—such as gender, race and family history. However, making healthy lifestyle changes can help you prevent hypertension. If you already have high blood pressure, these strategies can help keep it under control.

Get regular health exams. Blood pressure readings are a part of routine health exams. If your levels are high, your doctor may take repeated measurements to determine whether the hypertension is persistent or temporary. When hypertension is detected early, treatment may be more effective and complications may be prevented.

Maintain a healthy weight. Being overweight increases your risk of developing high blood pressure. In fact, losing just 10 pounds can help lower your blood pressure and reduce your risk of complications. Talk with your doctor about strategies for maintaining a healthy weight.

Exercise five days a week. Being physically active is one of the best ways to prevent and control hypertension. Just 30 minutes a day of moderate-level activity, such as walking, biking or swimming, can make a big difference. Talk with your doctor first if you've been inactive for a while, or if you have any other health concerns.

Eat healthfully. Any healthy diet should include plenty of fruits, vegetables and whole-grain foods. Avoid saturated fat and cholesterol. You also should reduce your salt and sodium intake. A simple step is to replace your salt shaker with tasty herbs and spices. But, also beware of processed foods. They often may contain high levels of sodium. Read nutrition labels carefully when shopping.

If you drink alcohol, do so in moderation. Drinking too much alcohol can raise your blood pressure. Alcohol also contains a lot of calories.

Monitor your blood pressure. Your doctor may recommend that you check your blood pressure at home. This can help you keep track of your progress. Monitor your blood pressure several times a week in a resting, non-hurried state. Don't take it right after a meal.

How is it treated?

Your doctor may prescribe medication to help keep your blood pressure under control. Keep in mind that you still should follow healthy lifestyle habits. Doing so will help your medication work better, and may reduce the amount you need.

Diuretics, also known as water pills, flush excess salt and water from your body. They're believed to reduce sodium in your small blood vessels, lowering your blood pressure through that mechanism. Unfortunately, most of these drugs also can remove another important mineral—potassium—from your body. You may need potassium supplements if you take diuretics. Take these only if your doctor directs you to do so.

Other blood pressure medications include:

Alpha blockers and central alpha agonists—block the activity of nerves that cause vessels to constrict.

Angiotensin-converting enzyme (ACE) inhibitors—expand blood vessels by decreasing the level of a hormone that causes blood vessels to constrict.

Beta blockers—cause the heart to beat more slowly and with less force.

Calcium channel blockers—help keep the arteries from narrowing.

Vasodilators—cause your arteries to relax.

Drugs can affect people differently. Side effects or levels of effectiveness may vary. Trial periods and changes in medication can be common. Your doctor may prescribe a combination of two or more drugs to achieve the best results for you.

If you have secondary hypertension, treating the primary health concern often helps your blood pressure return to normal.

Controlling hypertension is a lifetime commitment. But it's a worthwhile investment because it can help you prevent serious complications. Because hypertension generally doesn't cause any symptoms, follow your treatment plan even if you feel perfectly fine. Talk with your doctor if you have any concerns.

WHEN TO SEEK HELP

Seek emergency help if:

▶ You have high blood pressure and experience confusion or severe headache.

Call your nurse information service or doctor if:

▶ You have high blood pressure and experience dizziness, nosebleeds or headaches that last.

▶ You experience side effects from your blood pressure medications. These may include erectile dysfunction, fatigue, sedation, postural lightheadedness and gastrointestinal symptoms.

▶ You checked your blood pressure several times in a given week and the average reading is greater than 140/90, despite lifestyle changes or medication.

For related information, see: Congestive Heart Failure, Page 275; Coronary Heart Disease, Page 278; Dizziness, Page 92; Medications, Page 37; Nosebleed, Page 182; Staying Healthy, Page 17; Stroke, Page 305

MIGRAINE HEADACHE

What is a migraine?

A migraine headache is characterized by intense pain, typically on one side of the head. It often is accompanied by nausea, and sensitivity to light and sound. The pain of a migraine often is so severe that it interferes with daily activities. And, it can last for days.

Migraines are more common in women than men. They most frequently occur between ages 25 and 45. But, people of all ages get migraines—even a small percentage of children.

What are the causes?

The cause of migraines is unknown. They seem to be related to changes in blood flow in the brain. Attacks can occur suddenly and unexpectedly. But, there are a number of factors that seem to trigger migraines.

Stress is a trigger for many people. Even the stresses of everyday life—traffic, work or juggling your busy schedule—in combination, can contribute to a migraine. And, when migraine pain hits, your stress may seem even worse.

Hormones also are key triggers. Many women who suffer from migraines can predict when they're most likely to occur—just before, after or during their menstrual periods. Estrogen in hormone replacement therapy (HRT) or birth control pills may contribute to attacks.

Certain foods may trigger migraines, too—red wine, aged cheeses, chocolate, pickled herring, fava beans, processed meats, and peanut butter, to name a few. Caffeine and some food additives, such as monosodium glutamate (MSG), also may cause problems.

Migraines often are the result of a combination of factors. Other triggers may include changes in air pressure due to weather shifts or altitude; jet lag; changes in sleeping or eating patterns; or certain medications.

What are the symptoms?

Migraines can last from a few hours to a few days. Symptoms may vary. But they most commonly include throbbing or pulsating pain—usually starting on one side of the head—nausea or vomiting, and increased sensitivity to light and sound. The pain often is intense—and it typically starts suddenly.

Some people report visual disturbances—such as flashing lights, zigzag lines or even a temporary loss of vision—just before a migraine. This "aura" is a telltale sign that a migraine is about to occur. Migraines occasionally are accompanied by speech difficulty, confusion, or

290

tingling in an arm or leg. If this happens, seek emergency help.

Can migraines be prevented?

You may ward off some migraines by avoiding your triggers. A headache diary can help you notice patterns. Write down the day and time each headache starts, and how long it lasts. In addition, note possible triggers such as foods or sleeping habits. Women should be aware of any possible relation to their menstrual cycles.

Discuss your headache diary with your doctor. Together you may be able to pinpoint triggers and avoid them in the future. There also are some medications available that may help prevent migraines.

In the meantime, establish healthy habits. Learn stress management techniques. You can't escape stress altogether, but controlling your reactions can make a difference. Eat balanced meals and develop regular sleeping patterns. You also may want to get in touch with other migraine sufferers, through support groups. Their insight may be invaluable.

How are migraines treated?

There are a variety of prescription and over-the-counter medications that are effective in relieving migraine pain. Your doctor can help you determine which is best for you. You may want to retreat to a quiet, dark room while you wait for the medication to take effect. Apply gentle pressure or an ice pack to the painful areas of your head. Depending on your situation, your doctor may refer you to a specialist.

Relaxation techniques, such as deep breathing, biofeedback and visualization, also may be soothing. Some migraine sufferers find relief through complementary therapies, such as acupuncture, acupressure or yoga.

WHEN TO SEEK HELP

Seek emergency help if:

▶ **You have a sudden, severe headache accompanied by loss of consciousness; slurred speech; weakness; or numbness or tingling in the face, arm or leg.**

Call your nurse information service or doctor if:

▶ **You, or any member of your family, experience headaches that interfere with daily activities.**

For related information, see:
Complementary Medicine, Page 335;
Eye Pain, Page 110; Headache, Page
138; Medications, Page 37; Premenstrual
Syndrome, Page 316; Staying Healthy,
Page 17; Stress, Page 334

MULTIPLE SCLEROSIS (MS)

What is multiple sclerosis?

Multiple sclerosis, or MS, is a disease of the central nervous system. It affects twice as many women as men. It's most commonly diagnosed between ages 20 and 60. But, people outside that age group can get it, too.

MS can be a challenging and frustrating diagnosis. However, with a healthy regimen—including exercise and reduced stress—many patients are able to lead full and active lives.

What are the causes?

A tissue called myelin protects the nerve fibers of your brain and spinal cord. It's much like an insulating material covering a bundle of electrical wires. In MS, this myelin sheath is damaged and scarred. Signals are unable to transmit easily or completely across the "wires."

The cause of MS is unknown. Research suggests there may be a number of factors, including the possibility of viral or environmental triggers. There also may be a genetic component that makes some people more susceptible.

What are the symptoms?

Symptoms are varied and unpredictable. No two individuals will experience the same effects. Some people have symptoms that disappear just as mysteriously as they appeared. Others experience a progressive worsening of symptoms. Each case is unique, and getting an accurate diagnosis isn't always easy.

Most commonly, people with MS experience localized muscle weakness and spasms; trouble maintaining balance; bladder and bowel problems; numbness; double vision or vision loss; and vertigo. The nature of the symptoms is determined by the exact location of the lesions in the myelin sheath.

In the early stages of MS, you may experience numbness, tingling or fatigue. But, any of these symptoms—especially fatigue—can be caused by many other conditions. And, they may flare up and then fade. You may begin to question whether you're really even having symptoms. This can be very frustrating. It may take a number of neurological tests and exams to diagnose MS.

Can MS be prevented?

Because the cause of MS is a mystery, there's currently no way to prevent it. With the right treatment, however, the disease can be managed and its progression can be slowed. You may be able to avoid some of the setbacks that were once more common with MS.

292

How is MS treated?

Treatment goals for MS are three-fold—improve recovery from attacks, prevent or lessen the number of relapses, and halt disease progression. Usually medication is the best course of action. There are a variety of effective drugs available. And, new treatments are showing great potential. Take an active role. Work with your doctor to find out which is best for you. Ask questions, voice your concerns and try to stay positive.

Taking care of yourself, in general, is very important. You may feel like you have no control over your condition or your treatment, but your efforts can make a difference. Eat a balanced diet—you may help reduce some of the complications of MS. And, try to stay active.

Many people with MS also seek out alternative or complementary treatments, such as acupuncture or chiropractic care, to help manage their symptoms. You may find massage, meditation, yoga or other relaxation techniques helpful. Talk with your doctor before beginning any additional treatments.

How can I cope?

Living with MS can be stressful and challenging. Coping with the unpredictable nature of this disease can be tough. Reach out to your family and friends for strength. Be open and honest about your feelings. It may help to talk with a professional counselor. Or, you may want to seek out a support group. Talking with others who are going through the same thing can be reassuring. You may find that you can learn a lot from shared experiences. You don't have to face this alone.

For related information, see: Caregiver's Concerns, Page 331; Complementary Medicine, Page 335; Depression, Page 332; Dizziness, Page 92; Fatigue, Page 114; Numbness or Tingling, Page 184; Staying Healthy, Page 17; Stress, Page 334

OSTEOPOROSIS

What is osteoporosis?

Osteoporosis is a condition wherein calcium and phosphorous are lost gradually from the bones. The result is that bone mass or density also decreases. Most commonly, it affects bones in the spine, hips and wrists. Over time, your bones may become porous and weak. They may be more vulnerable to breaks or fractures. Some loss of calcium is a normal condition of aging for some people. However, as the loss becomes more significant, or goes untreated, problems can result.

Osteoporosis affects four times as many women as men. In severe cases, it may lead to pain, suffering or disability. These effects are due primarily to the loss of mobility, and health risks that may follow a bone fracture.

What are the causes?

As in other tissues, cells in the bones are being renewed constantly. With age, however, phosphorus and calcium are lost faster than the body can replenish them. Hormonal changes accelerate this imbalance between bone buildup and breakdown—particularly the loss of estrogen due to menopause. As men age, they also may be at risk due to the decline of testosterone—or male

hormone—levels. Bones that once were solid and sturdy may become brittle and full of empty spaces.

Diet is a very important risk factor. If you're not getting enough calcium, your body can't maintain strong bones. While exercise helps build bone, inactivity accelerates bone loss. Other risk factors include smoking; drinking alcohol; being underweight; being small framed; having a light complexion; having certain medical conditions such as hormonal deficiency associated with aging; using corticosteroids or excessive use of thyroid replacement hormones; and extended periods of bed rest.

What are the symptoms?

In its early stages, there are no symptoms of osteoporosis. As the disease advances, pain may develop in certain bones, especially in the lower back. Loss of bone mass may cause some bones to become compressed. This can lead to loss of height as well as an increasingly stooped posture known as "dowager's hump." Affected bones, especially in the wrist, hips or spine, are more likely to break or fracture—even from minor trauma. Osteoporosis won't show up on X-rays until approximately 30 percent of the bone has been lost. This is why a bone density test is needed to make a diagnosis.

Can it be prevented?

True prevention of osteoporosis begins in childhood and adolescence, when our most rapid period of bone development takes place. Getting plenty of calcium and weight-bearing exercise in these early years is crucial.

But even as an adult, there are things you can do. Get adequate calcium through diet or supplements. Your doctor can help determine how much is right for you. Calcium-rich foods include low-fat dairy products; leafy, green vegetables; beans; nuts; and fortified orange juice and cereals. Don't forget about vitamin D—it helps your body absorb calcium.

Regular, weight-bearing exercise also can help keep bones strong. Jogging, walking, dancing, low-impact aerobics and weight training are good choices. The risk of osteoporosis is higher in smokers. So, if you smoke, it's time to quit. Also, limit alcohol use.

As a preventive measure, many women benefit from starting hormone replacement therapy (HRT) right after menopause. This can help slow the rate of bone loss during therapy. But remember, HRT doesn't replace lost bone. HRT isn't right for all women. Discuss the risks and benefits with your doctor.

How is it treated?

Treatment of osteoporosis aims to slow down further loss of bone minerals, restore as much bone mass as possible and prevent fractures. The first step is to increase calcium and vitamin D intake through diet and supplements. Some doctors recommend treating osteoporosis with HRT. There also are medications such as bisphosphonates that may help.

Though weight-bearing exercise slows bone mineral loss, strenuous activity poses a risk of bone injuries. Talk with your doctor about developing a safe exercise routine.

One of the greatest dangers from this disease is injury from falls, including fractures. Take measures to prevent injury. Improve lighting and floor surfaces in your home. Add handrails in your bathroom. And, ask your doctor if you might benefit from using a cane or walker.

WHEN TO SEEK HELP

Seek emergency help if:

▶ **You have a fall or an accident that may have caused a bone fracture.**

Call your nurse information service or doctor if:

▶ **You have any risk factors for osteoporosis, especially if you're postmenopausal.**

For related information, see: Menopause, Page 317; Staying Healthy, Page 17

PARKINSON'S DISEASE (PD)

What is Parkinson's disease?

Parkinson's disease, or PD, is a disease of the central nervous system. It's progressive—which means signs and symptoms develop gradually over time. PD is slightly more common in men than women. Typical onset is at about age 60. However, a small percentage of cases are diagnosed in people younger than age 40.

What causes Parkinson's?

In PD, cells in part of the brain degenerate. These are cells that normally produce dopamine—a chemical that helps relay messages that control body movement. Everyone loses some of these neurons as a normal part of aging. But, people with PD lose a significantly greater amount. It's uncertain what causes this. Researchers have studied genetics, environmental factors, medications and toxins. No single cause has been found. Many scientists believe that a combination of factors may be at work.

What are the symptoms?

The earliest signs of PD may be subtle. You may have a slight tremor of your hand, arm or leg, which may stop when you make a deliberate movement. You may have one hand that doesn't swing like it used to when you walk. Or, your voice may be soft, you may mumble your words, or your handwriting may worsen and become smaller.

Because PD develops gradually, early signs and symptoms may go unnoticed. And, the disease may not be quickly or easily diagnosed. That's why it's important to report any possible signs of PD to your doctor. Some prescription medications can cause symptoms that mimic Parkinson's. So, be sure your doctor knows about all the medications you're taking, too.

As the disease progresses, you likely will experience one or more of the classic symptoms of Parkinson's. You may have a resting tremor on one side of your body. You may experience bradykinesia—a general slowness of movement. Your limbs may be stiff or rigid. Or, you may have trouble writing, walking, running or maintaining balance.

You may experience secondary symptoms, as well. These may include depression, anxiety, memory loss, dizziness, constipation or increased sweating. You may have difficulty sleeping, regulating your body temperature, or chewing or swallowing. And, sexual dysfunction can be common. You may have cramps, numbness, tingling or pain in your muscles.

You also may have slurred or soft speech. Yet, it's possible that you may not experience any of these symptoms.

Can it be prevented?

Because the cause of PD is unknown, there currently is no way of preventing or curing the disease.

How is Parkinson's treated?

There are treatments that are very effective in helping patients manage their symptoms as PD progresses. And, new research has been very promising.

A variety of drugs are available that may provide dramatic relief from your symptoms of PD. Unfortunately, most of these medications can cause side effects. So, it's important to work with your doctor to find the right balance between the benefits and side effects of a particular drug. Get involved in your treatment plan. Talk openly with your doctor about your concerns.

Taking care of your overall health may make living with PD easier. For instance, a balanced diet, including lots of fiber, can help prevent constipation. Eat plenty of fruits, vegetables and whole grains. If you have difficulty chewing or swallowing, take small bites and swallow each mouthful before taking another. Chop food in a blender or food processor. Eat slowly—a warming plate can help keep your food appetizing.

Regular exercise or physical therapy may help improve your mobility, flexibility, balance and range of motion. Talk with your doctor or therapist about developing a program that's right for you. Whether it's walking, swimming, gardening or dancing, staying active may improve your quality of life. Your energy level may go up and down, so pace yourself.

How can I cope?

Living with PD can be stressful and challenging. It's not unusual to feel sad, angry or depressed. Find a way to express these feelings. You may want to seek out a support group—a great outlet for laughing, crying and sharing stories with others who know just what you're going through. Reach out to your family and friends. Try to keep doing the things you love—a positive attitude can go a long way.

For related information, see: Anxiety, Page 330; Caregiver's Concerns, Page 331; Complementary Medicine, Page 335; Constipation, Page 80; Depression, Page 332; Dizziness, Page 92; Numbness or Tingling, Page 184; Staying Healthy, Page 17; Stress, Page 334

PEPTIC ULCER OR GASTRITIS

What is peptic ulcer or gastritis?

A peptic ulcer is an open wound or sore in the mucous membranes that line the stomach or duodenum—the upper portion of your small intestine. Ulcers in the stomach are called gastric ulcers. Those in the duodenum are called duodenal ulcers. Rarely, ulcers may occur in the esophagus. These aren't referred to as peptic ulcers. Ulcers typically affect more men than women. The risk is higher among smokers and people with a personal or family history of ulcers. Gastritis is a similar condition. However, rather than an ulcer, it's an inflammation of the stomach lining.

What are the causes?

The digestive system uses powerful chemicals, such as the enzyme pepsin, to break down food. The membranes that line the surface of the stomach and the intestine—-or the gastrointestinal (GI) system—secrete mucus to protect tissues against these corrosive agents. However, these membranes sometimes can become damaged. Then the acids and enzymes eat away at the unprotected tissue of the stomach and intestines.

Despite popular belief, stress and spicy foods don't cause ulcers or gastritis. Roughly four of five peptic ulcers— particularly duodenal ulcers—are caused by bacterial infection. The Helicobacter pylori, or H. pylori, bacterium is a common infection that affects people as they age. Doctors aren't sure how people become infected.

Long-term use of nonsteroidal anti-inflammatory drugs (NSAIDs) such as aspirin, ibuprofen and naproxen sodium also may be a factor in the development of peptic ulcers and gastritis. Other drugs such as cortisone or steroid medications also can break down the stomach lining and increase your risk. Smoking is a big risk factor. In rare cases, tumors may trigger excess production of gastrin, which can cause the stomach to produce too much acid.

What are the symptoms?

Not everyone with a peptic ulcer has symptoms. If the ulcer is in your stomach, you may feel a dull, aching pain that's relieved by certain foods—and made worse by not eating. Ulcers in the duodenum may produce a gnawing pain that occurs one to three hours after a meal—or in the middle of the night. The pain sometimes may radiate to your chest or back. It might be present for a few weeks, then subside for a while before recurring. Certain foods or antacids may bring some relief. Other symptoms may include indigestion, heartburn, nausea, vomiting and, in some cases, weight loss.

Severe cases may cause internal bleeding. You may have stools that appear black or tarry. Or, you may vomit bloody material that resembles coffee grounds. Often, signs of bleeding are noticed before there's any pain. Extreme pain could be a sign of a perforated ulcer—an ulcer that completely penetrates the lining or wall of the stomach or, more often, the duodenum.

Can they be prevented?

It's unclear how to avoid being infected by the bacteria that cause peptic ulcers and gastritis. But, the presence of the microbe doesn't result in these health conditions in everyone. Certain lifestyle changes—quitting smoking, limiting alcohol and avoiding long-term use of aspirin or other NSAIDs—may help. There's no strong evidence, though, that dietary strategies can prevent either peptic ulcers or gastritis.

How are they treated?

If you test positive for the H. pylori bacteria, your doctor may prescribe antibiotics. Additional treatment will focus on relieving symptoms. In mild cases of either peptic ulcers or gastritis, treatment with drugs that reduce stomach acid or coat the stomach lining can reduce pain. Many of these products are available over-the-counter. Antacids

must be taken in sufficient doses—and for a long enough period—to allow ulcers to heal. Talk with your doctor about an effective approach.

Most ulcers heal after six to eight weeks of treatment. But, there's a high risk that they'll recur within one year. Try to avoid alcohol and caffeine, which often is found in foods such as coffee, tea, cola and chocolate. If you smoke, quit. Smoking contributes to ulcer formation and delays healing. Talk with your doctor about other measures to help prevent recurrent ulcers.

WHEN TO SEEK HELP

Seek emergency help if:

▶ **You have any of the following symptoms: medium to large amount of bloody or black, tarry stools; severe abdominal pain; shock including cold, clammy skin or fainting; or vomiting bright-red blood.**

Call your nurse information service or doctor if:

▶ **You have symptoms of an ulcer or gastritis that last longer than three days after trying self-care.**

For related information, see: *Backache, Page 56; Chest Pain, Page 76; Heartburn, Page 144; Medications, Page 37; Nausea or Vomiting, Page 174; Staying Healthy, Page 17; Stomach Pain, Page 212; Weight Loss, Page 244*

PROSTATE CONDITIONS

What is the prostate?

The prostate is a gland of the male reproductive system. About the size and shape of a walnut, it's located just below the bladder and in front of the rectum, surrounding the urethra. The prostate secretes a fluid that, along with sperm, becomes part of semen.

What causes prostate conditions?

Benign prostatic hyperplasia (BPH), or enlarged prostate, is a typical part of aging for most men. Although it can cause some urinary problems, it isn't cancerous and usually is treatable.

Prostatitis is an inflammation of the prostate gland. It usually is caused by bacteria, though it isn't contagious. Microbes may enter the prostate through the urethra, possibly due to a backward flow of urine. Prostatitis sometimes develops following an infection of the urinary tract or bladder. You also may be at greater risk for this condition if you have BPH.

Prostate cancer—the most common type of cancer in American men—begins as a tumor that develops in the prostate. Over time, the tumor grows, usually very slowly. Cancerous cells can metastasize, or spread, to other body parts.

The exact cause is unknown, but male hormones and heredity seem to play a part.

What are the symptoms?

BPH may cause problems with urination. You may have weak, hesitant or interrupted urine flow. It may be difficult to stop, and you may experience dribbling. Or, you may not be able to empty your bladder completely. You also may feel a strong urge to urinate frequently, especially at night, which may disrupt your sleep.

Symptoms of prostatitis vary depending on the nature of the infection. You may experience blood in your urine or ejaculate, chills, fever, or pain in your lower abdomen or scrotal area. It also may be painful or difficult to urinate.

Prostate cancer usually causes no symptoms in its early stages. For this reason, it's important to have regular exams. Ask your doctor at what age you should have prostate screenings. As the tumor grows, urinary problems resembling those seen in BPH may develop. Prostate cancer that has metastasized can cause fatigue, weakness and pain in the back, ribs, hips, shoulders or other bones.

Can prostate conditions be prevented?

For most men, BPH is inevitable. But, there are some things you can do to reduce symptoms. Limit your intake of liquids in the evenings so you won't have to get up as often to use the bathroom. Empty your bladder as fully as possible each time. Talk with your doctor about the medications you're taking. Even some over-the-counter products may aggravate your condition, especially cold and allergy pills.

Prostatitis generally can't be prevented. But the sooner the infection is caught, the more likely it is to respond to treatment.

There are no proven strategies for preventing prostate cancer. Some evidence suggests that eating a low-fat diet rich in vegetables may provide some protection. But the most important thing you can do is have regular health exams—early detection is key.

How are prostate conditions treated?

Watchful waiting often is the first step for BPH. If your symptoms aren't severe, you and your doctor may agree to monitor your condition over time. If BPH becomes troublesome, medication usually is an option. There are a number of effective drugs on the market, but there are some possible side effects. Discuss the risks with your doctor. Don't be embarrassed to ask questions. Surgery may be required in more severe cases.

In benign prostatic hyperplasia (BPH), the prostate becomes enlarged. This squeezes the urethra and causes urination problems.

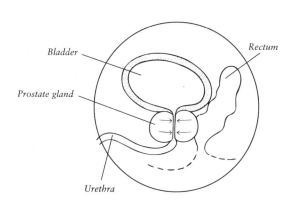

Enlarged view of hyperplasia

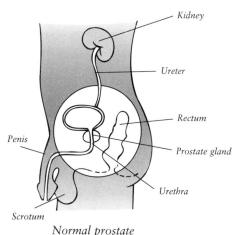

Normal prostate

Prostatitis caused by bacteria can be treated with antibiotics for a few weeks. If the inflammation is due to some other cause, treatment may be aimed at relieving symptoms with bed rest, increased fluid intake, or use of aspirin or other pain relievers. In cases where there is an obstruction, a catheter may be used to improve urine flow.

Prostate cancer treatment is a complex subject. In many cases, the tumor will grow so slowly that it may not pose a threat to your health or life. So, watchful waiting often is advisable.

If a follow-up exam shows that the cancer is growing rapidly, prostatectomy—removal of the prostate—is a possibility. Radiation therapy sometimes is used to destroy cancerous cells without surgery. Radioactive implants and cryotherapy also may be used as alternatives to surgery. But because the prostate remains in the body, it's impossible to know if the treatment is totally effective.

In advanced cases, the tumor spreads outside the prostate to nearby tissues or other places in the body. Hormonal therapy or radiation therapy often is used in the case of painful bone metastases. There also are a number of new procedures being developed, and research is ongoing.

Often, doctors will prescribe a combination of approaches. Choice of treatment depends on many factors—age, general health, cancer stage and personal preferences. There may be some risks involved. So, it's important to communicate openly and honestly with your doctor about any concerns you may have.

WHEN TO SEEK HELP

Seek emergency help if:

▶ **You're unable to pass any urine despite drinking plenty of fluids.**

▶ **You're passing very bloody urine, possibly with clots.**

Call your nurse information service or doctor if:

▶ **You have trouble urinating, get up often during the night to urinate, or notice blood in your urine or semen.**

For related information, see: Cancer, Page 264; Fatigue, Page 114; Fever, Page 116; Medications, Page 40; Prevention and Early Detection, Page 31; Sexual Health, Page 311; Staying Healthy, Page 17; Urination Concerns, Page 230; Urine, Blood In, Page 232

SINUSITIS OR ALLERGIC RHINITIS

What are sinusitis and allergic rhinitis?

These common conditions affect the mucous membranes that line your nose and sinuses—hollow spaces behind your forehead, nose and cheeks.

Sinusitis is a condition in which the sinuses become inflamed and blocked. The resulting pressure often is painful. Acute sinusitis typically follows a cold or flu. It usually disappears with treatment in one to two weeks. Chronic sinusitis often is milder but lasts longer. It also recurs throughout the year.

Allergic rhinitis, or hay fever, is a chronic condition. You may suffer from symptoms throughout the year or during particular seasons. It's triggered by sensitivity to airborne pollens and molds.

What are the causes?

Acute bacterial sinusitis often follows viral upper respiratory infections which can interfere with the drainage of mucus. A viral infection also may weaken the body's defenses and allow a subsequent bacterial infection to take hold. Chronic sinusitis may follow untreated or persistent acute sinusitis. But some cases arise from exposure to airborne irritants such as dust, chemicals, fumes or smoke. Smokers are especially susceptible. The same is true for people who have nasal polyps, unusually narrow sinus openings or an abnormality of the nasal passages, such as a deviated septum.

Allergic rhinitis develops due to sensitivities to allergens. These may include pollen, dust, mold, mites, animal dander, medications or foods.

What are the symptoms?

In sinusitis, the mucous membranes become inflamed. Swelling blocks drainage of mucus from the sinuses. Pressure builds up, causing headaches, or pain and more swelling. You may feel pressure above or behind your eyes, on the bridge of your nose, in your cheeks, or in your upper jaw or teeth. The pain may be worse when you first wake up. Your eyes may become watery, and your eyelids may swell. Typically, you'll have a thick, yellowish-green nasal discharge. You also may have a low-grade fever and chills. In some cases, you may lose your sense of smell and taste, or your voice might sound scratchy or nasal.

Symptoms of allergic rhinitis resemble those of the common cold—sneezing; nasal congestion and itching; itchy, red, watery eyes; cough; headache; or a persistent tickle in your mouth or throat. You also may have a lot of nasal discharge, which may be clear and watery.

Can they be prevented?

To reduce your risk of sinusitis, minimize your exposure to people with colds. Wash your hands frequently, and avoid touching your nose and eyes.

To minimize outbreaks of allergic rhinitis, try to avoid exposure to allergens. Use air conditioners or air-purification systems. Change the filters on these appliances and on furnaces regularly. Stay indoors during peak allergy season or when the pollen count is high. Try to avoid chores such as dusting, gardening or mowing the lawn. Keep pets clean and groomed—and don't allow them in your bedroom. Wash your hair at night and change pillowcases frequently.

How are they treated?

Most cases of sinusitis can be treated with over-the-counter products. Oral or nasal decongestants may reduce swelling and promote drainage. Use these with caution as directed by your doctor. Using a cool-mist vaporizer or humidifier, or saline spray may moisten and soothe your nasal passages. Pain relievers, ice packs or heating pads may help relieve sinus pain and headache. Antibiotics can help to eliminate an infection. Steroid nasal sprays can help reduce symptoms.

In severe cases, a diagnostic procedure called endoscopy can detect a sinus blockage. Surgery may be required to improve sinus drainage.

Allergy treatments often include antihistamines, short-term use of decongestants, eye drops and nasal corticosteroids. Other treatments include desensitization therapy, which involves a series of shots to reduce your response to allergens. Ask your doctor if this will work for you. Reducing exposure to allergens is still the best option for most people.

WHEN TO SEEK HELP

Seek emergency help if:

► **You have any sudden change in vision; you can't move your eye normally; or if you experience confusion, nausea, vomiting, severe head pain or high fever.**

Call your nurse information service or doctor if:

► **You've tried self-care but your symptoms haven't improved after three days—or if you notice a bloody nasal discharge.**

For related information, see: Cough, Page 84; Eye, Itchy or Red, Page 104; Fever, Page 116; Headache, Page 138; Medications, Page 37; Nose, Congested or Runny, Page 178; Sinus Pain, Page 202

STROKE

What is a stroke?

A stroke occurs when blood flow to the brain is interrupted. There may be an obstruction in an artery, or a broken blood vessel. Cells in the brain can become damaged very quickly if they're not getting oxygen. The damage often is serious and may be permanent. Strokes can be fatal. But when a stroke is recognized and treated in time, doctors can drastically reduce disabilities caused by strokes.

What causes a stroke?

There are two main types of strokes—ischemic and hemorrhagic. In an ischemic stroke, a blood vessel or artery in the brain becomes blocked, cutting off the supply of oxygen and other nutrients to parts of the brain. There may be a blood clot, plaque or other tissue obstructing the artery. About 80 percent of all strokes are ischemic.

In a hemorrhagic stroke, a blood vessel in the brain ruptures and bleeds. It may bleed until pressure stops it, or a clot forms and prevents blood from escaping.

A related condition, transient ischemic attack (TIA), occurs when an artery is temporarily blocked. TIAs sometimes are called "mini-strokes." They may cause some of the same symptoms. However, TIAs don't result in brain damage and permanent loss of function.

The leading risk factors for stroke are high blood pressure and heart disease. Your risk also increases if you smoke, have diabetes, sickle cell disease, high cholesterol, or a family or personal history of strokes or TIAs. Most strokes occur in people ages 65 and older, and they're somewhat more common in men. Oral contraceptives may increase the risk for some women—especially if you're age 35 or older and you smoke.

What are the signs of stroke?

Strokes occur suddenly and without warning. Symptoms may include:

- Numbness or weakness of the face, arm or leg
- Confusion, or trouble speaking or understanding
- Blurred or double vision, or loss of vision
- Difficulty walking, dizziness, or loss of balance or coordination
- Sudden severe headache with no known cause

Symptoms may affect only the right or left side of the body. The person having a stroke may not realize it's happening.

So, bystanders play an important role in recognizing the warning signs and getting emergency help.

Can a stroke be prevented?

The best way to prevent stroke is to maintain the healthiest possible lifestyle. Quit smoking. Get plenty of exercise. Eat a balanced diet low in saturated fats and cholesterol. Limit alcohol consumption to two drinks or fewer per day. Maintain a healthy weight. Get regular health exams, including blood pressure checks. If your doctor prescribes medication for high blood pressure, be sure to take it exactly as directed. Some people may benefit from the use of medications that prevent blood clots. In rare cases, surgery may be needed to help keep arteries clear. Talk with your doctor about your risk of stroke.

How is a stroke treated?

Timing is everything. The sooner a person gets treatment for a stroke, the better the chances for recovery. A drug called tissue plasminogen activator (t-PA) can dramatically reduce disability associated with some types of strokes. But, it needs to be administered within three hours of the onset of symptoms to be effective. Other treatments depend on the type and extent of damage caused by the stroke.

How can I cope?

Each stroke is different. The range and severity of effects depend on a number of factors, including the part of the brain that was injured, the person's age, and how quickly he or she was treated. The effects of a stroke may include weakness or paralysis on one side of the body; trouble with balance or coordination; problems using language or speaking; being unaware of or ignoring one side of the body; pain, numbness or odd sensations; problems with memory, thinking, attention or learning; being unaware of the effects of the stroke; trouble swallowing; incontinence; and fatigue. Depression is common in stroke survivors. Sudden bursts of emotion such as laughing, crying or anger also are common.

Learning to live with these new challenges can be stressful and frustrating. Everyday activities, such as bathing, dressing, eating and using the bathroom, suddenly may be difficult. You may have no trouble walking or talking, but you may find yourself confused when you try to write a check or drive a car. It's natural to feel discouraged. But help is available, and there are things you can do to regain some control over your life.

Reach out for assistance. There are excellent rehabilitation programs that may help you overcome some of the new challenges that you may face. They offer a wide range of therapies that can be suited to fit your needs.

Take care of your emotional health, as well. Professional counselors can help you work through some of the difficult feelings you may be dealing with. It also may be reassuring to talk with other people who know what you're going through. Ask your doctor for information about support groups in your area—these can be valuable for family members and caregivers, as well.

WHEN TO SEEK HELP

A stroke is always a medical emergency. Any of the signs of stroke noted on Page 305 indicate that immediate help is needed.

Because a stroke affects the brain, the person having one may not realize what's happening. Act quickly if you see any signs of stroke in someone around you.

For related information, see: Caregiver's Concerns, Page 331; Depression, Page 332; First Aid and Emergencies, Page 16; Hypertension (High Blood Pressure), Page 287; Staying Healthy, Page 17

THYROID CONDITIONS

What are thyroid conditions?

The thyroid is a small, butterfly-shaped gland below the Adam's apple. It controls your metabolism by producing hormones that tell your body how fast to work and how to use energy. When your thyroid doesn't produce the right amount of these hormones, your metabolism is thrown off balance. This can affect you physically and emotionally.

About 20 million people have thyroid conditions. Three common disorders are hypothyroidism, hyperthyroidism and Graves' disease. Although thyroid conditions can't be prevented, most can be diagnosed with blood tests, and effectively treated.

What is hypothyroidism?

Hypothyroidism, or underactive thyroid, results when the thyroid doesn't make and release enough hormones.

Causes. Some factors that can cause the thyroid to slow down hormone production include:

- Hashimoto's thyroiditis, an auto-immune disease
- Previous radiation therapy in the neck area

- Removal of part of the thyroid during surgery
- Certain medications

Symptoms. Early symptoms may be difficult to notice. You may start to feel tired and sluggish. As your metabolism continues to slow, you may notice:

- Increased sensitivity to cold
- Unexplained weight gain
- Pale, dry skin
- Drowsiness, even after a full night's sleep
- Thinning hair
- Heavier menstrual periods
- Depression
- Constipation

Treatment. See your doctor if you have symptoms of hypothyroidism. If you're diagnosed with this condition, he or she will prescribe synthetic thyroid hormones. This medication is taken by mouth and usually restores hormone levels successfully.

What is hyperthyroidism?

Hyperthyroidism, or overactive thyroid, results when the amount of hormones the thyroid makes and releases is too high.

Causes. Most cases of hyperthyroidism are associated with a disorder called

Graves' disease. Other causes include:

- Hyperfunctioning thyroid nodules—occurs when certain parts of the gland produce too much thyroid hormone

- Thyroiditis—occurs when the thyroid becomes temporarily inflamed; causes excess thyroid hormone to leak into the bloodstream

- Excessive treatment with thyroid hormone

Symptoms. Some symptoms of hyperthyroidism may resemble other health problems. And, symptoms such as elevated heart rate are very subtle. You also may notice:

- Progressive weight loss, even though your appetite may increase

- Nervousness or irritability

- Increased perspiration

- More frequent bowel movements

- Decreased menstrual flow

- Muscle weakness

- Heat intolerance

- Fine tremor

Hyperthyroidism in older adults may be difficult to recognize. There often are few symptoms. Fatigue and depression may be the most prominent—this is known as apathetic hyperthyroidism.

Treatment. Your doctor will consider your overall health, age and severity of your condition. Common treatments include:

- Radioactive iodine—taken orally and absorbed by the thyroid. This causes the thyroid to shrink. Symptoms may decrease in about three months. Sometimes, production of hormones may slow too much. If this happens, you may need medication to replace these hormones.

- Medications—lower the amount of thyroid hormone in the blood

- Surgery—a less common treatment option

What is Graves' disease?

Graves' disease is an autoimmune disorder. It's the leading cause of hyperthyroidism. As in other autoimmune diseases, your body attacks its own healthy cells and tissues. Graves' disease causes the body to produce antibodies against the thyroid. This stimulates the thyroid to overproduce hormones. Graves' disease is more common in women than men.

Causes. The cause of Graves' disease is unknown. However, factors may include heredity, gender and age. In some cases, it may follow pregnancy or a very stressful life event.

Symptoms. Graves' disease presents the same symptoms as hyperthyroidism. They include:

- Progressive weight loss

- Anxiety and irritability

- Rapid heartbeat

- Sensitivity to heat
- Increased perspiration
- Enlarged thyroid, or goiter
- Fine tremor

In some cases, you may experience Graves' ophthalmopathy. This occurs when the tissues and muscles behind the eyes swell. You may notice that your eyeballs are bulging, red or swollen. Other symptoms may include excessive tears, sensitivity to light, and blurry vision. If you have this condition, your doctor may prescribe medication or suggest surgery.

Treatment. Graves' disease often is treated with the same methods as hyperthyroidism. Radioactive iodine may be used to shrink the thyroid and slow hormone production. Medication also may be prescribed to lower the amount of thyroid hormone in the blood.

Will my thyroid condition affect me emotionally?

If you have a thyroid condition, you may feel anxious, irritable and depressed. These emotions often are associated with the condition itself and may interfere with your daily life. Talk with your doctor about how you feel. He or she may be able to treat these symptoms or help you connect with a support group. Also, be open with your family and friends. They may be good sources of love and support as you deal with your condition.

For related information, see:
Constipation, Page 80; Depression, Page 332; Fatigue, Page 114; Hair Loss, Page 132; Heartbeat, Rapid, Page 142; Medications, Page 37; Sweatiness, Page 218; Vision Problems, Page 238; Weight Gain, Page 242; Weight Loss, Page 244

Sexual Health

8

Our sexual health affects how we feel, emotionally and physically. Engaging in healthy sexual relationships—based on trust, self-respect and communication—and taking care of yourself can help you maintain your overall health and well-being.

Sexually Transmitted Diseases

Sexual activity can be enjoyable, but it also has its risks. Protecting yourself is extremely important. One possible consequence of sexual activity is becoming infected with a sexually transmitted disease (STD).

The most common STDs in the United States are herpes simplex virus type 2, chlamydia, gonorrhea, syphilis and genital warts. While infections such as HIV and hepatitis B aren't always referred to as STDs, they're commonly spread by sexual contact. They also can be spread by other means such as infected needles.

Symptoms

It's important to know that not all STDs show symptoms. When symptoms are present, they vary, depending on the type of infection. You may notice these signs around your genitals:

- Abnormal discharge, possibly from your rectum as well
- Bleeding
- Blisters

- Burning sensation
- Growths or warts
- Itching or irritation
- Foul-smelling odors
- Pain or tenderness
- Rashes
- Sores
- Swollen lymph nodes
- Urinary difficulties

If you think you may have been infected with an STD, talk with your doctor. Also, see your doctor to be evaluated if your sexual partner has, or has had, an STD—even if you don't have symptoms.

STDs increase your risk of other health concerns. Pelvic inflammatory disease (PID) is an infection of the female reproductive organs (see Page 236). It usually is caused by gonorrhea or chlamydia. PID can lead to complications such as ectopic pregnancy and infertility. The human papillomavirus (HPV) causes genital warts (see Page 124). Various strains of this virus are responsible for at least 95 percent of cervical cancer cases.

Treatment

Most STDs respond well to treatment, which varies depending on the type of infection. Some STDs, however, require lifelong management. Genital herpes, for example, can't be cured. The virus remains dormant in the nerves even when no symptoms are present. Work closely with your doctor. Follow all

instructions and take medication as prescribed. You also may be advised to avoid sexual activity while being treated. If you're diagnosed with an STD, notify all recent sexual partners. Urge them to get medical checkups.

Safer Sex

Safer sex can lower—but not necessarily eliminate—your risk of sexually transmitted diseases. The goal is to prevent contact with genital sores, and prevent exchange of body fluids such as semen, blood, vaginal secretions and saliva.

- **Abstinence.** The most effective way to prevent STDs is to not have sexual contact.
- **Mutual monogamy.** Have sex with only one partner who also is monogamous and free of STDs.
- **Condoms.** Consistently, and correctly, using latex condoms during oral, anal or vaginal sex can reduce your risk of exposure to STDs. But, they don't provide 100 percent protection.

If you're sexually active, these steps can help you stay healthy:

Talk with your partner about his or her sexual history. Have an honest discussion. Ask if he or she has an STD, has been exposed to one, or has any unexplained physical symptoms. You may be at risk for an STD if your partner engages in high-risk behaviors. This includes drug use or a history of multiple sexual contacts. Get a health exam.

Talking about this may be uncomfortable, but don't let embarrassment jeopardize your health.

Learn to recognize the signs of STDs. If you notice any symptoms—in yourself or your partner—don't have sex. Seek medical attention as soon as possible. Urge your partner to do so, too.

Have regular checkups for STDs—even if you don't have any symptoms. These can be done at regular preventive visits with your doctor. Use the opportunity to ask any other questions about your sexual health.

Men's Sexual Concerns

For some men, discussing sexual concerns can be difficult. But open communication with your partner and your doctor is crucial. It can help provide peace of mind and, in most cases, effective treatment.

Erectile Dysfunction

Erectile dysfunction (ED), or impotence, is the consistent inability to achieve or sustain an erection sufficient for sexual intercourse. An occasional episode of ED happens to nearly all men. It's perfectly normal and nothing to be concerned or embarrassed about. If it's persistent, however, your self-esteem and personal relationships may become affected. Fortunately, ED is often very treatable.

ED once was believed to be mainly a psychological problem. It's now known that physical factors also play a role in most cases. Psychological causes include stress, anxiety, fatigue, depression and relationship problems. Physical causes may include diabetes, heart disease, vascular disease, hormone disorders, cigarette smoking, excessive alcohol or other drug use, certain medications, surgery or other trauma.

With age, some men may notice that their erections take longer to develop or are less firm. These changes aren't the same as ED, which isn't a normal part of aging.

Many cases of ED resolve on their own. Talk with your doctor if the condition lasts for longer than two months, or is a recurring problem. He or she can help you determine the underlying cause. Treatment may include medication, surgery or counseling. Remember to talk openly and honestly with your partner. Treatment often is more successful that way.

Premature Ejaculation

A premature ejaculation is one that occurs before a man wishes it to, or too quickly to satisfy his partner. It's a common sexual complaint, particularly for young men and those involved in new relationships. The condition often can lead to great distress. It can cause feelings of guilt, embarrassment or frustration. It also may lead to relationship difficulties.

Premature ejaculation rarely is due to a physical condition. The excitement and anxiety of a new relationship can contribute to the problem. Other factors that affect mental and emotional health—such as stress and depression—

also may be involved. Talk openly with your partner to avoid any miscommunication. Also, try to avoid unrealistic expectations. If you consistently ejaculate before you wish to do so, talk with your doctor. He or she may be able to ease your fears, or suggest techniques to help you learn to delay ejaculation. If psychological factors are involved, your doctor may recommend professional counseling.

Loss of Sexual Desire

Loss of interest in sex affects everyone from time to time. You should consider it a problem only if it becomes a long-term condition, and if you or your partner is dissatisfied as a result. Loss of desire may have several underlying causes. Depression, fatigue, stress, pain or relationship difficulties may diminish your interest. However, there may be a physical cause—for example, a drop in the male hormone testosterone. If you experience loss of sexual desire, see your doctor for a diagnosis.

Long-Lasting Effects of Sexual Abuse

Not every sexual experience is welcome, or healthy. A history of sexual abuse or rape can continue to haunt survivors long after the crisis has passed.

If you're a survivor of abuse or rape, professional counseling can help you work through the events and issues you may be facing.

Women's Sexual Concerns

Many women feel embarrassed discussing their sexual concerns. While this is understandable, it's important to address difficulties early. Otherwise, they may become larger. Eventually, they may negatively impact your health or personal relationships. Talk with your doctor. Many conditions have physical causes that can be treated effectively once identified. Open communication between you and your partner also can help ease any frustration you may feel.

Vaginal Dryness

Lack of vaginal lubrication can cause painful intercourse. This condition can result from insufficient foreplay. If this is the case, learn what is pleasurable for you and gently talk with your partner about your desires. Vaginal dryness also can occur when the body produces less estrogen after a menstrual period or at menopause. You also may notice vaginal dryness when using a decongestant medication. An over-the-counter, water-based lubricant may help. Some lubricants can damage latex condoms and make them less effective, so check with your doctor or pharmacist. If you're postmenopausal, hormone replacement therapy (HRT), topical estrogen creams or estrogen vaginal rings may ease your symptoms. Talk with your doctor.

Loss of Sexual Desire

Many women go through periods when they don't desire sex. This is normal.

> ### The Importance of Gynecological Exams
>
> Women ages 18 or older, or who are sexually active, should have regular gynecological exams. These can help protect your sexual and reproductive health. Your exam may include a discussion of your personal, family, medical and sexual history, as well as laboratory tests and screenings. Your doctor also may perform a clinical breast and pelvic exam.

But, if the situation lasts a long time or causes problems in your relationship, you may want to seek help. Several medical conditions can cause diminished sexual interest and desire in women, as can certain medications. Other common causes include anger, relationship conflict, depression, stress, alcohol and fatigue. Talk with your doctor if you're concerned. Appropriate treatment for an underlying condition may resolve the problem.

Orgasmic Dysfunction

Some women never reach orgasm during sexual activity with a partner. Yet, they still have pleasurable sexual experiences. Others achieve orgasm only occasionally or with certain kinds of stimulation. Still others reach orgasm every time they have intercourse.

The causes of orgasmic dysfunction may be physical, psychological or both. Painful intercourse is a common physical cause. Psychological causes may include depression (see Page 332), anger (see Page 330) or other feelings that affect your ability to focus on pleasurable sensations. Certain medication side effects include orgasm difficulty. Talk with your doctor if you're concerned. Identifying the cause can help determine appropriate treatment. As you learn what is pleasurable for you and communicate this to your partner, you may find that this concern resolves itself.

Painful Intercourse

You may have pain or discomfort—either at the opening of your vagina or deeper inside—during vaginal penetration. Painful intercourse can be caused by several medical conditions including vaginal dryness or irritation, infection, pelvic inflammatory disease, growths and endometriosis. Other causes may include certain medications or psychological trauma. Although sexual intercourse may be uncomfortable at times—especially at first—it should never be painful. If you suddenly begin having pain before, during or after intercourse, see your doctor. A physical examination can help identify the cause.

Vaginismus

Some women may experience severe tightening of their vaginal muscles when they attempt to have sexual intercourse. Penetration even may become impossible. Vaginismus is an involuntary spasm of the muscles in the vagina. It's helpful to remember that this condition isn't deliberate or intentional. The origin of vaginismus may be physical, psychological or both. An examination by your doctor can help determine the cause and lead the way to treatment.

A Woman's Cycle of Life

The menstrual cycle occurs during a woman's reproductive years—from menarche to menopause. About once a month, blood and tissue are shed from the lining of the uterus. The onset of menstruation, or menarche, usually occurs between ages 12 and 14. But, many girls start earlier or later.

Talking openly with your daughter about menstruation before it occurs can help her understand and cope with her body's changes. During the first three years, irregular periods are normal. The menstrual cycle is measured from the first day of one period to the first day of the next. After the cycle stabilizes, it averages about 28 days. But it can vary widely—from 20 to 40 days—and still be normal.

Premenstrual Syndrome

In the week or two before their periods start, some women may experience a collection of physical, psychological and emotional symptoms known as premenstrual syndrome (PMS). This likely is related to cyclical hormonal fluctuations but the exact cause is unknown. Physical symptoms may

316

include bloating, breast tenderness, headaches, acne, backaches and weight gain from fluid retention. Psychological or emotional symptoms may include mood swings, irritability, depression, crying spells and difficulty concentrating.

Many women experience some premenstrual discomfort. A much smaller number have symptoms severe enough to disrupt their work and personal relationships. When symptoms are severe, this sometimes is called premenstrual dysphoric disorder (PMDD).

Talk with your doctor if your symptoms significantly interfere with your daily activities. He or she may want to discuss your medical history and perform a physical exam. Treatment will depend on the severity of your symptoms. Your doctor may recommend lifestyle changes, or prescribe medication.

Even though the exact cause of PMS is unclear, some lifestyle changes may help ease your symptoms. Eating smaller, more frequent meals can help reduce bloating. Choose fruits, vegetables and whole grains. Limit your salt intake. Avoid caffeine and alcohol, especially right before your period. Regular exercise can help improve your health and overall sense of well-being. Reducing stress and getting enough sleep may help prevent headaches and mood swings. Keeping a journal of your symptoms and possible causes can help you minimize your personal PMS triggers.

Many women experience PMS every month until menopause. Others notice that their symptoms lessen after age 35. Whether your symptoms are mild or severe, open communication with your loved ones can help them understand what you're going through. By taking care of yourself and working closely with your doctor, you can help control the impact PMS has on your life.

Menopause

The end of menstrual periods, or menopause, is a natural biological process. Most women experience it, on average, at age 51, but it can occur any time between ages 40 and 60.

The time prior to menopause is called perimenopause. It may last four to five years, or more. During perimenopause, you may begin to experience the symptoms typically associated with menopause:

- Irregular periods—lighter or heavier
- Hot flashes
- Insomnia
- Mood changes
- Night sweats
- Changes in sexual desire
- Extreme sweating
- Frequent urination
- Vaginal dryness
- Difficulty concentrating
- Headaches

These symptoms, while often unpredictable, are normal for many women. But, you should see your doctor if you start to notice them. He or she may be able to help reduce your symptoms—and rule out other possible causes. Some women don't experience any symptoms.

When one year has passed since your last period, you're considered postmenopausal. Your ovaries no longer release eggs, nor produce enough of the hormones estrogen and progesterone to induce menstruation.

It's important to have regular checkups once you're postmenopausal. A significant long-term effect of decreased estrogen during menopause is an increased risk of osteoporosis (see Page 294). A woman's risk of heart disease also increases after menopause.

Is HRT Right for You?

Because it's a natural part of a woman's life cycle, menopause itself doesn't need to be treated. However, treatments can relieve symptoms and help reduce the risk of chronic conditions that may occur. Hormone replacement therapy (HRT) provides a low dose of estrogen, typically in combination with progestin. HRT can help reduce many symptoms of menopause, including vaginal dryness, hot flashes and painful intercourse. HRT also helps protect against bone loss, and lowers cholesterol levels.

However, there are some risks. HRT may increase a woman's risk of breast cancer, blood clots and gallstones. Talk with your doctor to determine if HRT is right for you.

Your doctor also may prescribe medications to help prevent osteoporosis and other chronic conditions. He or she can help you weigh the benefits and risks of any treatments you may be considering.

Self-Care Can Help

Self-care may help ease your symptoms. If you have hot flashes, dress in layers and try to identify what spurs them. For many women, triggers include spicy food, hot beverages, alcohol or a warm room. Water-based lubricants can help ease vaginal dryness and discomfort. Staying sexually active also helps reduce these symptoms. If you have trouble sleeping, avoid caffeinated beverages before going to bed. Relaxation techniques also may help. If urinary incontinence is a problem, ask your doctor to recommend exercises to strengthen your pelvic floor muscle. An overall healthy lifestyle can reduce your symptoms as well as preserve your long-term health. Eat a balanced diet, don't smoke, exercise regularly and get regular health exams.

Menopause is a significant point in a woman's life. It can be frightening or depressing for some women. For others, it's liberating. Your feelings and experiences are important. Identify sources of support that can provide you with information as well as comfort. Developing partnerships with other women, family members and your doctor can help you stay in charge of your health.

Contraceptives

Contraception is a personal decision that should be made in the context of your own personal beliefs and concerns. There are a variety of options available—each with its own risks and benefits to be considered. This chart shows some of the most commonly used methods of contraception. Your doctor can give you detailed information and help you choose what's right for you.

Method	Effectiveness	Risks	Protection From STDs	Convenience	Availability
Male latex condom	86%	Irritation and allergic reactions	Except for abstinence, latex condoms are the best protection against STDs	Applied immediately before intercourse; used only once and discarded	Nonprescription
Female condom	79%	Irritation and allergic reactions	May give some protection against STDs	Applied immediately before intercourse; used only once and discarded	Nonprescription
Diaphragm with spermicide	80%	Irritation and allergic reactions; urinary tract infection	Protects against cervical infection	Inserted before intercourse and left in place at least six hours after; can be left in place for 24 hours, with additional spermicide for repeated intercourse	Prescription
Cervical cap with spermicide	60-80%	Irritation and allergic reactions; abnormal Pap test	None	May be difficult to insert; can remain in place 48 hours without reapplying spermicide for repeated intercourse	Prescription
Spermicides alone	74%	Irritation and allergic reactions	None	Instructions vary; usually applied no more than one hour before intercourse and left in place at least six to eight hours after	Nonprescription

Method	Effectiveness	Risks	Protection From STDs	Convenience	Availability
Oral contraceptives (combined pill)	Over 95%	Dizziness; nausea; changes in menstruation, mood and weight; rarely, cardiovascular disease, including high blood pressure, blood clots, heart attack and strokes	None, except some protection against pelvic inflammatory disease	Must be taken on a daily schedule, regardless of frequency of intercourse	Prescription
Oral contraceptives (progestin only)	95%	Irregular bleeding, weight gain, breast tenderness, slightly increased chance of ectopic pregnancy	None, except some protection against pelvic inflammatory disease	Must be taken on a daily schedule, regardless of frequency of intercourse	Prescription
Emergency contraceptives	75%	Nausea, vomiting, menstrual changes, breast tenderness	None	Taken in two doses	Prescription
Injection (Depo-Provera®)	Over 99%	Irregular bleeding, weight gain, breast tenderness, headaches	None	One injection every three months	Prescription
Implant (Norplant®)	Over 99%	Irregular bleeding, weight gain, breast tenderness, headaches, difficulty in removal	None	Implanted by health care provider; minor outpatient surgical procedure; effective for up to five years	Prescription
Intrauterine device (IUD)	98-99%	Cramps, bleeding, pelvic inflammatory disease, infertility, perforation of uterus	None	After insertion by physician, can remain in place for up to one to 10 years, depending on type	Prescription
Periodic abstinence	About 75% (varies, based on method)	None	None	Requires frequent monitoring of body functions (e.g., body temperature for one method)	Instructions from health care provider
Surgical sterilization (male or female)	Over 99%	Pain, bleeding, infection, other minor postsurgical complications	None	One-time surgical procedure	Surgery

Source: Adapted from the U.S. Food and Drug Administration

Taking Care: Self-Care for You and Your Family

Pregnancy

9

Parenthood is an exciting journey—one that starts long before you change that first diaper. Preparation can help you and your partner feel more confident.

Before You're Pregnant

If you're planning to conceive soon, consider a pre-pregnancy health exam. Talk with your doctor about your health history including chronic conditions; medications, vitamins or supplements you may be taking; sexually transmitted diseases; and genetic concerns.

You'll increase your chances of getting pregnant and minimize risks to your baby if you start practicing healthy lifestyle habits now. Quit smoking, and don't drink or use drugs. Exercise regularly and get enough sleep.

Nutrition is crucial if you're planning to have a baby. Eat foods that contain folic acid to help prevent birth defects. You should get a total of 400 micrograms each day. Oranges, nuts and beans are good sources of folic acid. Ask your doctor if you need a supplement.

Getting the Good News

Finding out that you're pregnant is an exciting moment. The most commonly recognized symptom is a missed menstrual period. But some women may experience unusually light periods. Others may notice spotting during the time of the month they normally would menstruate. Other common signs include nausea or vomiting, tender breasts, or feeling tired or bloated.

A roller coaster of feelings. Pregnancy is an emotional time. So many changes are happening—to your body and your life. You and your partner may be thrilled, fearful and worried all at once. This is perfectly natural. Expecting a baby is a big event. Don't try to absorb it instantly. Take your time to adjust. Talk with your doctor for reassurance.

Prenatal care. From the first days of pregnancy, your baby's brain and other major organs are beginning to develop. With good prenatal care, you're more likely to have a healthy, full-term baby:

■ Focus on nutrition. Eat balanced meals that include lots of calcium, protein and iron. You will need about 300 extra calories a day. Choose healthy snacks. Try to avoid too much sodium and sugar. Take your prenatal vitamins faithfully.

■ Follow your doctor's recommendations regarding healthy weight gain. Most women gain 25 to 35 pounds.

■ Stay active. Exercise is important for your baby and it can help you feel better. It also may result in an easier delivery. Many women can continue the exercises they were doing before becoming pregnant. However, some sports may be prohibited. Check with your doctor.

■ Get lots of sleep. You may feel very tired—don't fight it. Get the rest that both you and your baby need.

■ Don't miss any prenatal appointments. During these visits, your baby's development will be monitored. Your blood pressure, weight and some blood levels will be checked, too. This is the perfect time to ask the many questions you and your partner probably have.

■ Be aware that your baby may be affected by things that posed no problem for you before you became pregnant. Talk with your doctor before you eat raw fish, handle your cat's litter box, or use cosmetics—such as acrylic nails or hair color—with potentially harmful chemicals, to name a few concerns.

Your Pregnancy

Here's a look at what you may expect during your pregnancy:

First Trimester—0 to 14 weeks

During the first trimester, you may not look pregnant, but there's a good chance you'll feel it. In these early months of pregnancy, about half of all expectant women experience morning sickness.

Infertility

A couple is considered infertile after one year of regular, unprotected intercourse. A diagnosis of infertility can be devastating. Decisions about fertility treatments, adoption—or neither—sometimes can take a toll on relationships. Work closely with a doctor in whom you can confide. He or she can help you connect with valuable resources.

This actually can occur any time of day. Nausea or vomiting may be triggered by certain smells or tastes. Sometimes, your queasiness may not seem related to anything at all. Eating small, frequent meals may help. Try munching on some plain crackers before getting out of bed each morning. Drink plenty of clear liquids—dehydration is a serious risk associated with vomiting. Call your doctor if nausea or vomiting are severe.

You may begin to notice changes in your body. Your breasts may become fuller and tender. Your nipples may become more prominent.

Exciting developments are happening for your baby, as well:

- The heart begins to beat.
- Bones appear—head, arms, fingers, legs and toes are formed.
- Major organs and the nervous system form.
- The placenta forms.
- Hair starts to grow.
- Twenty buds for future teeth appear.

By the end of the first trimester, the fetus is about 4 inches long and weighs between 1 and 2 ounces.

Depending on your situation, your doctor may recommend an ultrasound test. Ultrasound tests commonly are done to monitor the baby's development as needed. The test may be done either externally, over the abdomen, or internally through the vagina.

Thinking About Breast-Feeding?

One very important and personal decision you'll make during your pregnancy is whether or not to breast-feed your baby.

Breast milk is a powerhouse of short- and long-term health benefits. Babies who are breast-fed have less diarrhea, vomiting, colds, infections and pneumonia. Breast milk also can improve neurologic development, and reduce the risk of diabetes and various cancers later in life. It even can protect premature babies from some serious complications.

The American Academy of Pediatrics recommends breast milk for at least the first year of life. While this is ideal, remember, even breast-feeding for a shorter period of time can give your baby tremendous health advantages.

Learn as much as you can ahead of time. Talk with your doctor or a lactation specialist. Ask about the importance of colostrum—the yellowish fluid that flows a few days after delivery; what is proper "latch on"; and how to avoid sore nipples and address other breast health concerns. Also, discuss breast pumping, especially if you intend to do so when you return to work.

Being well-prepared to breast-feed can help make it a successful and fulfilling experience for both you and your baby.

Second Trimester—14 to 28 weeks

By now, your morning sickness probably has eased. However, some women experience it into their second trimesters. Your abdomen may begin to swell. Stretch marks may appear on your breasts or abdomen. Moisturizing lotion can help soothe dry skin. You may notice a dark line going from your navel, down the middle of your abdomen. You also may develop brown, uneven marks on your face, and your nipples may darken.

At around 16 to 20 weeks, you may start to feel the fetus move. Your baby may kick, sleep and wake, swallow, hear sounds and pass urine. Your baby now begins to grow quickly. Some developments include:

- Organs develop further.
- Eyebrows and fingernails form.
- Skin is wrinkled and covered with fine hair.

The fetus grows to about 11 to 14 inches, and weighs between 2 and 2 1/2 pounds by the end of the second trimester.

At this point, your doctor may recommend certain tests and screenings for birth defects or genetic diseases. Certain factors, such as your age or pregnancy history, may be considerations. Ask about the benefits and risks. Some tests, such as amniocentesis, slightly increase the risk of miscarriage.

This a good time to start looking ahead. Talk about delivery options with your doctor or midwife. Learn about the advantages breast-feeding offers you and your baby. Consider enrolling in childbirth or breast-feeding classes. Connecting with other expectant parents can be helpful. Check with your hospital or birthing center for information about resources in your area.

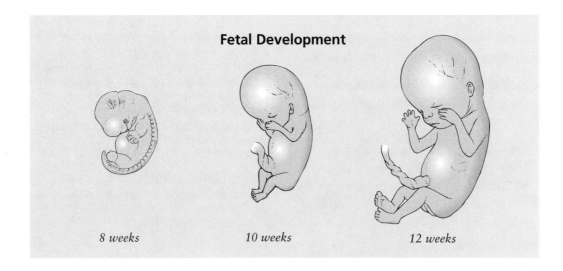

Fetal Development

8 weeks   10 weeks   12 weeks

Third Trimester—28 to 40 weeks

As you enter your third trimester, the fetus may be very active—kicking, stretching and running out of room to move. He or she will continue to grow and develop at a rapid pace:

- Fine body hair disappears.
- Bones harden—except for some skull bones, which remain soft and flexible for delivery.
- Fetus typically settles into a head-down position for birth.

At 40 weeks, the fetus is full term—about 20 inches long and 6 to 9 pounds.

As your due date approaches, start getting ready for the arrival of your baby.

Choose a doctor. Find a pediatrician or family physician before your baby is born. Check with your insurance provider to find someone who's covered by your plan. Or, ask your primary care doctor or obstetrician for a referral. Discuss with your doctor issues such as circumcision, child care arrangements, return-to-work concerns and breast-feeding resources for those times when questions arise.

Get a car safety seat. You'll need one to get your baby home safely. Be sure your car seat meets current requirements. Follow all installation instructions. Some police, fire or public health departments can check it for you to make sure it's installed correctly.

Pack your suitcase. Don't forget phone numbers of family and friends and a coming-home outfit for your baby.

Have a game plan. Plan your route to the hospital or birthing center. Familiarize yourself with the facility, including parking and check-in procedures. Arrange for someone to watch your other children, or pets.

Labor and Delivery

While false labor is certainly a possibility, especially with first babies, call your doctor or midwife if:

- Contractions occur at regular intervals and last 60 seconds. They don't stop even when you move around.

Postpartum Depression

This is a serious illness, not to be confused with the "baby blues." About 10 percent of new mothers are affected.

Seek emergency help if you have thoughts of hurting yourself or your baby.

Call your doctor if you have prolonged sadness, loss of interest in your baby, or any other signs of depression (see Page 332).

Partners and loved ones should realize that a woman experiencing postpartum depression might not recognize the severity of her symptoms. She may not be capable of reaching out for the help she needs.

- Your water breaks or leaks.
- You have "bloody show"—a blood-tinged mucus plug—with or without pain.

If you are more than six weeks from your due date and have more than six contractions in an hour, or if there are less than 10 minutes between contractions, you may be experiencing pre-term labor. Call your doctor right away.

Once you're home with your new son or daughter, savor every precious moment. Your journey as a parent will continue to amaze you—and it likely will go faster than you ever can imagine. Hold on tight—and enjoy the ride!

For related information, see: Backache, Page 56; Breast Pain, Page 66; Constipation, Page 80; Depression, Page 332; Faintness, Page 112; Fatigue, Page 114; Heartburn, Page 144; Hemorrhoids, Page 194; Nausea or Vomiting, Page 174; Sexual Health, Page 311; Staying Healthy, Page 17; Vaginal Bleeding, Page 234; Vaginal Discharge, Page 236; Working with Your Doctor, Page 43

WHEN TO SEEK HELP

Warning signs during first trimester

Call your doctor if you have:

▶ **Vaginal bleeding**

▶ **Change in vaginal discharge**

▶ **Pain or burning during urination**

▶ **Very bad or frequent headaches**

▶ **Severe vomiting**

▶ **Increasing pelvic pressure**

Warning signs during second and third trimesters

Seek emergency help if you have:

▶ **Contractions—six or more an hour when you're less than 37 weeks pregnant**

▶ **Heavy vaginal bleeding**

▶ **Marked swelling of hands and face**

▶ **Severe headache not relieved with acetaminophen**

▶ **Blurred or double vision, or seeing white lights like shooting stars**

▶ **Absent fetal activity**

Call your doctor if you have:

▶ **Bleeding causing a stain larger than a quarter**

▶ **Any fluid leaking from your vagina**

▶ **Decreased fetal activity**

▶ **Pain or burning during urination**

Mental and Behavioral Health

10

You may not think about it every day, but your state of mind has a lot to do with your overall health. It affects how you feel, how successfully you perform your job and how you treat others. It also influences how you live and make decisions.

We all experience emotional or mental health concerns from time to time. It's natural and part of being human. But, you don't have to deal with personal worries alone. If you think something is affecting your well-being and peace of mind, seek help from friends, family or a medical professional. Remember, taking a proactive approach to your mental health can help you lead a happier, more fulfilling life.

The mental and behavioral health concerns in this chapter are listed alphabetically for convenient reference.

Addictive Behavior

Addiction is a powerful physical or psychological dependence on a substance or activity. It can be so overpowering that the individual may not even realize that he or she has a problem. In fact, many people resist intervention and refuse to accept help. But, without help, people with addictions may experience serious consequences—including legal or financial trouble, shattered personal relationships and job loss. If you think you or someone you know has an addiction, don't delay seeking help.

Professional help is necessary—only rarely can addictions be beaten alone. Some may benefit from individual treatment programs or therapy. Others find that support groups are lifelines to staying strong and determined. If you're a family member trying to cope with a loved one's addiction, you also may find comfort in support groups or counseling.

Dealing with an addiction is a lifelong struggle—and some people relapse and fall back into dangerous habits. The risk of relapse is always there—often, people attend support groups and counseling for many years. But, with continuing support systems in place, many people can avoid relapse.

Alcohol

People with alcohol addiction crave alcohol so much that drinking far outweighs everything else significant in their lives. Family, friends, work and health lose importance—even the possibility of death may not be a concern. The only thing that may matter is where the next drink comes from.

Alcohol dependence also has physical effects. If the person addicted to alcohol hasn't had a drink in a long time, he or she may start to feel withdrawal symptoms that indicate a medical emergency—including shaking, rapid pulse and breathing, and fever. These effects, combined with the psychological need to drink, make alcohol extremely difficult to give up.

Someone may have an alcohol addiction if he or she:

- Drinks alone or secretly
- Experiences impaired judgment and ability to function
- Needs a drink first thing in the morning or to fight a hangover
- Feels guilty about drinking
- Has blackouts
- Has mood or personality changes when drinking

You can't treat alcohol addiction by yourself. If you or someone you know has a problem with drinking, seek help. Therapy and support groups such as Alcoholics Anonymous are good resources. Friends and family may find strength and comfort in support groups, too. With continued encouragement, alcohol addiction can be controlled. But remember—the battle must be fought one day at a time.

Drugs and Other Substances

Some drugs, when used properly, can save lives. But when drugs are abused, they can destroy or kill. People who are addicted to or abuse drugs endanger their own health, as well as the safety of those around them.

People can become addicted to any kind of drug—illegal, prescription, over-the-counter and tobacco. It's even possible to be addicted to substances you might not think of, such as chemical inhalants like aerosol sprays. Drug addiction has many physical and emotional effects, including:

- Slurred speech
- Impaired judgment
- Agitation and irritability
- Depression
- Decline in hygiene and health

As with alcohol, drug addiction needs to be treated by a medical professional. If you or someone you know abuses or is addicted to drugs, seek help immediately.

Often, treatment includes steps to control withdrawal symptoms, counseling, and self-help or support groups. It's not unusual to relapse into drug use. But, persistence, determination and a strong support system can make your effort toward success worthwhile.

Other Addictions

Eating. Shopping. Gambling. Sex. When done in a healthy manner, participating in these activities can be an enjoyable part of life. But for individuals who

Substance Abuse and Your Child

As parents, we'd like to think that substance abuse won't affect our children. The reality is, it can happen to anyone, at any age. Recognizing the signs of substance abuse—especially during the turbulent teen years—isn't always easy. Some moodiness and reluctance to communicate can be normal.

However, pay attention to any dramatic changes in your child's behavior:

- Noticeable slip in grades
- Sudden loss of interest in school or other activities
- Different group of friends
- Change in sleep patterns
- Change in appetite
- Sudden bursts of anger or dramatic mood swings
- Dilated pupils and red eyes

An important clue to your child's emotional health can be how he or she interacts with peers at school. Talk with the teachers. Make sure your child isn't isolating himself or herself. Be aware that headaches and stomachaches are often stress related. Becoming sedentary—watching more television or focusing only on computer games—may be signs of personal turmoil. Do you know who your child hangs out with? How his or her friends behave may be the way your child acts when you're not around.

Typically, children have a hard time asking for help. And, parents sometimes have a hard time acknowledging that their children may need it. If you think your child is abusing drugs, seek help immediately. If your child is experiencing any emotional difficulty, continue to reach out even if he or she pushes you away. Remember, you are your child's strongest lifeline.

are addicted to these things, they're no longer fun—they're overpowering.

Addictions to these and other behaviors can have some of the same negative effects on one's life as alcohol and drugs. Self-esteem may suffer, your relationships can be torn apart, financial problems may develop and your job may be jeopardized. Seeking help for any type of addictive behavior is important for your overall health and peace of mind. Support groups are available for many types of addictions. Talk with your doctor about helpful resources. You're not alone—don't delay getting help.

Anger

Anger is a normal and often powerful emotion. While there are many constructive ways to deal with this feeling, at times it can be difficult to control. Letting anger consume you may lead to problems at work, in relationships and with your overall health. Just think of how your body reacts when you're enraged. For these reasons, it's important to learn techniques that can help you express your anger constructively.

These tips may help calm you down:

- Breathe deeply and slowly.
- Count to 10, or repeat a calming word such as "peace."

- Imagine yourself in a stress-free environment.
- Walk away from the situation to regain your composure.

Practicing these types of techniques can help some people. For others, controlling anger can be a bigger challenge. If your anger is disruptive to you or upsets those around you, talk with your doctor or a counselor. You also may consider joining an anger management group.

For some people, anger can result in violence or abuse. If your anger is out of control—or if you're dealing with a loved one's uncontrolled anger—seek help right away.

Anxiety

Anxiety is a natural reaction to stress. Perhaps you feel butterflies in your stomach before a date. Or, maybe your palms get sweaty when you give a presentation at work.

Some people experience mild anxiety. Common symptoms include a racing heart (see Page 142), sweaty palms, mild shaking and a general feeling of nervousness. For others, anxiety can be more severe—resulting in constant feelings of powerlessness and fear.

Anxiety disorders take many forms. Some include:

Generalized anxiety disorder—a condition that causes people to suffer from persistent feelings of worry

Panic disorder—frequent episodes of intense fear that strike without any warning; also called panic attacks

Phobia—an extreme, disabling fear of a situation or object

Post-traumatic stress disorder—persistent physical and emotional symptoms that occur after a recent or past traumatic event

If you have periods of anxiety that interfere with your daily life, see your doctor. The first step is to determine if your anxiety is caused by a physical condition or even a side effect of a medication you're taking. Your doctor also may recommend treatment to reduce your symptoms. Some options include individual counseling and medication. Support groups also can be very helpful—you may find it reassuring to know that you're not alone.

If your anxiety is mild, there are things you can do to cope:

- Change the way you think. Don't dwell on negative thoughts. And, don't jump to conclusions.
- Meditate or practice deep breathing exercises.
- Exercise regularly.

Caregiver's Concerns

A caregiver provides assistance to someone—often a family member—who is aging, sick, or has a physical or mental disability. While caregiving can be a rewarding experience, it also can be exhausting.

If you're a caregiver, it's important to take care of your own physical and emotional health, too. Try to eat well and get enough sleep. Exercise also can help increase your energy and lift your spirits. These tips may help:

- See your doctor regularly to maintain your own health.
- Ask friends and family for help so you can have an occasional break.
- If your budget allows, hire a home health aide or nurse.
- Look into community resources that offer respite care.
- Learn to say, "No." You aren't superhuman, and you can't do everything.

Also, check for caregiver support groups in your area. It may be helpful to share your frustrations—and joys—with others in similar situations. You also may learn more about additional resources.

- Reduce caffeine and alcohol intake.
- Express your feelings.

Remember, occasional anxiety isn't unusual. Taking a proactive approach can help you better manage your feelings.

Depression

Everyone feels sad from time to time. But when those feelings don't go away and begin to interfere with everyday life, they may signal a more serious condition—depression.

Depression can affect you physically and emotionally. It's important to remember that it's not a character flaw or sign of weakness. In fact, depression is an extremely common condition that can affect men, women and children of all ages. If you have depression, you can't just snap out of it. But, treatment often helps and can get you back on track.

Symptoms can vary, but people who suffer from depression may experience:

- Persistent sadness or emptiness
- Feelings of hopelessness, guilt, helplessness or pessimism
- Loss of interest in once-pleasurable activities
- Difficulty concentrating
- Decreased energy (see Page 114)
- Change in appetite (see Page 54), weight, or sleep patterns (see Page 154)
- Thoughts of death or suicide

Don't take threats or thoughts of suicide lightly. Seek emergency help.

If you have any of these symptoms, talk with your doctor. He or she first will try to rule out any physical causes such as medication side effects or a health condition. Your doctor then may refer you to a professional counselor.

People with depression often find it therapeutic to talk about their feelings with a counselor or a loved one. Prescription medication can ease symptoms for some people. Your doctor or counselor can recommend an appropriate treatment for your situation. In addition to following recommended treatment, practice healthy lifestyle habits (see Page 17). Eating well and exercising can help boost your energy and spirits.

Remember, depression can be treated. So, if you or your loved one has symptoms, seek help right away.

Mental Health and Your Child

Many mental health conditions may seem like adult issues. But, children also experience everyday and serious concerns that affect their well-being. This is especially true during the sometimes-tumultuous adolescent and teen years.

Talk with your child about his or her thoughts, fears or ambitions. More importantly, listen to what your child says. He or she may not express concerns directly. However, you may notice behavioral changes that will give you clues that something may not be right.

If you notice any symptoms that could signal a mental health concern, seek help immediately. You're the most important advocate for your child's health and well-being.

Eating Disorders

Eating disorders are characterized by serious disturbances in eating behavior. Teens and younger women most commonly suffer from them, though they can affect men and women of all ages. It's important to get help right away. If left untreated, they can lead to serious health problems—even death. If you think you or someone you know has an eating disorder, seek help right away.

Anorexia Nervosa

People with anorexia nervosa fear getting fat. They believe they're overweight even if they're dangerously thin. They become obsessed with the idea they're eating too much. Unusual eating habits, such as skipping meals, weighing and portioning food, or avoiding food altogether are characteristics of anorexia. These habits may be accompanied by periods of intense exercise or purging—forced vomiting or intentional, inappropriate use of laxatives.

Anorexia can have deep physical and emotional effects. For some people, the condition can be a brief, isolated episode that might have been the result of a stressful event. For others, it may be a chronic condition. Either way, if you or someone you know has anorexia nervosa, don't delay getting help. Treatment varies, but may include counseling and medication.

Bulimia Nervosa

Bulimia nervosa is characterized by recurrent episodes of binge eating and purging—forced vomiting or intentional misuse of laxatives. Individuals with bulimia fear gaining weight and are unhappy with their bodies. However, unlike people who have anorexia, those with bulimia usually have body weights that are normal or slightly high.

People with bulimia may feel ashamed or guilty. They don't feel in control of their actions. This condition can have physical effects such as tooth decay and erosion from repeated vomiting, low blood pressure, hormonal changes and dehydration. Seek help right away if you or someone you know has bulimia. Treatments such as counseling and medication can help.

Grief

Any major life change—such as death of a loved one, illness, loss of a job, divorce or relocation—can cause a wide range of emotions. You may feel stress, shock, confusion or anger. Or, you may feel sadness and despair. These are all normal, but nonetheless painful, stages of grief.

Grieving is a physical or emotional expression of how you feel. It's important to let your feelings out. Keeping them to yourself can result in stomach problems, insomnia (see Page 154), fatigue (see Page 114), loss of appetite (see Page 54), or depression.

Each person deals with grief in his or her own way. Some people grieve for a few weeks, others for several months or longer. These tips may help you get through a difficult time:

- Share your feelings with friends or family. Connecting with a support group also can be helpful.

- Don't neglect your own health. Eat balanced meals. Exercise regularly. It can help you feel—and sleep—better.

- Be patient—the stages of grief take time and don't necessarily flow in any particular order.

If your grief interferes with everyday life, or if you're concerned that it's lasting longer than you expected, seek professional help. Don't feel embarrassed. Acknowledging that you need help is a sign of strength.

Stress

Stress is a part of everyday life. Juggling the demands of work, family and personal responsibilities can be challenging. The stress you feel and how you cope with it is unique to you. What may cause you stress may not be a problem for someone else.

Stress often causes symptoms that can affect your physical and emotional health, relationships and job performance. You may experience muscle tension, fatigue (see Page 114), headaches (see Page 138), anger, anxiety, irritability or insomnia (see Page 154).

It can be difficult to control stress. You may have a tight deadline at work or concerns about your family's well-being. But, making some adjustments in your lifestyle and the way you look at things can help you cope (see Page 28).

- No one can do everything. Learn to prioritize and say, "No" without feeling guilty.

- Exercise. It's a great stress-buster.

- Meditate. Take 10 minutes to breathe deeply and relax.

- Get organized. Use checklists. Toss out the clutter at work and home.

- Ask for help. Your friends or loved ones may have some time to assist you—or give you the emotional support you need.

Complementary Medicine

11

Some people find complementary—or alternative—medicine beneficial, while others say it's a hoax. But whatever you think, it seems to be here to stay.

Complementary medicine includes therapies or health practices designed to enhance the effectiveness of conventional medical treatments. There are many types, including physical movements and exercises, meditation and herbal supplements. Some claim to reduce stress and tension, or enhance memory. Others may help diminish aches and pains. Healthy people also may see benefits, such as improved health and emotional well-being.

If you choose to try a complementary therapy, talk with your doctor first. Whether you have an existing health condition or a new concern, your doctor needs to know what treatments you're considering. He or she also may guide you toward therapies that are appropriate for your situation.

Therapeutic Exercises

Some forms of complementary medicine seek to enhance the balance between body and mind. Others simply strive to relieve stress or pain without the use of medication. Some well-known therapies include:

Acupuncture and acupressure. Acupuncture originated in China more than 2,500 years ago. It's based on the theory that energy flows along channels throughout the body. If something disturbs this movement of energy, pain or injury may result. In acupuncture, very fine needles are inserted into the skin. This is designed to stimulate acupoints. These specific places on the skin are thought to be energetically connected to each other—and to certain organs and body systems. The needles may be twirled, or energized, by very mild electrical currents to create a tingling sensation.

Acupuncture most commonly is used to ease pain. It also is used to treat allergies, headaches, carpal tunnel syndrome, premenstrual syndrome, stress, insomnia and many other health concerns.

Acupressure sometimes is considered "acupuncture without needles." In this technique, deep finger pressure is used to stimulate the body's acupoints. This ancient practice is used to relieve neck and backaches, headaches, sinus problems and arthritis.

Chiropractic. This practice focuses on joint manipulation. It's used to treat illnesses of the nerves, muscles, bones and joints. The back is usually, but not always, the main emphasis—and techniques can vary.

Typically, a chiropractor applies pressure to the affected joint to restore it to its correct position. You may hear a popping noise as pressure is relieved. Chiropractic is used to relieve low back and neck pain, headaches, carpal tunnel syndrome, arthritis and sport injuries. Certain conditions shouldn't be treated with chiropractic, such as bone fractures and herniated disks (see Page 176).

Through the initial screening process, your chiropractor should determine if this therapy is right for you. People often find that one session isn't enough to produce long-lasting results. They may need several weeks of treatment.

Massage. This therapy involves the manipulation of muscle tissues by a skilled practitioner. It aims to ease muscle spasms, pain, discomfort and stress. Massage also may help reduce heart rate and blood pressure, relax muscles and increase endorphins—the body's natural painkillers.

Of course, some people get massages simply because they feel wonderful. There are several forms, including Swedish, pressure point therapy and sports massage. The technique that's right for you depends on several factors, including your overall health and desired results.

Tai chi. This ancient Chinese martial arts exercise focuses on creating a balance of body, mind and spirit. To achieve good overall health, qi—or life energy—should flow freely throughout the body. Tai chi uses slow, smooth body movements, meditation and deep breathing to help strengthen body and mind. These three components produce many

Popular Herbal Supplements

Herbal Supplement	Possible Benefits	Precautions
Echinacea	May help strengthen the immune system to fight bacteria and viruses—particularly the cold virus.	Not recommended for long-term use or for those with certain health conditions including autoimmune diseases.
Flaxseed	May reduce cancer risk and help improve cardiovascular health.	May cause upset stomach if taken in large quantities.
Ginkgo Biloba	May increase blood flow to the brain, therefore slowing mental decline or memory loss. May protect the central nervous and cardiovascular systems from damage and the effects of aging.	Rarely, may cause headaches, dizziness and gastrointestinal upset. Interacts with blood-thinning agents.
Ginseng	May contain antioxidant properties, helping to fight viral, bacterial, emotional and physical stresses placed on the body.	Not recommended for pregnant women or people with hypertension. Shouldn't be used with caffeine or other stimulants.
St. John's Wort	May help treat mild depression, anxiety and sleeplessness.	May cause side effects such as abdominal problems, nausea and vomiting, dizziness and dry mouth. Also may cause sun sensitivity. Not recommended for women who are pregnant or breast-feeding.

desired effects including improved balance and muscle tone, enhanced concentration, lowered blood pressure, and increased lung capacity.

Because it's a low-impact exercise that easily can be modified, tai chi is safe for almost everyone. It may be especially beneficial for people with chronic pain, heart disease, hypertension, osteoporosis, sleep disorders and respiratory conditions.

Yoga. Yoga means "to join together." It's built on three structures—exercise, breathing and meditation. There are more than 100 types of yoga. Hatha yoga is the most commonly practiced form. Hatha combines physical movements and postures with special breathing techniques. It strives to create an invigorating experience for the body and mind. Some physical and mental benefits that yoga provides include stronger muscles, improved circulation, better posture, heightened concentration, reduced stress and focus, and an overall feeling of relaxation.

Yoga is a non-impact form of exercise. So, most people can practice it safely—regardless of age or physical condition.

However, some of the more strenuous movements may not be recommended for women who are pregnant.

Herbal Supplements

Herbal supplements have been around for centuries. While most are safe, you still should be careful when taking herbals. Some can cause side effects. They also can interact with prescription or over-the-counter medications. Learn as much as possible about any supplement you're considering.

Always ask your doctor if it's safe for you to use an herbal supplement—especially if you're having surgery, taking medication for a diagnosed illness, or if you have a chronic condition.

Be a Wise Consumer

Don't be disappointed or discouraged if you don't see or feel immediate results from the exercises or herbal supplements you try. Work closely with your doctor to find a therapy that may benefit you.

If you decide to try complementary therapy, choose only certified professionals or instructors. Check out related organizations and associations. They may provide referrals or information about instructors' credentials. Your doctor may have some recommendations, too. Also, it's important to keep in mind that not all insurance or health plans cover complementary therapies. Be sure to check your coverage beforehand.

If you choose to include complementary medicine in your personal approach to health care, be an inquisitive researcher. Information isn't always readily available on the effectiveness of every supplement or therapy. Do your homework and seek out reliable sources. Keep up on new developments and findings so that you can make educated decisions about your health.

Workplace Health

12

What you do for a living is more than just a way to pay the bills—it's an integral part of who you are. We often define ourselves by our jobs, and take pride in being part of a team. Whether you're in an office, factory or at your home computer, chances are you spend many of your waking hours on the job.

Work can place demands on both your physical and mental health. But, with a proactive approach and positive point of view, you can minimize the stress and maximize the rewards.

Time Management

Do you sometimes feel as if there aren't enough hours in the workday?

Managing your time to fulfill each day's obligations can be challenging. If you feel as if the day gets away from you before you can accomplish your goals, try these hints:

Get organized. Make daily, weekly or monthly task lists. This will help you know exactly what's expected. Break down each project into manageable steps. As you complete each step, cross it out so you have a clear inventory of your progress. Use a calendar to list all deadlines and meetings. Include important personal obligations, such as doctor appointments, to prevent scheduling conflicts. Take a few minutes at the end of each day to organize your workstation for the following day.

Prioritize. When you're juggling a lot of tasks at one time, it can be easy to feel overwhelmed. Rank projects, tasks or events according to what's most urgent. Stay focused on your highest priority tasks. While most of your day might be spent on meeting immediate deadlines, make time each day for some of your long-term goals, too. This can help keep your workload under control.

Communicate. If you're having problems with managing your time at work, talk with your supervisor. Discuss the most efficient way to manage your workload. There may be a solution that you haven't considered.

Undermining Stress

Not all stress is bad. As human beings, we thrive on little bits of suspense and up-to-the-minute pressures. Some of the most moving moments in our lives—weddings, births and holidays—can be very stressful events. But, we certainly wouldn't want to do without them.

Stress comes in many forms—and it's different for everyone. Some people may find it stressful to have a lot of deadlines, for instance. Others may feel stressed without them. Stress can be a driving force and, ultimately, motivate you.

However, stress also can have negative effects if it starts to take over. You may feel aggravated, tense or worried. You may have trouble sleeping or suffer from headaches. Prolonged, unchecked stress can make you susceptible to more serious conditions, such as high blood pressure, heart disease and depression. Although you can't eliminate stress from your life, you can change the way you respond.

Try some deep breathing. One of the easiest things you can do to deal with pressure is to take a few deep breaths. Inhale slowly and hold the air in your lungs for five seconds. Then exhale as completely as you can. Let the stress flow out of your body. Do this through-out the day.

Have a sense of humor. It often is said that laughter is the best medicine. When things go wrong or start to get out of hand, step back and try to find humor in the situation. Learn to laugh at your-self and look on the lighter side. It can help you stay relaxed.

Fuel up on healthy foods. It's easy to let healthy eating habits slip when you're swamped. But, nutritious foods make you feel better and more energized. Tempted to grab fast food on your way to work? Cereal bars and breakfast shakes are just as quick. No time to make lunch? Stock up on soup or frozen meals to bring to work. Look for brands that limit sodium and fat. Or, make extra helpings of dinner and pack left-overs for lunch. Satisfy your afternoon munchies with a snack that can keep you fueled—fruits, nuts or whole-grain crackers are good choices.

340

Keep moving. Exercise is a terrific stress-buster. It gives you a chance to burn off some energy and may take your mind off things for a while. Working out also helps lower blood pressure and keeps your heart healthy—great defenses against stress. Make time for exercise. Try walking or jogging during your lunch breaks. Find a workout buddy to help keep you motivated.

Get some help. There may be times when the stress in our lives is more than we can handle alone. Seek help if you feel your stress is interfering with your daily activities. Many employers and health plans can connect you with helpful resources—such as employee assistance programs or resources in your community. Check with your supervisor or benefits department.

Health and Safety on the Job

No matter what your workplace environment is like, safety should be your top priority. Depending on the nature of your work, you may be at risk for repetitive motion injuries, such as carpal tunnel syndrome (see Page 134), backaches (see Page 56) or eyestrain (see Page 110). Take some time to consider the possible hazards—big and small—that you may face each day. Make a few changes to ensure your safety and comfort:

Watch your position. Bending or hunching over puts strain on your lower back. Keep your head high and your shoulders down to improve your posture.

Keep things within reach. Are you constantly grabbing for the same clipboard, stapler or piece of equipment? Set up your workstation so that frequently used objects are within comfortable reach.

Adjust your surroundings. Make sure your chair is the right height for you—you should be able to sit up straight with your feet flat on the floor. Position your computer keyboard so that you can type with your wrists held parallel to the floor. If you spend a lot of time on the phone, consider using a headset so you won't strain your neck leaning into the receiver.

Change your position often. Occasionally stand up and stretch your arms. Shrug your shoulders or rotate your neck to keep your muscles from tightening up. Alternate sitting and standing if possible. Be sure to wear comfortable shoes with good support if you spend a lot of time on your feet.

Lift carefully. Put the strain on your legs, not your back (see Page 56). Always keep objects close to your body when lifting. Be realistic—if something is too heavy for you to move by yourself, get some help.

Reduce eyestrain. Working on a computer for long periods may tire your eyes. Don't stare at the screen nonstop.

Focus on something else every 10 minutes or so. And, don't forget to blink.

Wear appropriate safety gear. If your job requires helmets, goggles, dust masks or other protective items, wear them faithfully. Don't take chances with your safety by thinking you can do without them "just this once."

Whether you spend your time standing behind a counter, driving heavy equipment or working at a desk, be sure you aren't putting yourself or someone else in danger. Safety is everyone's responsibility. Do your part—keep walkways clear. Clean up spills and keep sharp objects in a secure place. Be aware of and follow all safety rules in your workplace. Talk with your supervisor or co-workers about other things you can do to keep your work area safe.

Workplace Relationships

In many ways, co-workers are like a family. You spend a great deal of time together—growing and learning through shared experiences. In the workplace, many different personalities and work styles come together. It can be challenging sometimes to keep all of your work relationships going smoothly.

Do your part—develop good relationships. Communicate clearly with your co-workers. Be fair and patient. You won't always agree, but you can try to learn from your differences. Keep your

emotions in check. Don't get defensive when you're given feedback from supervisors or co-workers. Your opinions will be considered more valuable when you go the extra mile to be courteous and professional.

Practice good workplace etiquette. Be considerate of the people around you. Keep your voice low if you work close to others. Don't play your radio too loudly. Make any personal calls from a private location during your break. Think before you send that e-mail. If you reply hastily to something that's upsetting, you may regret it later.

Address problems openly. There may be times when co-workers disagree or just don't get along. Try to talk problems through before they become more complicated. Ask your supervisor for advice or assistance if you need it. Occasionally, problems escalate to a more serious nature. Many organizations have conflict resolution resources—such as employee assistance programs—available for these situations. Your supervisor or human resources department can help.

Beware of workplace pitfalls. You work hard every day to meet your job-related goals as well as your personal objectives. Keeping your own morale up is key to your success. One way to do this is to avoid the "water cooler syndrome." No workplace is immune to gossip and rumors. And, there are always people who prefer to focus on anything that's going wrong. Negativity is extremely contagious and can leave you feeling miserable. If you have legitimate concerns about problems in your workplace, take a constructive approach toward problem solving whenever possible.

Be flexible. Today's work force is continuously changing. At some point, most workers experience transitions in their workplaces. Be prepared by staying flexible. Keep expanding your skill set so that you can adapt to new responsibilities. When change comes along, look for new opportunities. Don't be shy about asking questions and making suggestions.

Finding Balance

We live in a very busy world. Many businesses operate 24 hours a day, seven days a week. At any given time, clients and colleagues may be just a phone call or an e-mail away. Many of us take our jobs with us wherever we go. Then, we spend much of our free time running errands, keeping up with household chores, advancing our education, and tending to our families.

With so much going on, you may feel like a candle that's burning at both ends. It may seem like there's no time left to take a moment alone or to relax. Striking a balance in your life can be a challenge. But, it's crucial to your peace of mind and your health. Look for little ways

to make the most of your time away from work:

Find shortcuts. There are small changes you can make that might free up some of your time. Start buying groceries in bulk so you won't have to shop as often. Make meals ahead of time and freeze them. Let dinner cook in a crockpot while you're at work. Get everyone in the household involved in chores. Get rid of the clutter that makes clean up more difficult.

Take time out. Schedule a little time for relaxation each day. Even five or 10 minutes can make a difference. Keep it simple. Grab a mug of warm tea and work on a crossword puzzle. Do a few stretches. Write your thoughts in a journal. Or, just close your eyes and unwind. You'll feel refreshed and energized after a well-deserved mental break.

Cherish your personal relationships. Family and friends can be an oasis of comfort when life is busy and stressful. Talk with your significant other; laugh with your children; call an old friend just to say hello. Connecting with those you love can give you the inner peace and strength you need to meet the challenges of the day ahead.

Your Health Forms

Personal Health History

(Use this form to make as many copies as you and your family need.)

Name:_____

Date of Birth:_____ **Blood Type:**_____

History of Childhood Diseases

Disease	Date of Illness	Disease	Date of Illness
Chickenpox	_____	Measles	_____
Ear infection	_____	Mononucleosis	_____
German measles (rubella)	_____	Mumps	_____
Hepatitis	_____	Polio	_____
		Scarlet fever	_____

History of Chronic Diseases

(may include anemia or other blood disorder, arthritis, asthma, cancer, cataracts, diabetes, epilepsy, gastrointestinal disorder, glaucoma, heart disease, high cholesterol level, high blood pressure, kidney disease, mental illness, sexually transmitted disease or ulcer)

Disease: _____ **Date Diagnosed:** _____

Treatment: _____

_____

_____

Disease: _____ **Date Diagnosed:** _____

Treatment: _____

_____

_____

Disease: _____ **Date Diagnosed:** _____

Treatment: _____

_____

_____

Disease: _____ **Date Diagnosed:** _____

Treatment: _____

_____

Family Health History

(Use this form to make as many copies as you and your family need.)

Knowing your family's health history is important to your own health. Record all known health conditions of your immediate relatives. Include your grandparents, parents, siblings, aunts and uncles. While you should note conditions such as heart disease, high blood pressure, epilepsy and liver disease, be sure to include conditions such as cataracts, glaucoma, allergies, asthma and ulcers. The more complete your history is, the better your doctor can assess your health risks.

Mother: _____

Conditions: _____

Cause of Death: _____ **Age at Death:** _____

Father: _____

Conditions: _____

Cause of Death: _____ **Age at Death:** _____

Grandparent: _____

Conditions: _____

Cause of Death: _____ **Age at Death:** _____

Grandparent: _____

Conditions: _____

Cause of Death: _____ **Age at Death:** _____

Other Relation: _____

Conditions: _____

Cause of Death: _____ **Age at Death:** _____

Other Relation: _____

Conditions: _____

Cause of Death: _____ **Age at Death:** _____

Other Relation: _____

Conditions: _____

Cause of Death: _____ **Age at Death:** _____

Screenings and Immunizations

(Use this form to make as many copies as you and your family need.)

Regular screenings are vital to your continued good health. Ask your doctor about screenings for cholesterol, blood pressure, cancer and osteoporosis. Find out which are appropriate for you, and how often you should have them.

Regular Screenings	Date	Results or Comments	Next Due

Immunizations can help keep you going strong. Follow your doctor's recommendations regarding annual flu shots and immunizations against pneumonia, tetanus, diphtheria and other preventable illnesses.

Immunizations	Date	Results or Comments	Next Due

Healthful lifestyle actions recommended by your doctor: _____

_____

_____

Medication Record

(Use this form to make as many copies as you and your family need.)

Record all medicines you take—including prescription and over-the-counter drugs. Remember that vitamins and supplements such as herbal remedies can affect the medicines you take, so be sure to include those, too. Keep this chart in your medicine center. Take it with you when you visit your doctor.

Drug or Supplement: _____

Purpose: _____

Dose: _____

Instructions: _____

Date started: _____

Drug or Supplement: _____

Purpose: _____

Dose: _____

Instructions: _____

Date started: _____

Drug or Supplement: _____

Purpose: _____

Dose: _____

Instructions: _____

Date started: _____

Drug or Supplement: _____

Purpose: _____

Dose: _____

Instructions: _____

Date started: _____

Drug or Supplement: _____

Purpose: _____

Dose: _____

Instructions: _____

Date started: _____

Drug or Supplement: _____

Purpose: _____

Dose: _____

Instructions: _____

Date started: _____

Drug or Supplement: _____

Purpose: _____

Dose: _____

Instructions: _____

Date started: _____

Drug or Supplement: _____

Purpose: _____

Dose: _____

Instructions: _____

Date started: _____

Resources

General Health and Well-Being

American Academy of Family Physicians

11400 Tomahawk Creek Parkway
Leawood, KS 66211-2672
(913) 906-6000
www.aafp.org

American Association of Poison Control Centers

3201 New Mexico Avenue, Suite 310
Washington, DC 20016
(202) 362-7217
For poison emergencies:
(800) 222-1222
www.poison.org

American College of Surgeons

633 N. Saint Clair Street
Chicago, IL 60611-3211
(312) 202-5000
Fax: (312) 202-5001
www.facs.org

American Medical Association

515 N. State Street
Chicago, IL 60610
(312) 464-5000
www.ama-assn.org

American Red Cross

811 Gatehouse Road
Falls Church, VA 22042
(703) 206-6000
To donate blood: (800) GIVE-LIFE
To donate money: (800) HELP-NOW
www.redcross.org

Centers for Disease Control and Prevention

1600 Clifton Road
Atlanta, GA 30333
(800) 311-3435
www.cdc.gov

Hotlines:

National AIDS Hotline
(800) 342-2437

National HIV/AIDS Hotline (Spanish)
(800) 344-7432

National Immunization Information
Hotline (English) (800) 232-2522

National Immunization Information
Hotline (Spanish) (800) 232-0233

National STD Hotline (800) 227-8922

SafeUSA Federal Safety
(888) 252-7751

Traveler's Health (877) 394-8747

Healthfinder

An online guide to reliable consumer health and human services information, developed by the U.S. Department of Health and Human Services

www.healthfinder.gov

National Institutes of Health

Building 1
Center Drive
Bethesda, MD 20892
(301) 496-4000
www.nih.gov

Includes:

National Cancer Institute

National Eye Institute

National Heart, Lung and
Blood Institute

National Human Genome
Research Institute

National Institute on Aging

National Institute on
Alcohol Abuse and Alcoholism

National Institute of Allergy
and Infectious Diseases

National Institute of Arthritis and
Musculoskeletal and Skin Diseases

National Institute of Biomedical
Imaging and Bioengineering

National Institute of Child Health and
Human Development

National Institute on Deafness and Other
Communication Disorders

National Institute of Dental
and Craniofacial Research

National Institute of Diabetes and
Digestive and Kidney Diseases

National Institute on Drug Abuse

National Institute of Environmental
Health Sciences

National Institute of
General Medical Sciences

National Institute of Mental Health

National Institute of Neurological
Disorders and Stroke

National Institute of Nursing Research

National Library of Medicine

Aging

AARP

601 E Street, N.W.
Washington, DC 20049
(800) 424-3410
www.aarp.org

Centers for Medicare & Medicaid Services

(800) MEDICARE
www.medicare.gov

National Institute on Aging Information Center

P.O. Box 8057
Gaithersburg, MD 20898-8057
(800) 222-2225
TTY: (800) 222-4225
www.nia.nih.gov

AIDS/HIV

CDC National AIDS Hotline

P.O. Box 13827
Research Triangle Park,
NC 27709-3827
(800) 342-AIDS
Spanish: (800) 344-SIDA
TTY: (800) 243-7889
www.ashastd.org/nah

HIV/AIDS Treatment Information Service

P.O. Box 6303
Rockville, MD 20849-6303
(800) HIV-0440
TTY: (888) 480-3739
www.hivatis.org

Project Inform

205 13th Street, Suite 2001
San Francisco, CA 94103
(800) 822-7422
www.projectinform.org

Alzheimer's Disease

Alzheimer's Association

919 North Michigan Avenue, Suite 1100
Chicago, IL 60611-1676
(800) 272-3900
www.alz.org

**Alzheimer's Disease Education
and Referral Center**

P.O. Box 8250
Silver Spring, MD 20907-8250
(800) 438-4380
www.alzheimers.org

Arthritis

Arthritis Foundation

P.O. Box 7669
Atlanta, GA 30357-0669
(800) 283-7800
www.arthritis.org

**National Institute of Arthritis and
Musculoskeletal and Skin Diseases**

Information Clearinghouse
1 AMS Circle
Bethesda, MD 20892-3675
(877) 22-NIAMS
TTY: (301)5652966
www.niams.nih.gov

Asthma and Allergies

**American Academy of Allergy,
Asthma and Immunology**

611 East Wells Street
Milwaukee, WI 53202
(800) 822-2762
www.aaaai.org

**Asthma and Allergy Foundation
of America**

1233 20th Street, N.W., Suite 402
Washington, DC 20036
(202) 466-7643
www.aafa.org

**National Institute of Allergy
and Infectious Diseases**

Office of Communications
Building 31, Room 7A-50
31 Center Drive, MSC 2520
Bethesda, MD 20892-2520
(301) 496-5717
www.niaid.nih.gov

Cancer

American Cancer Society

1599 Clifton Road, N.E.
Atlanta, GA 30329-4251
(800) ACS-2345
www.cancer.org

Cancer Care Inc.

275 Seventh Avenue
New York, NY 10001
(800) 813-HOPE
www.cancercare.org

National Cancer Institute

Public Inquiries Office
Building 31, Room 10A31
31 Center Drive, MSC 2580
Bethesda, MD 20892-2580
(800) 4-CANCER
www.nci.nih.gov

National Coalition for Cancer Survivorship
1010 Wayne Avenue, Suite 770
Silver Spring, MD 20910-5600
(877) NCCS-YES
www.cansearch.org

Susan G. Komen Breast Cancer Foundation
5005 LBJ Freeway, Suite 250
Dallas, TX 75244
(972) 855-1600
National Toll-Free Breast Cancer Helpline
(800) 462-9273
www.komen.org

Caregiver Advocacy

Family Caregiver Alliance
690 Market Street, Suite 600
San Francisco, CA 94104
(415) 434-3388
www.caregiver.org

National Family Caregivers Association
10400 Connecticut Avenue, Suite 500
Kensington, MD 20895-3944
(800) 896-3650
www.nfcacares.org

Children's Health

American Academy of Pediatrics
141 Northwest Point Boulevard
Elk Grove Village, IL 60007-1098
(847) 434-4000
www.aap.org

Chronic Pain

American Chronic Pain Association
P.O. Box 850
Rocklin, CA 95677
(916) 632-0922
www.theacpa.org

Complementary Medicine

**American Academy of
Medical Acupuncture**
4929 Wilshire Boulevard, Suite 428
Los Angeles, CA 90010
(323) 937-5514
www.medicalacupuncture.org

American Association of Oriental Medicine
433 Front Street
Catasauqua, PA 18032
(888) 500-7999
www.aaom.org

American Chiropractic Association
1701 Clarendon Boulevard
Arlington, VA 22209
(800) 986-4636
www.amerchiro.org

American Massage Therapy Association
820 Davis Street, Suite 100
Evanston, IL 60201-4444
(847) 864-0123
www.amtamassage.org

American Yoga Association
P.O. Box 19986
Sarasota, FL 34276
(941) 927-4977
www.americanyogaassociation.org

International Chiropractors Association
1110 N. Glebe Road, Suite 1000
Arlington, VA 22201
(800) 423-4690
www.chiropractic.org

**National Center for Complementary and
Alternative Medicine**
NCCAM Clearinghouse
P.O. Box 7923
Gaithersburg, MD 20898
(888) 644-6226
TTY: (866) 464-3615
www.nccam.nih.gov

Dental Health

American Dental Association

211 E. Chicago Avenue
Chicago, IL 60611
(312) 440-2500
www.ada.org

Diabetes

American Diabetes Association

1701 North Beauregard Street
Alexandria, VA 22311
(800) DIABETES
www.diabetes.org

National Institute of Diabetes and Digestive and Kidney Diseases

National Digestive Diseases
Information Clearinghouse
2 Information Way
Bethesda, MD 20892-3570
(800) 891-5390
www.niddk.nih.gov

Epilepsy

Epilepsy Foundation of America

4351 Garden City Drive
Landover, MD 20785-7223
(800) 332-1000
www.efa.org

Fertility

RESOLVE—The National Infertility Association

1310 Broadway
Somerville, MA 02144
(617) 623-0744
www.resolve.org

Fitness

American Council on Exercise

4851 Paramount Drive
San Diego, CA 92123
(800) 825-3636
www.acefitness.org

Headache

American Council for Headache Education

19 Mantua Road
Mt. Royal, NJ 08061
(800) 255-2243
www.achenet.org

National Headache Foundation

428 W. St. James Place, 2nd Floor
Chicago, IL 60614-2750
(888) NHF-5552
www.headaches.org

Hearing

International Hearing Society

16880 Middlebelt Road, Suite 4
Livonia, MI 48154-3367
(800) 521-5247
www.ihsinfo.org

Self-Help for Hard of Hearing People Inc.

7910 Woodmont Avenue, Suite 1200
Bethesda, MD 20814
(301) 657-2248
TTY: (301) 657-2249
www.shhh.org

National Institute on Deafness and Other Communication Disorders

Information Clearinghouse
1 Communication Avenue
Bethesda, MD 20892-3456
(800) 241-1044
TTY: (800) 241-1055
www.nidcd.nih.gov

Heart Disease

**American Heart Association
National Center**

7272 Greenville Avenue
Dallas, TX 75231
(800) AHA-USA1
www.americanheart.org

Lung Disease

American Lung Association

1740 Broadway
New York, NY 10019
(800) LUNG-USA
www.lungusa.org

Mental Health

American Psychological Association

750 First Street, N.E.
Washington, DC 20002-4242
(800) 374-2721
TDD/TTY: (202) 336-6123
www.apa.org

American Psychiatric Association

1400 K Street, N.W.
Washington, DC 20005
(888) 35-PSYCH
www.psych.org

National Alliance for the Mentally Ill

Colonial Place Three
2107 Wilson Boulevard, Suite 300
Arlington, VA 22201-3042
(800) 950-NAMI
www.nami.org

National Institute of Mental Health

6001 Executive Boulevard,
Room 8184, MSC 9663
Bethesda, MD 20892-9663
(301) 443-4513
TTY: (301) 443-8431
www.nimh.nih.gov

National Mental Health Association

1021 Prince Street
Alexandria, VA 22314-2971
Resource Center: (800) 969-NMHA
TTY: (800) 433-5959
www.nmha.org

Multiple Sclerosis

Multiple Sclerosis Association of America

706 Haddonfield Road
Cherry Hill, NJ 08002
(800) 532-7667
www.msaa.com

Multiple Sclerosis Foundation

6350 N. Andrews Avenue
Ft. Lauderdale, FL 33309-2130
(888) MS-FOCUS
www.msfocus.org

National Multiple Sclerosis Society

733 Third Avenue
New York, NY 10017
(800) FIGHT-MS
www.nmss.org

Nutrition

American Dietetic Association

216 W. Jackson Boulevard
Chicago, IL 60606-6995
ADA Consumer Nutrition Information Line
(800) 366-1655
www.eatright.org

**Food and Nutrition Information Center
Agricultural Research Service, USDA**

National Agricultural Library
10301 Baltimore Ave., Room 105
Beltsville, MD 20705-2351
(301) 504-5719
TTY (301) 504-6856
www.nal.usda.gov/fnic

Osteoporosis

National Osteoporosis Foundation
1232 22nd Street, N.W.
Washington, DC 20037-1292
(202) 223-2226
www.nof.org

National Institutes of Health
Osteoporosis and Related Bone Diseases—
National Resource Center
1232 22nd Street, N.W.
Washington, DC 20337-1292
(800) 624-BONE
TTY: (202) 466-4315
www.osteo.org

Parkinson's Disease

American Parkinson Disease Association
1250 Hylan Boulevard, Suite 4B
Staten Island, NY 10305-1946
(800) 223-2732
www.apdaparkinson.com

National Parkinson Foundation
Bob Hope Parkinson Research Center
1501 N.W. 9th Avenue
Miami, FL 33136-1494
(800) 327-4545
www.parkinson.org

Parkinson's Disease Foundation
William Black Medical Building
Columbia-Presbyterian Medical Center
710 W. 168th Street
New York, NY 10032-9982
(800) 457-6676
www.parkinsons-foundation.org

Sleep Disorders

National Sleep Foundation
1522 K Street, N.W., Suite 302
Washington, DC 20005
(202) 347-3471
www.sleepfoundation.org

Stroke

National Institute of Neurological Disorders and Stroke
NIH Neurological Institute
P.O. Box 5801
Bethesda, MD 20824
(800) 352-9424
www.ninds.nih.gov

National Stroke Association
9707 E. Easter Lane
Englewood, CO 80112-3747
(800) STROKES
www.stroke.org

Substance Abuse

Alcoholics Anonymous
General Services Office
Grand Central Station
P.O. Box 459
New York, NY 10163
(212) 870-3400
www.alcoholics-anonymous.org

Al-Anon
1600 Corporate Landing Parkway
Virginia Beach, VA 23454
(888) 4AL-ANON
www.al-anon.org

Narcotics Anonymous
P.O. Box 9999
Van Nuys, CA 91409
(818) 773-9999
www.na.org

National Institute on Alcohol Abuse and Alcoholism
National Clearinghouse for Alcohol
and Drug Information
P.O. Box 2345
Rockville, MD 20847-2345
(800) 729-6686
TTY: (800) 487-4889
www.niaaa.nih.gov

National Institute on Drug Abuse

6001 Executive Boulevard, Room 5213
Bethesda, MD 20892-9651
(301) 443-1124
www.nida.nih.gov

Thyroid Conditions

American Thyroid Association

P.O. Box 1836
Falls Church, VA 22041-1836
(703) 998-8890
www.thyroid.org

National Graves' Disease Foundation

P.O. Box 1969
Brevard, NC 28712
(828) 877-5251
www.ngdf.org

Thyroid Foundation of America Inc.

Ruth Sleeper Hall, RSL 350
40 Parkman Street
Boston, MA 02114
(800) 832-8321
www.allthyroid.org

Urological Disorders

American Foundation for Urologic Disease

1128 N. Charles Street
Baltimore, MD 21201
(800) 242-2383
www.afud.org

Vision

American Academy of Ophthalmology

P.O. Box 7424
San Francisco, CA 94120-7424
(415) 561-8500
www.aao.org

American Optometric Association

243 North Lindbergh Boulevard
St. Louis, MO 63141
(314) 991-4100
www.aoanet.org

National Eye Institute

2020 Vision Place
Bethesda, MD 20892-3655
(301) 496-5248
www.nei.nih.gov

Women's Health

American College of Obstetricians and Gynecologists

P.O. Box 96920
Washington, D.C. 20090-6920
(800) 762-2264
www.acog.org

Other Resources

DoD Health Affairs (TRICARE)

Skyline 5, Suite 810
5111 Leesburg Pike
Falls Church, VA 22041-3206
www.tricare.osd.mil

Environmental Protection Agency

National Service Center for
Environmental Publications
P.O. Box 42419
Cincinnati, OH 42419
(800) 490-9198
www.epa.gov

Indian Health Services

Parklawn Building, Room 6-35
5600 Fishers Lane
Rockville, MD 20857
(301) 443-3593
ww.ihs.gov

Veterans Health Administration

Health Benefits and Services
(800) 827-1000
www.va.gov/vbs/health

Glossary

abscess: infected area where pus has collected

acute: usually severe, starting suddenly or lasting a short time; compare to *chronic*

adrenal glands: pair of organs above the kidneys that produce hormones to help control heart rate, blood pressure, metabolism and other bodily functions; key to the "fight or flight" response

analgesic: medication that relieves pain

anemia: condition in which the blood doesn't have enough red blood cells or hemoglobin—reducing its ability to adequately supply the body's cells with oxygen. It may cause fatigue, weakness, palpitations and headache.

anesthesia: loss of feeling. Local anesthesia is limited to part of the body. General anesthesia affects the entire body and involves loss of consciousness; also may refer to the medications used to cause anesthesia—anesthetics.

antibiotic: medication used to treat bacterial infections but ineffective against viral infections

anticoagulant: medication or toxin that reduces or impairs blood clotting

anti-inflammatory: medication that counteracts inflammation—the body's response to illness or injury, usually marked by pain, redness, heat and swelling

antioxidant: substance that protects cells from the damaging effects of oxidation—the normal chemical reaction of oxygen on blood or tissues; counteracts the free radicals that cause the damage; may possibly reduce the risk of cancer—though not yet proven—and age-related macular degeneration

arteriosclerosis: abnormal thickening and hardening of the walls of the arteries

artery: blood vessel that carries blood away from the heart

atrophic vaginitis: thinning of the vaginal lining due to the lack of estrogen that occurs after menopause or removal of the ovaries

autoimmune disorder: disease process in which the immune system attacks the body's own cells

avascular necrosis: death of body tissue due to poor blood supply

benign: mild, or nonthreatening to health or life. Benign also can refer to an abnormal growth that isn't cancerous; compare to *malignant*

biofeedback: process in which a person learns to monitor and influence his or her bodily processes such as heartbeat, temperature and brain wave activity

bisphosphonate: medication that inhibits calcium loss thereby helping to prevent bone loss and breakdown; used to treat osteoporosis

blood vessel: artery, vein or capillary through which blood flows

bronchiectasis: chronic dilation or enlargement of the bronchi—the main airway branches in the lungs—often due to tissue destruction from recurrent infection

capillary: tiny, thread-like blood vessel that connects arteries to veins

cardiomyopathy: disease of the heart muscle; sometimes caused by poor blood supply, but often the cause is unknown

cellulitis: spreading inflammation just under the skin's surface; usually caused by a bacterial infection; the extremities, especially the lower legs, most often are affected

central nervous system: body system that consists of the brain and spinal cord. It coordinates the activity of the entire nervous system.

cervical spondylosis: degenerative joint disease in the neck, also known as osteo-arthritis, or wear-and-tear arthritis

cervicitis: inflammation of the cervix—the neck-like opening to the uterus

chalazion: cyst caused by the blockage of a gland in the eyelid

cholinesterase inhibitor: medication that improves the transmission of nerve impulses by reducing the ability of cholinesterase—an enzyme or chemical—to break down acetylcholine—a neurotransmitter in the brain; used to help maintain function in people with mild or moderate Alzheimer's disease

chronic: lasting a long time; compare to *acute*

chronic fatigue syndrome: long-term condition marked by unexplained fatigue, weakness, muscle aches, swollen glands, difficulty concentrating and trouble sleeping

corticosteroid: hormone made in the adrenal glands; also, synthetic hormone often used to treat inflammation and other disorders

cryotherapy: use of cold to relieve pain, reduce swelling, slow down cellular metabolism or destroy abnormal cells such as warts and other skin growths

cystitis: inflammation of the bladder wall, usually caused by bacterial infection

degenerative joint disease: also known as osteoarthritis or wear-and-tear arthritis

deviated septum: a condition in which the wall between the nostrils isn't straight. It may partially block the airway, making it difficult to breathe.

diabetic retinopathy: complication of diabetes in which the retina is damaged. The retina is the thin membrane that covers the back of the eye and is responsible for vision. If untreated, it can cause blindness.

diaphragmatic irritation: undue sensitivity or inflammation of the diaphragm—the muscle separating the chest cavity from the abdomen. The diaphragm is primarily responsible for breathing. Diaphragmatic irritation can cause pain in the shoulder or abdomen. It also can cause hiccups.

diphtheria: acute, bacterial infectious disease marked by weakness, high fever and the formation of a tough membrane in the upper respiratory tract, especially the throat, making it difficult to breathe and swallow. It can be fatal, but is now rare due to immunizations.

dyshidrosis: dry, cracked skin eruption on the sides of the fingers, palms or soles

eighth nerve tumor: abnormal growth on the nerve coming from the brain, and responsible for hearing

ejaculation: discharge of semen from the penis

electrolyte: electrically charged particle, or an essential chemical in the blood. Examples include sodium, potassium and chloride.

encephalitis: inflammation of the brain, usually caused by a viral infection. By comparison, meningitis is an inflammation of the membrane covering the brain, and may be caused by viruses or bacteria.

endometriosis: condition in which tissue that normally lines the inside of the uterus forms and grows outside the uterus—usually elsewhere in the abdomen. It can cause pain and infertility.

endoscopy: procedure in which the inside of the body is inspected using a lighted, flexible instrument called an endoscope

epinephrine: substance produced by the adrenal gland that, among other things, opens up airways and causes the heart to beat faster and stronger. It can be used to counteract severe allergic reactions; also called adrenaline.

fibromyalgia: disorder marked by chronic fatigue, pain and stiffness in the muscles and joints

fifth disease: mild, contagious, childhood disease characterized by a lace-like rash, symmetrically distributed on the hands, arms and legs

gastrin: hormone secreted by the stomach that stimulates acid production

gentian violet: dark-green dye used to treat bacterial, fungal and parasitic infections. This is a very old treatment and its use is limited to surface fungal infections of the skin or vagina.

giardiasis: infection of the small intestine caused by the parasite Giardia lamblia

Gilbert's syndrome: harmless, inherited form of jaundice in which the body has difficulty disposing of bilirubin—a substance formed when old or damaged red blood cells are broken down

hemochromatosis: inherited disorder in which the body absorbs too much iron

hemophilia: inherited disorder in which blood clotting is impaired

hepatitis: inflammation of the liver, usually caused by a viral infection, toxin or drug

hernia: bulging of part of an organ or tissue through the wall that normally contains it—usually the intestines bulging through the abdomen

herpetic corneal ulcer: sore on the cornea— the transparent tissue covering the front of the eye—caused by the herpes virus

histamine: substance released by the body during allergic reactions

hyperhidrosis: excessive sweating

iliotibial band syndrome: condition in which the thick fibers that run along the outer thigh and the knee become irritated and inflamed. It's a common cause of knee and leg pain among runners.

immunocompromised: having a weakened or impaired immune system

immunosuppressant: medication that reduces the ability of the body to protect itself from disease

infectious arthritis: joint inflammation caused by an infection, usually from a bacterium

influenza: acute viral infection of the respiratory tract usually marked by fever, headache, chills, muscle aches, sore throat and fatigue; also called the flu

interferon: substance produced by the body that helps fight viral infections

interleukin: substance produced by the body that helps stimulate disease-fighting blood cells

kidney stone: hard mineral deposit that forms in the kidney and then usually passes through the urinary tract. It may cause pain, block the flow of urine, and result in other urinary problems.

laryngitis: inflammation of the larynx, or voicebox

leukemia: type of cancer in which there's an increased number of abnormal white blood cells

lymphoma: any of a group of diseases characterized by enlarged lymphoid tissue due to rapidly multiplying malignant lymphoid cells

malabsorption: poor absorption of nutrients by the digestive system

malignant: harmful; when referring to an abnormal growth, it implies the presence of cancer; compare to *benign*

metabolism: the whole range of biological processes that occur within any living organism. It commonly refers to the breakdown of food and its transformation into energy.

monoamine oxidase inhibitor: medication that slows the breakdown of certain brain chemicals called neurotransmitters. Also called MAOIs, they're used primarily to treat depression.

monoclonal antibodies: identical antibodies produced in a laboratory and derived from a single cell

mucus: thick, slippery fluid produced by mucous membranes—tissues that line internal surfaces, for example, airways, and gastrointestinal, vaginal and urinary tracts; offers moisture and protection

multi-infarct dementia: significant loss of intellectual capacity brought on by a series of small strokes

mumps: acute viral disease marked by fever and swollen salivary glands

myocarditis: inflammation of the muscular walls of the heart

optic neuritis: inflammation of the optic nerve, which connects the eye to the brain

osteomyelitis: inflammation of bone, usually caused by bacterial infection

palpitations: sensation of abnormally rapid or forceful beating of the heart

paralysis: complete or partial inability to move a body part

parasite: organism that lives in or on another organism, and which relies on that organism for nourishment and survival

peripheral neuropathy: condition in which the nerves that supply sensation to the arms and legs are injured or impaired

peripheral vascular disease: condition in which the flow of blood to the blood vessels outside the chest, especially the arms or legs, is partially or completely blocked

permethrin cream: insecticide and insect repellant applied to the skin. It's used to treat scabies and lice.

pinched nerve: injury to a nerve that's been compressed or constricted. Its effects can range from a temporary feeling of "pins and needles" to permanent nerve damage.

pneumonia: inflammation of the lungs, usually caused by an infection. It can range from mild to severe, and can be fatal, especially in those very young or old.

polyp: mass of tissue that develops on the inside of a hollow organ, such as the colon or nose

postnasal drip: flow of mucus from the back part of the nasal cavity down the throat

puberty: stage in life when secondary sexual characteristics develop and sexual reproduction becomes possible. Also called adolescence, puberty usually occurs between ages 13 and 15 in boys, and 9 and 13 in girls.

pustule: small bump in the skin that contains pus—yellowish-white fluid containing white blood cells, produced in response to certain infections

respite care: patient care provided in the home or an institution to give temporary relief to a family caregiver

Reye's syndrome: sudden, sometimes fatal, disease of the brain and liver that occurs after a viral infection. Almost always linked to the use of aspirin-containing products, it most commonly affects those ages 19 or younger.

rheumatic fever: disease that causes inflammation of the joints and heart; usually occurs in children after a streptococcal infection and may lead to permanent heart damage.

rigidity: abnormal stiffness or inflexibility of muscles

salicylates: a group of medications often used to help reduce inflammation, pain and fever

semen: whitish fluid containing sperm and other secretions released from a man during ejaculation

sickle cell disease: inherited condition in which the body produces abnormal, sickle-shaped red blood cells due to abnormal hemoglobin—the part of the blood that carries oxygen. It primarily affects people of African descent.

spinal stenosis: narrowing of the spinal canal, often caused by progressive degenerative changes of the spine, ligaments and disks, in the neck or low back

sputum: mucus coughed up from the lungs, usually in response to airway irritations, for example, from infection or cigarette smoke

strep throat: infection caused by a type of bacterium called streptococcus. It can lead to serious complications if left untreated.

stress fracture: small, or hairline, break in a bone, usually caused by repeated stress due to sports, strenuous exercise or heavy physical labor. It's most common in the foot and lower leg.

styptic pencil: substance that stops minor bleeding, shaped into a small stick

temporal arteritis: inflammation of the artery on either side of the head at the temples, or other arteries in the head, causing headache, often in people age 50 or older. If left untreated, it may lead to blindness or stroke.

tetanus: acute infectious disease caused by the bacterium Clostridium tetani, which usually enters the body through a puncture, deep cut or other dirty wound. It may lead to painful muscle spasms, "locking" of the jaw; also may lead to death.

thyroiditis: inflammation of the thyroid gland, which is located at the front of the neck

tourniquet: any device—often a bandage— used to control or stop the flow of blood. *Note: the use of tourniquets is strongly discouraged.*

toxin: poisonous substance from a plant, animal or bacterium

trauma: injury—may be physical or emotional

tremors: abnormal, involuntary shaking or quivering

tuberculosis: highly contagious bacterial infection usually affecting the lungs; also called TB

vaginitis: inflammation of the vagina from a bacterial or fungal infection, allergic reaction or irritation

vascular insufficiency: condition in which the blood flow to or from tissue is impaired

vasculitis: inflammation of a blood vessel

vein: blood vessel that carries blood toward the heart

visualization: act of creating peaceful or positive pictures in one's mind. This technique is used to help manage pain and anxiety, and enhance health and well-being.

wet macular degeneration: condition caused by the deterioration of the macula—the critical part of the retina responsible for visual acuity. It's less common than dry macular degeneration, but more likely to cause severe vision loss.

Index

A

ABCDE (Asymmetry, Border, Color, Diameter, Elevation) rule, 35, 168
ABCs (Airway, Breathing and Circulation), 4-5
abdominal cramping, 48-49, 122, 212, 261-263
abrasions, 198-199
abscess, 357
    gum, 130, 226
    perirectal, 196
abstinence, sexual, 125, 312
abuse, sexual, 235, 314
accidents:
    automobile, 26, 29, 136-137
    swimming, 8-9
    see emergency care
acetaminophen, 40
Achilles' tendinitis, 52, 146
"acid rebound," 41
acne, 50-51
acupuncture and acupressure, 156, 335-336
acute, 357
acute respiratory illness, 70
addictive behavior, 327-330
adrenal glands, 357
aerobic activity, 21
aging and:
    appetite loss, 54
    dry skin, 204
    hearing loss, 140
    vision problems, 238
AIDS, *see HIV*
air travel, 98, 99, 100
alcohol consumption, 25-26, 27, 154, 328
alcoholism, 25-26, 328
allergic rhinitis, 303-304
allergies and:
    anaphylactic shock, 15, 70, 150
    dermatitis, 88
    eye discharge, 108-109
    eye irritation, 104-105
    food, 90, 150-151
    itchy skin, 150-151, 204

    medications, 40
    nosebleeds, 182
    runny nose, 178, 303-304
    sinus pain, 202
alopecia areata, 132
alpha blockers, 289
Alzheimer's disease, 78, 252-254
anal fissures, 194, 195, 196
analgesic, 357
analgesic ointments, 148
anal itch, 196-197
anal warts, 240
anaphylaxis, 15, 70, 150
androgen, 132
anemia, 112, 114, 115, 232, 357
anesthesia, 357
anger, 330
angina, 11, 76, 77, 278, 279
angioplasty, 280
angiotensin-converting enzyme (ACE) inhibitors, 276, 289
animal bites, 60-61
ankle pain or swelling, 52-53
anorexia nervosa, 23, 54, 244, 333
antacids, 41, 144, 298-299
antibiotic, 357
anticoagulant, 357
antidiarrheals, 41
antihistamines, 40, 84, 150, 190
anti-inflammatory drugs, 39-40, 242, 256, 260, 298-299, 357
antioxidant, 357
antitussives, 40-41
anxiety, 114, 330-331
appendicitis, 48
appetite loss, 54-55, 114
arm, dislocated, 102-103
arrhythmias, 275
arteriosclerosis, 357
artery, 357
arthritis, 134, 148, 158, 160, 162-163, 176, 200, 224, 248, 252-254, 255-257
asbestos, 30

aspirin, 39-40, 76, 98, 198, 299
asthma, 70, 258-261
asymptomatic seropositivity, 285
atherosclerosis, 278
athlete's foot, 41, 120-121
atrophic vaginitis, 357
autoimmune disease, 110, 256, 309, 357
automobile safety, 26, 29, 136-137
avascular necrosis, 357

B

"baby acne," 51
bacitracin, 206
backache, 56-57, 116
bacteria:
    mouth, 68, 69, 130
    skin, 50
bacterial conjunctivitis, 108-109
bacterial infections, 84, 100, 108-109, 110-111, 116, 160, 174-175, 186, 188, 194, 202, 216, 222, 248, 298-299, 300, 302
balanitis, 186
baldness, 132-133
barotrauma, 98-99
bed-wetting, 58-59
bee stings, 210
benign, 357
benign hematuria, 232
benign prostatic hyperplasia (BPH), 40, 300, 301
benzocaine, 214
benzoyl peroxide, 50
beta blockers, 202, 276, 280, 289
bile duct obstruction, 156
bilirubin, 156
binge eating, 23, 244, 333
biofeedback, 98, 357
biological therapy (immunotherapy), 266
birth control, 132, 234, 319-320
bisphosphonate, 358

Taking Care: Self-Care for You and Your Family

HIV infection, 284-286
hives, 150-151
hoarseness, 152-153
hormonal changes, 50, 132, 235, 290, 294
hormone replacement therapy (HRT), 132, 228, 295, 318
hormone therapy, 266, 302
human papillomavirus (HPV), 124, 240, 312
hyperglycemia, 281-283
hyperhidrosis, 360
hypertension, 287-289
hyperthyroidism, 218, 308-309
hyperventilation, 70
hypoglycemia, 282-283
hypotension, 112
hypothermia, 8
hypothyroidism, 114, 132, 242, 308

I

ibuprofen, 40
iliotibial band syndrome, 360
immunizations, 31-33, 348
immunocompromised, 360
immunosuppressant, 360
immunotherapy (biological therapy), 266
incontinence, urinary, 228-229
infections:
    bacterial, 84, 100, 108-110, 116, 127, 160, 174, 175, 186, 188, 194, 216, 222, 248, 298-299, 300-302
    bladder, 228, 230, 232
    chronic, 244
    diarrhea and, 90
    ear, 92, 100-101
    fatigue and, 114
    foot, 172-173
    fungal, 41, 88, 120, 132, 170, 172-173, 188, 196
    respiratory, 70, 84, 141, 152, 216, 223, 303-304
    sinus, 68, 178
    swollen glands from, 126-127
    viral, 92, 114, 116-117, 126-127, 216
infectious arthritis, 360

infertility, 312, 322
inflammatory bowel disease (IBD), 261-262
influenza, 360
ingrown nails, 172, 224-225
injuries:
    compression, 102
    head, 9-10, 78, 92, 136-37, 139
    repetitive motion, 134, 248, 341
insect repellents, 211
insomnia, 154-155
insulin, 281-283
interferon, 360
interleukin, 360
intermittent claudication, 164
intracranial hematoma, 136
intrauterine device (IUD), 234, 320
iron deficiency, 114-115
irritable bowel syndrome (IBS), 48-49, 212, 262
ischemia, 278
itching:
    anal, 196-197
    eye, 104-105, 108-109
    groin, 128-129
    rashes, 190-191
    skin, 150-151, 204-205
    vaginal, 236-237

J

jaundice, 156-157
jaw pain, 158-159
jock itch, 128
joint pain, 160-161
juvenile rheumatoid arthritis (JRA), 256

K

Kaposi's sarcoma, 286
Kegel exercises, 229
keratitis, 104-105
ketoacidosis, 282
kidney infection, 116, 230
kidney stones, 232, 360
knee pain, 162-163

L

labor pains, 325-326
labyrinthitis, 92

lactase, 122
lactose intolerance, 18, 122
laryngitis, 152-153, 222, 360
laxatives, 23, 41, 48, 244, 333
"lazy eye," 239
lead paint, 30
leg pain, 163, 164-165
leukemia, 62, 130, 360
leukotriene modifiers, 260
lice:
    body, 166
    head, 166-167
    pubic, 128, 166-167
lifestyle, healthy, 17-30, 114, 265, 279, 287-288
liver, 156
low-density lipoproteins (LDLs), 18
L-tryptophan, 155
Lyme disease, 192
lymph nodes, swollen, see glands, swollen
lymphoma, 360

M

macular degeneration:
    dry, 238
    wet, 362
malabsorption, 360
male pattern baldness, 132
malignant, 360
mallet toe, 224-225
massage, 336
mastitis, 66
medications, 37-42
    abuse of, 26-27, 328-329
    antifungal, 41, 120, 132
    anti-inflammatory, 39-40, 256, 260, 298-299
    bismuth-containing, 194, 232
    blisters from, 64
    cough, 40-41, 76, 84
    groin itch from, 128
    nosebleeds from, 182
    over-the-counter (OTC), 39-42
    pain, 39-40
    prescription, 26-27, 37-39
    rapid heartbeat from, 142
    record of, 348
    side effects, 39
    storage of, 38-39, 41-42

PRICE (protect, rest, ice, compression and elevation), 52, 102, 118, 134, 162-163 208
proctalgia fugax, 196
prostatectomy, 302
prostate gland, 228, 300-302
prostatic hyperplasia, benign (BPH), 40, 300-301
prostatitis, 300
pruritis, 204
psoriasis, 88, 192
puberty, 361
pupils, dilation of, 136
pustule, 361

R

rabies, 60
radiation therapy, 265, 302, 308
radioactive iodine, 309, 310
radon, 30
rash, 120-121, 124-125
    diaper, 188-189
    itchy, 190-191
    non-itchy, 192-193
Raynaud's disease, 184
"rebound" insomnia, 154
rectal bleeding, 80, 194-195
rectal pain, 196-197
relaxation techniques, 28, 154, 274, 335-338
repetitive motion injuries, 134, 248, 341
repetitive strain disorder (tenosynovitis), 118
resources, health, 349-356
respiratory illnesses, 70-71, 270-272
respiratory infection, 70-71, 84-85, 141, 152-153, 216, 222-223, 303-304
respite care, 331, 361
retinal detachment, 238
Reye's syndrome, 40, 361
rheumatic fever, 361
rheumatoid arthritis, 104, 158, 162-163, 256-257
rigidity, 361
ringworm, 41, 132
Rocky Mountain spotted fever, 192
rosacea, 50, 192-193

S

safety concerns, 28-30, 341-342
salicylates, 361
scabies, 128
scalp infections, 126
scrapes, 198-199
screenings, preventive, 31-36, 347
seborrheic dermatitis, 88
seizures, 14-15, 117
self-exams, 33-36, 66
semen, 361
sexual desire, loss of, 314
sexual health, 311-320
sexual intercourse:
    painful, 316
    urination before and after, 230
sexually transmitted diseases (STDs), 64-65, 124-125, 170, 186, 230, 236-237, 240, 284-286, 311-313
shinsplints, 164
shock, 15-16
shock, electrical, 9
shoulder pain, 200-201
sickle cell disease, 361
sinus infections, 68, 178
sinus pain, 178, 202-203
sinusitis, 92, 138, 178, 202, 303-304
sitz baths, 195, 236
skin:
    inflammation of, 120-121, 124-125, 188-189, 190-193
    itchy or dry, 150-151, 204-205, 190-191
skull fractures, 136
sleep, 27, 94-95, 114-115, 138, 154-155
sleep apnea, 27, 94, 154
smoke detectors, 29
smoking, 25, 27, 84, 142, 152, 154-155, 202, 264, 270-271, 279, 298, 303
sneezing, 178, 180, 202
snoring, 27, 94, 154
sodium, 276
sores:
    genital, 124-125
    mouth, 170-171, 191
spider bites, 210-211

spinal injuries, 12-13
spinal stenosis, 362
spleen, 126
splinters, 206-207
sprains, 52-53, 134, 162-163, 208-209, 248
spurs, heel, 146
sputum, 362
sties, 110-111
stings, insect, 210-211
stomach-acid reflux, 144
stomach pain, 212-213
stool softeners, 41
strains, 176, 208-209
strength training, 21
strep throat, 222, 362
stress:
    coping with, 28, 334, 340-41
    fatigue and, 114, 115
    headaches from, 138, 291
    rapid heartbeat and, 142
stress fracture, 362
stretching, 21
stroke, 16, 92, 184, 305-307
sty, 110
sunburn, 29, 75, 169, 214-215
sun protection factor (SPF), 29, 75, 169, 214-215, 265
sunscreen, 29, 75, 169, 214-215, 265
superficial thrombophlebitis, 164
supplements, nutritional, 19, 54, 115, 194, 337-338
suppressants, cough, 40, 84
swallowing difficulty, 216-217
sweatiness, 218-219
swimmer's ear, 100
syphilis, 124

T

tai chi, 336-337
tattoos, 156, 284
T cells, 284-286
teeth, brushing, 68-69, 130, 170, 226-227
teething, 227
temporal arteritis, 362
temporomandibular disorders (TMD, also TMJ), 100, 158
tendinitis, 118, 134-135, 200